Macleod's
Clinical Examination

Benjamin Black

Barts & the London.

Macleod's
Clinical Examination

Edited by

John Munro

OBE MB ChB FRCPE

Former Consultant Physician, Eastern General Hospital,
Edinburgh
Former Consultant Physician, Edenhall Hospital,
Musselburgh
Honorary Fellow, Department of Medicine,
Western General Hospital, Edinburgh

Christopher Edwards

MD FRCPE FRCP FRSE

Professor of Clinical Medicine, University of Edinburgh
Dean of the Faculty of Medicine, University of Edinburgh

Illustrations by Robert Britton

NINTH EDITION

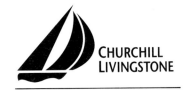

EDINBURGH LONDON MADRID MELBOURNE
NEW YORK AND TOKYO 1995

CHURCHILL LIVINGSTONE
Medical Division of Pearson Professional Ltd.

Distributed in the United States of America by
Churchill Livingstone Inc., 650 Avenue of the Americas, New York,
N.Y. 10011, and by associated companies, branches and representatives
throughout the world.

First edition 1964
Second edition 1967
Third edition 1973
Fourth edition 1976
Fifth edition 1979
Sixth edition 1983
Seventh edition 1986
Eighth edition 1990
Ninth edition 1995
  Reprinted 1996
  Reprinted 1997

ISBN 0443 048568

International Student edition of 9th edition 1995
Reprinted 1997
ISBN 0443 056331

British Library Cataloguing in Publication Data
A catalogue record for this book is available
from the British Library.

Library of Congress Cataloguing in Publication Data
A catalog record is available from the Library of Congress.

For Churchill Livingstone:
Publisher: Laurence Hunter
Project Edition: Barbara Simmons
Production Controller: Nancy Arnott
Design direction: Erik Bigland
Sales Promotion Executive: Marion Pollock
Indexer: June Morrison

The
publisher's
policy is to use
**paper manufactured
from sustainable forests**

Printed in Singapore

PREFACE

The practice of medicine is constantly changing. Some diseases are controlled, or even eradicated, while others increase in frequency and significance. New diagnostic techniques are developed and therapeutic regimens introduced. There is an increasing awareness of the importance of preventative medicine within the community, and also of the special needs of patients, relatives and carers. A ninth edition of this textbook is designed to keep abreast with changes in medical practice and to maintain the impetus for change in medical education.

The new edition has provided the opportunity to alter the previous text extensively. Seven new contributors have joined to create a balanced team of specialists in medicine and surgery. Much of the book has been rewritten. There is an additional chapter on the examination of the eye and numerous new sections have been added, for example the presentation and breaking of bad news, the diagnostic process, the examination of the skin and the peripheral vascular system. We have taken the opportunity to add many new tables, figures and colour photographs.

The basic aim of the book remains unchanged, namely to describe the various skills involved in taking a history, performing a physical examination and providing the patient with an explanation. These are attributes that every clinician requires in order to form satisfactory relationships with patients and to manage them appropriately. The book is intended to complement the information available in standard surgical and medical textbooks.

Throughout the book emphasis is placed on the method of obtaining an accurate history and of performing a physical examination appropriate to the clinical problem. The main chapters conform to a basic pattern. Each starts by describing the relevant symptoms and by discussing their significance. The normal findings in physical examination are detailed and related to important aspects of applied anatomy and physiology. The examination sequence is then described in detail. Thereafter, the relevance of abnormal signs is discussed. The advantages and limitations of the investigations are described and the chapters conclude by giving examples of the methods in practice. Throughout the text 'Key Points' are highlighted.

The book is intended primarily for undergraduates in their clinical years. It has proved to be of value to general practitioners and postgraduates, particularly for those working for a higher clinical examination or returning to clinical medicine after a period of research or working in a highly specialised field.

The ninth edition of *Clinical Examination* is closely integrated with *Davidson's Principles and Practice of Medicine,* to which many of the contributors participate. Both titles have established a wide international appeal and are available in low-priced editions in many overseas countries.

Edinburgh 1995   JFM
                                                                CRWE

ACKNOWLEDGEMENTS

The editors are very aware of their debt to Dr John Macleod and to other contributors to previous editions. We have had generous help from many sources and are grateful to those students and doctors from all over the world who have provided constructive suggestions towards the development of the book.

The editors thank Miss Elaine Anderson for her contribution to the section on the examination of the breast and Dr Patricia Sime for assisting with illustrating various examination techniques. They are indebted to Andrew Medford and Scott Adams for their photographic modelling and to Christine Stewart, Gary MacClean and George MacIntyre for taking the clinical photographs. We would like to express our thanks to Robert Britton, who produced the new line drawings.

Acknowledgements are made in the text to the source of the original photographs which have been kindly provided. Finally, the editors are particularly grateful to Rona Stevenson of Office Oveflow for all her secretarial assistance and to Laurence Hunter and Barbara Simmons of Churchill Livingstone. Their cheerful support and encouragement was very greatly appreciated.

CONTRIBUTORS

Peter J. Abernethy MB ChB FRCSE
Consultant Orthopaedic Surgeon, Royal Infirmary and
Princess Margaret Rose Orthopaedic Hospital,
Edinburgh

Graham K. Crompton MB ChB FRCPE
Consultant Physician Respiratory Diseases Unit,
Western General Hospital, Edinburgh; Part-time
Senior Lecturer, University Departments of Medicine,
Western General Hospital and Royal Infirmary,
Edinburgh

Roger E. Cull BSC (Hons) PhD MB ChB FRCPE
Consultant Neurologist, Royal Infirmary, Edinburgh;
Senior Lecturer in Neurology, University of Edinburgh

David P. de Bono MA MD FRCP
British Heart Foundation Professor of Cardiology,
University of Leicester; former Consultant
Cardiologist, Royal Infirmary, Edinburgh

Christopher R. W. Edwards MD FRCP FRCPE FRSE
Professor of Clinical Medicine and Dean of the
Faculty of Medicine, The Medical School, Edinburgh

Michael J. Ford MB ChB (Hons) MD FRCPE
Consultant Physician and Honorary Senior Lecturer,
Department of Medicine, Eastern General Hospital,
Edinburgh

David W. Hamer-Hodges MS (London) FRCS FRCSE
Consultant Surgeon, Western General Hospital,
Edinburgh

John A.A. Hunter BA MD FRCPE
Professor of Dermatology, University of Edinburgh;
Honorary Consultant Dermatologist, The Royal
Infirmary, Edinburgh

Nigel P. Hurst BSC FRCPE PhD (Edin)
Consultant Rheumatologist, Western General
Hospital, Edinburgh; Part-time Senior Lecturer,
University of Edinburgh

Robert E. Kendell CBE MD FRSE
Chief Medical Officer, The Scottish Office; former
Professor of Psychiatry and Dean of the Faculty of
Medicine, University of Edinburgh

Margaret Macdonald FRCSE FRC OPhth
Consultant Ophthalmologist, Queen Margaret
Hospital, Dunfermline, Fife

D. Symon Macpherson MA MD FRCS
Consultant Surgeon, Leicester General Hospital,
Leicester

John F. Munro OBE MB ChB FRCPE
Former Consultant Physician, Eastern General
Hospital, Edinburgh and Edenhall Hospital,
Musselburgh; Honorary Fellow, Department of
Medicine, Western General Hospital, Edinburgh

Stephen J. Nixon MB ChB FRCSE
Consultant Surgeon, Western General Hospital,
Edinburgh; Part-time Senior Lecturer, Department of
Surgery, Western General Hospital, Edinburgh

Hamish Simpson MB ChB MD FRCP FRCPE DCH DObst
RCOG
Professor of Child Health, Department of Child
Health, University of Leicester, Leicester

Ian R. Whittle MD PhD FRACS FRCSE
Reader in Surgical Neurology and Honorary
Consultant Neurosurgeon, University of Edinburgh;
Department of Clinical Neurosciences, Western
General Hospital, Edinburgh

CONTENTS

C. R. Edwards • R. E. Kendell • J. F. Munro

The principles of a clinical examination

The clinical consultation comprises three components: the history, the physical and mental examination, and the explanation, during which the clinician discusses the nature and implications of the clinical findings.

Patients seek medical help for three principal reasons: for diagnostic purposes, for treatment or for reassurance. Often a combination of these factors may be present. To be effective, the clinician offering reassurance or support must enjoy the trust and respect of the patient. The foundation for the development of a satisfactory 'patient–doctor' relationship is based on the rapport that is established during history-taking and physical examination. In this context, the importance of the first meeting with the patient continues long after the interview has been completed.

THE HISTORY

The history is arguably the most important aspect of the clinical examination. A carefully taken history should give a clear indication of the nature of the problem and may in itself provide the diagnosis. The art of history-taking is the most fundamental skill in medicine. It is an ability which not all doctors acquire, for the skill is not acquired automatically with practice. It can be acquired as a result of good teaching before and after qualifying, careful observation of how others take histories, a willingness to invite or accept comments and criticism and constant self-scrutiny. One effective way of gaining insight is the use of audiovisual records of interview situations. The contribution which textbooks can make to the acquisition of history-taking skills is limited to describing the basic procedures and principles and to providing useful hints.

The conduct and detailed content of the diagnostic interview vary enormously. They depend upon many factors, including whether or not the doctor and patient have met before, how much background information the doctor already possesses, the patient's state of mind and the nature of the presenting complaint. For example, the most acutely ill require urgent resuscitation and detailed history-taking is inappropriate. Nevertheless a number of fundamental principles are applicable in most circumstances.

Principles of history-taking

1. Put the patient at ease

At all times the clinician should treat the patient with respect and courtesy. It is important to know and remember the patient's name. Unless the patient is previously well known, clinicians should always introduce themselves by name and explain who they are. 'Good morning Mrs Blake. My name is Dr Paul Jones and I work for your consultant, Dr Susan Morrison.' A warm welcome, accompanied by a firm handshake, will help to put the patient at ease. The clinician should then explain the primary purpose of the interview. This is particularly important if the patient has already seen another member of the medical team. 'Dr Andrew Young, who also works for Dr Morrison, has asked me to see you to check up on some aspects of the problem before we start treatment.' Any other members of staff present should also be introduced. If there are students, it is essential that patients be asked if they are agreeable to their involvement in such a way, and at such a time, that the patient can decline without feeling either embarrassed or pressurised.

2. Choose an appropriate setting

When patients are being interviewed in bed, it is important to ensure that they are as comfortable as possible and that their privacy is respected. This can be achieved in a single room; in a ward situation it may be necessary to postpone asking some questions until the patient is fit enough to be interviewed elsewhere. A degree of privacy can be achieved by the use of bed screens, and these should always be drawn round the bed at the onset of the interview, not the physical examination. The clinician should sit on a chair, not the bed, facing the patient.

Mobile patients are best interviewed in a consulting room. Both the clinician and the patient should be seated on similar and comfortable chairs. It is inappropriate to talk across a desk (Fig. 1.1). The physical barrier created by the desk also sets up emotional barriers between the clinician and the patient. It is satisfactory to sit at the side of a desk or table (Fig. 1.2) and to use the surface for note-taking. However, if the interview is likely to be prolonged, an alternative and possibly ideal arrangement is for both patient and doctor to sit in comfortable chairs and for the latter to use a clipboard as a writing surface (Fig. 1.3).

3. Start by eliciting the presenting complaint

Once the introductions have been completed and the clinician has checked or obtained basic information such as age and address, the priority is to establish the nature and duration of the presenting complaint. There is no ideal method of obtaining this information. Some questions such as 'What brought you to

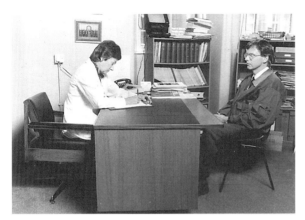

Fig. 1.1 **The desk as a defence mechanism.**

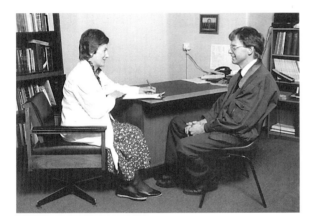

Fig. 1.2 **A more appropriate arrangement of doctor and patient designed to put the patient at his ease.**

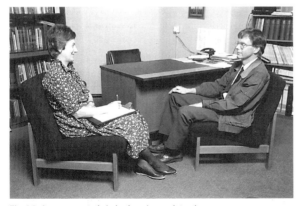

Fig. 1.3 **Arrangement of chairs for a longer interview.**

hospital?' or 'What are you complaining of?' invite retorts such as 'An ambulance' or 'I'm not the complaining type'. Something like 'Tell me what's troubling you and when did it start?' or 'When were you last in your usual state of health and what has happened since then?' will prove effective in most circumstances. It is also important to establish if the patient has been unwell in any other way. Patients may have several symptoms which may or may not be related, and each of these and their duration should be elicited.

4. Encourage the patient to give an uninterrupted history

Once the presenting complaint or complaints have been identified, the patient should be encouraged to recount the history with a minimum of interruption. This is the only way of determining the patient's own account of events and of the relative importance that the patient places on various happenings. At this stage the prerequisite is to keep the patient talking so that the narrative is provided as a whole, rather than stopping to clarify certain events; this comes later. The clinician should prompt the patient with remarks such as 'And what happened next?'. Many patients naturally stop giving the history once they reach that time when medical attention was first sought. However, the process should be continued right up to the moment of interview. Key phrases used by the patient should be reported verbatim. 'The least effort exhausts me' is more informative than 'complaining of (c/o) exertional dyspnoea' and 'a boring pain just here over my left eye' is more revealing than 'c/o left frontal headache'.

There are many reasons why this ideal pattern of history-taking cannot be achieved. They include learning problems, deafness, natural reticence, failing memory, the severity of the illness or the nature of the complaint, for example breathlessness. In such situations, the clinician has to help the patient to a greater or lesser extent by asking specific questions.

5. Use selective questions to clarify the presenting history further

Once the patient has completed the history the clinician will almost invariably wish to ask further questions to clarify the story. For example, a patient may have described in detail the onset, duration, site and character of a pain (p. 29) without mentioning whether or not there were any associated symptoms. It is important to fill in the gaps in the story by asking such questions. It is equally important to avoid asking questions, the answers to which have already been volunteered by the patient. To do so implies to the patient lack of either experience, concentration or interest.

6. Use further questions of diagnostic relevance

Much of the skill of history-taking consists in knowing what are the most useful and important questions to ask in each specific situation. This is a skill that is developed with experience and knowledge. The questions are used to focus on the range of diagnostic possibilities suggested by the history and also to assess the severity of the condition and the development of complications. Although these questions are of critical importance in some patients, they are not relevant to many others. They include, for example, enquiry about heat intolerance, a common feature of thyrotoxicosis in patients presenting with weight loss; recent contact with birds – a source of psittacosis – in patients presenting with pneumonia; or of the passage of air in the urine (pneumaturia), a feature of vescicocolic fistula, which is sometimes a complication of severe diverticular disease or pelvic malignancy.

7. Ask cardinal questions while reviewing the systems

It is always wise to check that the patient does not have symptoms referable to other bodily systems indicating additional or more widespread pathology. These may have been omitted from the history either because they have been forgotten, or dismissed by the patient as unimportant, or for a variety of emotional reasons, including embarrassment, anxiety or guilt. The cardinal symptoms for each of the major systems are described in the relevant chapters and summarised in Table 1.1.

Table 1.1 Systemic enquiry: 'cardinal' symptoms

1. *Cardiovascular system*
   Ankle swelling
   Palpitations
   Breathlessness when lying flat (orthopnoea)
   Attacks of nocturnal breathlessness (paroxysmal nocturnal dyspnoea)
   Chest pain on exertion
   Pain in legs on exertion

2. *Respiratory system*
   Shortness of breath: exercise tolerance
   Wheezing
   Cough
   Sputum production (colour, amount)
   Chest pain related to respiration or coughing
   Blood in sputum (haemoptysis)

3. *Alimentary*
   Condition of mouth (infected tongue or bleeding gums)
   Difficulty with swallowing (dysphagia)
   Indigestion
   Heartburn
   Abdominal pain
   Weight loss
   Change in bowel habit
   Colour of motion (e.g. pale, dark, black, fresh blood)

4. *Urogenital*
   Pain on passing urine (dysuria)
   Frequency of passing urine by day or night (nocturia)
   Abnormal colour of urine (e.g. blood)
   Number of sexual partners

   Males
   If appropriate age, prostatic symptoms such as difficulty in starting to pass urine, poor stream, terminal dribbling
   If appropriate, mental attitude to sex (libido), morning erections, frequency of intercourse, ability to maintain erections, ejaculation, urethral discharge

   Females
   If premenopausal, age of onset of periods (menarche), regularity of periods (e.g. 28-day cycle), length of period, blood loss (e.g. clots, flooding), date of last period, contraception if relevant, presence of vaginal discharge
   If post-menopausal, bleeding
   Stress and/or urge incontinence
   If appropriate, libido, pain during intercourse (dyspareunia)

5. *Central nervous system*
   Headaches
   Fits
   Faints
   Tingling (paraesthesiae)
   Numbness
   Muscle weakness
   Hearing symptoms (e.g. deafness, tinnitus)
   Excessive thirst
   Sleep patterns

6. *Visual*
   Appearance of eyes
   Pain
   Disturbance of vision

7. *Locomotor*
   Joint pain or stiffness
   Muscle pain or weakness

8. *Endocrine*
   Heat intolerance
   Cold intolerance
   Change in sweating
   Prominence of eyes
   Swelling in neck

8. Use language the patient understands

It is important to use a vocabulary that the patient understands. For example, 'Do you have problems with micturition?' may suit a medical colleague, but in most circumstances it is preferable to say 'Do you have any difficulties passing urine?' and sometimes it might be better to ask 'Do you have any trouble when you go for a pee?'.

The use of lay terminology such as 'wind' or 'indigestion' has the advantage of being fairly all-embracing, yet both the patient and the doctor then have to clarify what 'indigestion' comprises. Likewise, if patients use medical terms it is necessary to confirm that they are using them correctly. An episode of 'flu' three weeks ago might indeed have been influenza, but might be more suggestive of a transient bacteraemia subsequently resulting in infective endocarditis. 'Gastric flu' can be almost anything!

9. Avoid suggesting symptoms or answers to the patient

Some symptoms are so specific that they have considerable diagnostic significance. For example, there are many causes of chest pain, but retrosternal pain that radiates up into the root of the neck or into the left arm is highly suggestive of myocardial ischaemia. For this reason it is important to establish in patients complaining of chest pain whether or not it spreads into the neck or left arm. If the patient mentions this spontaneously or when asked 'Does it spread any-where?', it is very likely that they are describing the symptom of myocardial ischaemia. This would be far less probable, however, if the patient merely agreed when asked if the pain ever spread into the neck or down the left arm.

This illustrates an important principle. Symptoms which are described spontaneously, or in response to open-ended enquiries, are likely to be genuine; but there will always be doubt about those which are only elicited in response to specific questions which come close to putting words into the patient's mouth. Initial questions should be unbiased and as general as possible. Highly specific questions may eventually be necessary, but little weight can be placed on a mere assent ('yes, that happens sometimes'). A negative response, however, provides important information.

Another pitfall is the use of questions in such a way as to reveal the expected answer. 'You don't have a family history of heart disease, do you?' implies that the interviewer is expecting the answer 'no', and so invites that answer. It is particularly important to avoid this when asking about topics that may be difficult or embarrassing for the patient. There is a difference between the question 'You haven't ever had gonorrhoea, have you?' and 'Have you ever had gonorrhoea or anything similar?'.

10. Write notes while the patient is talking

It is much easier to observe patients' behaviour and to show genuine interest in what they are saying by maintaining eye-to-eye contact, as occurs in a normal conversation. On the other hand, it is usually bad practice, except in very brief interviews, not to take notes or to make only rough jottings. Notes made in retrospect are less complete and less accurate, and are liable to be distorted by the interviewer's diagnostic assumptions. It may, of course, be necessary later to add to the notes in the patient's absence. If the patient is emotionally upset by the interview or is describing a traumatic experience, such as sexual abuse, it is best to stop writing and to give undivided attention to the patient.

Because of the need to write and observe simul-taneously, it is important to sit in a position that permits note-writing while facing the patient. In practice, this usually means sitting with the chair at an oblique angle to the desk as in Figure 1.2 or using a clipboard instead of a desk for lengthy interviews (Fig. 1.3).

Other informants

Sometimes it is vital to obtain a history from someone other than the patient. The need is most obvious in infants and small children, or if the patient is coma-tose, unconscious or aphasic. Loss of memory prevents many elderly patients recalling recent events accurately.

The clinician who speaks to, and listens to, relatives obtains additional information which may prove in-valuable. For example, it may be apparent that a patient is no longer capable of coping without support, or conversely that the symptoms are much more long-standing and less incapacitating than the patient has implied. Relatives and friends may also be the primary source of important information in the social history. This may alert the clinician to such problems as concealed grief, marital disharmony, previous suicide attempts, lack of drug compliance (a common prob-lem, especially in the elderly) or increasing reliance on alcohol or other drugs. Whenever there is a possibility of abuse of alcohol or other drugs, it is very important to obtain information from such sources, preferably in the presence of the patient, if the patient is denying the existence of a problem.

Problem patients

Various categories of patients present special problems. These include the shy and uncommunicative, the garrulous, the touchy or irritable and the distressed. The astute clinician will not only recognise the problem early in the interview but may also identify an underlying explanation. For example, patients who appear angry may be using anger to conceal anxiety, and relatives who appear angry may in reality feel guilty. It is particularly important to make every effort to put such individuals at ease from the outset, to treat them with respect and courtesy and to show genuine concern for their welfare. This alone may resolve the situation. Doctors, however, need to develop the skills required to cope with any situation which threatens to prevent them obtaining the information needed to help the patient.

Garrulous patients seem incapable of giving short or simple answers to the plainest of questions. They may go into endless and often inappropriate detail, digress and repeat themselves. Such behaviour may relate to an underlying obsessional personality, or to anxiety. They have to be guided, but this can usually be achieved politely and without causing offence. 'Thank you very much; I would now like to ask you some specific questions to help clarify one or two aspects of the story.'

Uncommunicative patients. Many such patients answer questions hesitantly and in whispers or monosyllables. This behaviour may suggest embarrassment or may occur in patients who feel pressurised into seeking medical help against their will. The best approach is to be understanding and to say something which implies a knowledge of how they feel. 'It's not easy to talk to someone you have never met before, is it?' It may prove necessary, however, to obtain the history during a series of interviews once the patient has gained trust in the clinician.

Tearful patients. It is not uncommon for patients or their relatives to start weeping while discussing a painful topic or memory. The patient is often embarrassed and may vainly search for a handkerchief. The first requirement is to be sympathetic and to allow the patient time to regain composure. It is useful to have a box of paper hankies near at hand. It is then important to encourage patients to explain why they were so upset and to express the feelings they were trying to bottle up. Doctors who avoid discussing distressing topics, sometimes because they themselves feel too embarrassed to do so, miss an opportunity of helping their patients.

One common cause of distress is grief. Once this has been expressed, the clinician should take whatever action seems appropriate. For example, the doctor could explain that grief is a very 'normal' emotion and one that everybody experiences from time to time. The doctor can then continue by suggesting that grief is a mixture of different emotions and that prolonged grief is sometimes in part caused by guilt, though in the clinician's experience that guilt is almost invariably inappropriate or misplaced. Such an approach may encourage patients to talk about any aspect of the bereavement that has caused distress, thereby helping them to come to terms with their grief.

Angry patients. From time to time every clinician will encounter an angry patient. The patient may express anger about being kept waiting before the consultation, or being seen by 'yet another doctor'. These explanations are rarely the underlying cause of the emotion, especially if the clinician has already apologised for keeping the patient waiting and explained the purpose of the consultation. Sometimes the patient has a justifiable grievance relating either to the clinician or to a previous medical experience or to one involving a close friend or relative. Often such grievances are the product of inadequate communication. On other occasions, the anger conceals some other underlying emotion. Indeed, the normal response to bad news, or the anticipation of bad news, comprises shock followed in turn by disbelief, anger, resignation and finally acceptance.

Once the clinician has become aware of the situation, it is important to try to deal with it. If the patient has a genuine grievance then clearly the doctor should apologise and try to resolve the problem. If the cause of the anger is unknown then the clinician should explore the problem by asking questions: 'I have the impression that you are not finding this interview very satisfactory. Can you help me by explaining what is going wrong?' or 'Are you upset with me personally, or is it something else that is distressing you?'. Such an approach will provide patients with an opportunity to express their anger, and this itself may diffuse the problem. However, no clinician can expect to achieve satisfactory relationships with every patient. If there is personal antagonism then it is best to offer the patient an alternative consultation with a colleague, preferably of the patient's choice. Effective medical care requires mutual trust and respect.

Handling sensitive situations

Patients will provide information to doctors about their bodily functions and social life that they may never have discussed with a close relative. They do so in the belief that the matter is strictly confidential and that the questions have been asked because they are relevant to helping with the current problem. Some situations are particularly sensitive and need to be handled with discretion. These include enquiry into sexual activity, both past and present. The delicacy of the question depends largely upon the patient. For example, it may be perfectly appropriate to ask a single patient in their thirties, fully aware of the implications of HIV infection, 'How many sexual partners have you had in the last 12 months?'. Such a direct approach to a married patient in their middle fifties may cause offence and embarrassment.

Likewise, where there is a possibility of childhood sexual abuse it is usually advisable to prompt the patient by first asking 'Do you look back on your childhood with happiness?' and then 'Was there any particular event in your childhood that caused distress?' followed by 'Were you ever subjected to bullying, physical abuse or sexual abuse?'. Such questions should only be asked if they are clearly relevant.

The special role of the student

Students are disadvantaged when they are taking a history for one major reason. In most instances the primary purpose of the exercise is to benefit the student, not the patient. Most patients are very willing to help with this educational activity, particularly if they are asked. 'Good morning, Mrs Brown. My name is Sally Mitchell. I am a senior medical student. I wonder if you could help me in my training by going over your history with me.'

The skill of history-taking is not acquired overnight, and it is not appropriate for a student to ask highly personal or potentially sensitive questions. If such matters are volunteered by the patient, the student is best advised to listen without interruption and then to ask permission to convey the essence of the conversation to a senior doctor.

The explanation is an integral component of clinical examination (p. 18). However, it should be undertaken by a doctor who has clinical responsibility for the patient. This excludes students and doctors with postgraduate attachments from active involvement. Indeed, if patients solicit their advice, the situation is best handled by saying that they do not have the necessary background information to offer help. The student should suggest to the patient that a member of the medical staff would be in a better position to explain the situation – and then, with the patient's approval, discuss the problem with that staff member. Undergraduate training sometimes fails to give recent graduates the necessary skills to handle these aspects of the doctor–patient relationship with confidence. Students and recent graduates should therefore try to avail themselves of any opportunity to 'sit in' during such a consultation.

KEY POINTS

- The history is important for two reasons. In most instances it provides a clear indication of the nature of the problem. It also forms the foundation of a satisfactory patient–doctor relationship.

- It is essential to use a flexible method of history-taking.

- The patient should be encouraged to give the account of the presenting history without interruption.

- The supplementary questions are of two kinds: those required to fill in gaps in the patient's account and specific questions designed to clarify the diagnostic alternatives.

- Terms used by the patient or clinician should be understood by both.

- Information volunteered by the patient is more valuable than that obtained by questioning.

- Open-ended questions are preferable to leading questions.

- A supplementary account from a third party is often of great value.

- 'Problem patients' require special consideration.

Psychiatric histories

There is no fundamental difference between a psychiatric history and any other medical history. However, psychiatric histories generally need to be more detailed, and therefore take longer, because more information is needed about the patient's personal life and family and social background. This is partly because laboratory tests and other investigations contribute so little to diagnosis. A more fundamental reason is that many of the stresses that contribute to the genesis of psychiatric disorders are highly personal. An understanding of why one patient was so devastated at being passed over for promotion, or why a couple were already at the end of their tether when their daughter announced that she was pregnant, requires a knowledge of the patients' previous lives – their upbringing, their careers and their marriages, their hopes and their fears.

In addition, the symptoms which have led to the consultation often themselves interfere with the conduct of the interview. The patient may be abnormally anxious, suspicious, deeply depressed or retarded, or muddled and forgetful. Patients may be tempted to conceal vital information because they are embarrassed or ashamed, or because they are reluctant to divulge family secrets. Sexual abuse in childhood, for example, is rarely revealed until patients are sure they can trust the doctor not to be censorious and not to pass the information on to other people. Some patients are so psychotic or demented that they are not capable of giving a history and this has to be obtained from someone else. Even when the patient can give a coherent account, it is often wise to obtain a further history from a relative or close friend. This may significantly differ from the patient's, and the discrepancies between the two accounts may provide important information about the relationship between the people concerned as well as about the clinical problem.

THE MENTAL STATE EXAMINATION

Examination of the patient's mental state is the psychiatric equivalent of the physical examination, though this does not imply that patients whose symptoms are primarily psychiatric do not need to be examined physically. Physical and psychiatric disorders coexist more commonly than can be explained by chance.

The ability to carry out and interpret a mental state examination should be within the competence of all practising clinicians. Depressions and phobic anxiety states are extremely common, and all doctors should be able to diagnose them. Dementing illnesses are common in old age, and anyone dealing with the elderly must be able to decide whether or not they show evidence of early dementia. Organic mental disorders (delirium and confusional states) may complicate a wide range of illnesses including ischaemic heart disease, pneumonia and various kinds of drug intoxication or withdrawal. These can only be effectively treated if they are recognised.

The amount of time and attention devoted to examining the patient's mental state will vary considerably depending upon the history, which itself provides a form of assessment. No further examination is needed if the patient's symptoms do not suggest psychiatric illness, the history has not raised the possibility of memory impairment or disorientation and the patient's behaviour has been unremarkable.

When a mental state examination is indicated, the time devoted to different components of the examination should depend on the diagnostic possibilities. Just as there is little point in carrying out a detailed neurological examination in a man with a history of duodenal ulcer, so there is little point in asking questions about orientation and memory in a young woman whose symptoms suggest that she has a depressive illness. Making the best use of limited time is achieved by focusing on relevant topics and possibilities. Even so, it is important for students and other trainees to conduct a comprehensive mental state examination as often as possible. This will provide the opportunity to become fluent in the testing of concentration, orientation and memory and to become familiar with the wide range of normal responses.

Although the mental state examination need not be conducted in any set order, it is common practice to record the information in sequence, under the following headings.

General behaviour

The interviewer should observe, and record, anything about the patient's behaviour, demeanour or dress which seems unusual, or may have diagnostic significance, either during the consultation or in other settings which provide an opportunity to observe the patient (e.g. on the ward or in the waiting room). The range of possibilities is extremely wide. Patients may weep, or their eyes may fill with tears. They may be restless and incapable of sitting still for longer than a few minutes. They may be agitated, sitting in a tense posture on the edge of their chair and twisting a handkerchief in their hands or constantly adjusting their rings or some article of clothing. They may be shy or sullen, deferential or over-familiar, flirtatious or aggressive.

The clinician needs to be familiar with the patient's cultural background in order to know what is abnormal and therefore potentially significant. Claims to hear the voice of God or the Devil would be strong presumptive evidence of psychosis in a native-born Scot but might have little psychiatric significance in a West Indian member of a Pentecostal sect. A willingness to discuss sexual matters might be unremarkable in a young British woman but would suggest pathological disinhibition in a woman from a Muslim community.

Despite their brevity, technical terms are best avoided. It is more informative to describe someone as 'sitting woodenly with almost no facial expression' than as being 'retarded', and to describe a woman as 'wearing a low-cut dress, and describing her life story and symptoms in rather sensational terms' than as being 'attention seeking' or 'histrionic'.

Speech

Speech is one aspect of behaviour, but its importance is so great that it is convenient to treat it separately.

Some patients are so garrulous that the interviewer is forced to interrupt. Others seem incapable of giving straightforward replies to simple questions; others reply with monosyllables and almost never make spontaneous remarks. Such verbal behaviour may provide important clues to diagnosis. Pressure of speech may suggest hypomania, monosyllabic replies may be a manifestation of retardation or resentment and remarks which are consistently vague and off the point may suggest a schizophrenic thought disorder. A sudden change in the patient's verbal style may also indicate an emotionally sensitive topic requiring further exploration.

Any particularly striking remarks, especially those that may indicate a disorder of the form of speech (p. 204), should be recorded verbatim.

Mood

Mood is a subjective state and information about it can only be obtained by questioning patients, or noting their spontaneous comments. People who are depressed, anxious or perplexed often have characteristic facial expressions or behave in characteristic ways. However, subjects may look depressed without being depressed or feel anxious without appearing anxious. It is therefore important not to confuse subjective description and observed behaviour, particularly if the two are in conflict.

Mood states are extremely variable and our language has a great range of adjectives to describe them – happy, sad, dejected, miserable, anxious, panic-stricken, ecstatic, euphoric, suspicious, perplexed, and so on. The commonest abnormal mood states in patients are depression and anxiety. Routine enquiry about these is best done by asking open-ended questions such as 'How have your spirits been recently?' or 'How have you been feeling in yourself?'. If the patient admits feeling anxious or miserable further questions should be asked to determine how consistent this feeling is, its duration and severity and if this fluctuates during the day.

Anyone who appears to be significantly depressed should be asked whether life still seems worth living and whether they have had thoughts of suicide. The notion that this may put the idea into the patient's mind is mistaken. The deeply depressed have almost invariably experienced transient thoughts of suicide and it is often a relief to be able to talk about these. Equally important, the management of a depressive illness is strongly influenced by the clinician's assessment of the risk of suicide. Direct questions are needed to establish this. Fleeting thoughts are of little con-

sequence, but the risk is much greater in anyone who is preoccupied with thoughts of suicide, is planning how to kill themselves, or frightened that they might do so.

The symptoms of an underlying anxiety state may range from a vague feeling of being ill at ease to uncontrolled terror. Patients who describe bouts of anxiety or episodic physical symptoms such as palpitations, dizziness or breathlessness, which commonly accompany anxiety, should be questioned closely about where they are when the attacks occur, and whether they avoid particular places or situations in case they develop these symptoms. Unpleasant sensations, subjective or somatic, which occur only in crowded or enclosed places, or when the subject is alone, are highly suggestive of phobic anxiety. A confident diagnosis of a phobic state can often be made from the history. This is preferable to reaching the diagnosis by exclusion as it saves the patient from unnecessary investigations.

It is valuable to record the patient's replies to key questions verbatim in the case notes. For example:

How have you been feeling recently?
    Pretty low, I'm afraid.
Every day the same?
    More or less, yes.
Life worth living nowadays?
    Well, sometimes I've wondered recently.
Have you thought of suicide?
    Well, I've thought about it.
Have you seriously considered taking your life?
    Not really; I don't think I'd ever have the courage.

Thought content

The patient's preoccupations should be recorded. Often the history will have revealed these, and questions like 'What is your biggest worry?' may reveal others.

Some people are troubled by *obsessional symptoms*, stereotyped ideas or impulses which they strive unsuccessfully to resist. Obsessional thoughts are invariably distressing either because they are frightening, obscene or blasphemous, or simply because they are so obviously pointless. This is why they are resisted, albeit unsuccessfully. Obsessional rituals involve behaviour like repetitive handwashing and usually represent a symbolic defence against an underlying idea (e.g. 'I am dirty or guilty and must wash to cleanse myself'). With early dementia some subjects will develop coping strategies such as double checking that the door has been locked at night. These must not be confused with obsessional rituals.

Only a small minority of patients are deluded. A *delusion* is a private, firmly held belief which is erroneous, often but not necessarily absurd, and un-influenced by logical argument, for example that the neighbours are using electromagnetic rays to poison the environment. A delusion must be distinguished from an overvalued idea. This is an unusual and sometimes bizarre conviction which the patient shares with other people and has been acquired in circum-stances that are comprehensible (e.g. belief in witch-craft or a conviction that eating carrots improves night vision). The distinction is important. A delusion implies that the patient has a psychotic illness whereas over-valued ideas are evidence only of personal eccentricity or 'cultural pressure'.

It is pointless asking patients if they are deluded. Sometimes delusional ideas are expressed during the interview; others may have to be sought. This requires knowledge of the kind of delusions particular patients are likely to experience. For example, if delusions of persecution are suspected, the clinician might ask 'Are other people ganging up against you?' or 'Are you in danger at present?'. It is important to record the patient's replies and to explore any abnormal pheno-mena elicited.

Perceptual abnormalities

Hallucinations are apparently normal perceptions occurring in the absence of the appropriate stimulus. They may involve any of the five senses – vision, hearing, touch, taste and smell. *Pseudohallucinations* are similar except that the subject is able to recognise them as false perceptions and therefore responds quite differently. A man who hears a voice threatening to kill him may attack and even kill his neighbour but, if he recognises that he is 'hearing voices', he is more likely to consult his doctor. *Illusions* are misinterpretations of genuine perceptual stimuli, e.g. being convinced that a pyjama cord on the floor is a snake.

The commonest hallucinations are visual or auditory, the latter usually, though not necessarily, taking the form of human voices. Visual hallucinations occurring in the absence of auditory hallucinations are nearly always organic in origin, particularly if they are noctur-nal. The classic example is delirium tremens, in which the patient is terrified by imaginary insects or reptiles crawling around the room. Such hallucinations often start as illusions, e.g. as a misinterpretation of the pattern on the wallpaper or a stain on the bedspread.

Attention and concentration

Impairment of concentration occurs in confusional states and dementias. It is also a characteristic depressive symptom, and depressed patients often complain, or admit, that they are no longer able to read. They read a paragraph and do not take it in, so they read it again with no more success and eventually give up. They may wrongly conclude that they have lost their memory and are dementing. A simple and widely used test of concentration is to ask the patient to subtract 7 from 100 serially and see how far they get and how many errors they make in 60 seconds. Patients who cannot subtract, or simply panic when asked to do mental arithmetic, can be asked instead to list the days of the week in alphabetical order which is surprisingly hard. It is necessary to learn by experience the range of normal responses to these tests. Most people complete serial 7s within the minute and make no more than two mistakes.

Orientation

There are three components to orientation – place, time and person. One or more of these may be dis-turbed in organic mental states. Indeed, disorientation is a cardinal feature of confusional states and dementias and has considerable diagnostic significance. Orientation is tested by asking a few simple questions about the day, the month, the year and the time of day, and the building and city in which the patient is residing. Obviously, replies have to be interpreted in the light of recent events and 'normal' responses. Patients taken to hospital by ambulance in the middle of the night may not know the name of the hospital but should know that they are in a hospital. Similarly, many people do not know the exact date but do know the month, year and day of the week. Disorientation in person is commonly revealed by the patient misidentifying a nurse as their daughter, or a visiting grandson or nephew as their son or husband.

Memory

There are many different types of memory impair-ment. The most important is a loss of recent memory with a relative preservation of distant memory. This is a common feature of dementias. A simple and widely used test of recent memory is to give patients a name and address to remember, preferably written on a card in bold type, and then, after explaining the nature of the test, ask them to repeat the information 5 minutes later. Distant memory can be tested by asking the dates and salient facts of some well-known but distant public event. It is important only to ask questions to which the patient once knew the answers, and to which the clinician also knows the answers. Questions such as 'What did you have for breakfast this morning?' or 'Where were you born?' should be avoided if there is no immediate means of knowing whether the replies are true or false.

Dementing patients often have a remarkably detailed memory of their early lives but very little memory for the last few years. They characteristically make statements that were true some years ago, for example that Margaret Thatcher is Prime Minister.

General knowledge

Questions such as 'Who is the Prime Minister?', 'Who preceded him?', 'Who is the President of the USA?', 'What has been in the news recently?' and 'What is the cost of a first-class stamp?' may reveal important deficiencies, though it is sometimes difficult to distinguish between failing memory and loss of interest. It is important to know the range of normal responses before drawing conclusions from the replies. People who cannot name the Chancellor of the Exchequer may be able to tell you last Saturday's football scores, and vice versa.

Other cognitive tests

Patients suspected of brain damage or localised brain disease may need to be given a variety of tests to establish whether they have an expressive or a receptive dysphasia (see Ch. 7, p. 205), and whether they have dysgraphia, dyslexia or apraxias or agnosias of various kinds. Different components of memory (e.g. visual and auditory, short term and long term, retention and recall) may also need testing individually. Although the tests are quite simple, they are normally only used by neurologists, psychiatrists and clinical psychologists.

Formal tests of intelligence or personality are similarly best left to specialists. They rarely make a significant contribution to diagnosis.

One simple method of assessing the overall severity of intellectual impairment in chronic brain failure is the abbreviated mental test (AMT) shown in Table 1.2.

Insight

It may be important to ask patients if they consider that they are ill and, if so, whether the illness is physical or mental. The replies may have diagnostic significance and may also place important constraints on treatment.

Table 1.2 Abbreviated Mental Test

Score 1 for each correct response.

1. What is your name?
2. What is the name of this place? (Where are we now?)
3. What year is this?
4. What month is this?
5. What day of the week is it today?
6. How old are you?
7. What is the name of the Prime Minister (President)?
8. When did World War I start?
   Remember the names of the following, *three* items; I will ask you to recall them in a few minutes' time. (Use standard items within the room and ask the patient to repeat their names before proceeding.)
9. Count backwards from 20 to 1. (Score 0 for any uncorrected error.)
10. Repeat the names of the three items I asked you to remember. (Score if only *one* item is remembered.)

Normal score	8 or more
Mild–moderate dementia	4–7
Moderate–severe dementia	less than 4

KEY POINTS

- Symptoms that lead to a psychiatric referral often influence the conduct of the interview.

- The history is of special diagnostic importance in patients with psychiatric problems.

- All practising clinicians require the skill to perform and interpret a mental state examination.

- Observed behaviour may, but does not necessarily, reflect mood.

- Impaired concentration is a characteristic symptom of depression.

- The potential risk of suicide should always be assessed in the severely depressed.

- A confident diagnosis of a phobic anxiety state can be made from the history, thereby eliminating unnecessary investigation of the symptoms.

- Delusions are a feature of psychotic illness.

- Dementia is commonly associated with loss of recent memory but preservation of distant memory.

- The selection of questions used to test memory and general knowledge must be appropriate to the individual patient.

- The AMT provides a simple method of assessing severe intellectual impairment.

PUTTING PRINCIPLES INTO PRACTICE

It is now time to apply the principles of history-taking. In practice, this will depend on many factors such as the mental and physical condition of the patient. The approach to a psychiatrically disturbed patient will obviously be different from the approach taken to a patient with a normal mental state. Similarly, it would be inappropriate to take a full history from someone with a medical emergency. Clinicians must learn to be flexible in their approach and to adapt their questions to the individual patient. However, in many situations the following method is suitable.

Personal details

Name
Age and date of birth
Occupation

In hospital it is important also to ascertain the patient's address and telephone number, and the name and address of their general practitioner.

Presenting complaint

This should be recorded using the patient's words rather than medical terms. At this stage 'chest pain on walking uphill' should not be translated into 'angina of effort' or 'attacks' of breathlessness at night' into 'paroxysmal nocturnal dyspnoea'. The danger of substituting medical terms is that they may bias the critical evaluation of the history.

The aim is to get a clear chronological history of the presenting complaint. The principal symptoms must be analysed as described in Chapter 2. Thus, if a patient complains of chest pain on walking uphill, it is necessary to know when the pain first started, the location and nature of the pain and its radiation, its frequency and its relationship to exercise and any associated symptoms or relieving factors. Some of these points will have been mentioned by the patient. Others may need to be elicited by specific questioning. It is often useful to get the patient to describe in detail the first time that they experienced their symptoms. It is important not to ask unnecessary leading questions because a positive reply is of limited diagnostic value.

Illustrative case

The following history was obtained from a patient with chest pain.
Mr A.P.T. – age 40, DoB 11.3.1954, salesman for carpet company
Presenting complaint
Chest pain.

History of presenting complaint (HPC)
Six months ago (3 January 1994)
Onset of lower retrosternal chest pain after walking about half a mile uphill to buy the newspaper.
Pain
- felt like a heavy weight or a band around chest
- radiated to jaw and inner aspect L arm
- relieved by resting for 5 minutes
- no associated palpitations or shortness of breath.
Over next 3 months
Two further similar episodes, both related to walking uphill into a strong wind.
Three months ago
Increased frequency of pain:
- now brought on by walking 200 yards on the flat or by climbing one flight of stairs
- character of pain, radiation and relief with rest as before
- worse after heavy meals.
Two months ago
Visited general practitioner. Diagnosis of angina. Prescribed glyceryl trinitrate tablets for pain. These produced effective relief.
One week ago
Chest pain as before but on three occasions has occurred at rest.
Day of admission
Occurred while watching the television and lasted for 10 minutes in spite of using glyceryl trinitrate.

This history provides a clear account of the chronological development of the condition from the onset to the date of interview. In some instances patients may be able to give precise dates and these should be recorded. It is important to try to avoid statements such as 'a few weeks ago' or 'last Saturday'.

Elderly or ill patients may tire during the initial history-taking. The process should then be curtailed and completed on another occasion.

Past history

The past history often contains useful clues regarding the nature of the presenting complaint. Because of this, some clinicians ask the patient to describe in detail any previous illness before they enquire about the presenting symptoms. This approach provides a chronological logic to history-taking.

All available information about the patient's previous illnesses, operations and accidents should be recorded in chronological order. The patient's recollection of the past history may be incomplete. Patients may forget previous admissions to hospital or illnesses at home. They may think that something that happened many years ago, such as rheumatic fever, is not relevant. Sometimes they may fail to mention episodes such as a history of sexually transmitted disease because of embarrassment or guilt.

It is important to note the following: chronic conditions, conditions that may recur, conditions that may give rise to long-term complications, surgical history, residence or travel abroad, obstetric and gynaecological history and other sources of information.

Chronic conditions

These include diabetes mellitus, heart disease, epilepsy, hypothyroidism and chronic bronchitis. If a positive response is elicited then further questioning will be required. In diabetics these would include:

- 'What diet and other treatment are you receiving (insulin, tablets, none)?'
- 'Have there been any complications (hyperglycaemic coma, hypoglycaemia, infections, eye, kidney or neurological problems, etc.)?'
- 'How do you monitor the control of your diabetes?'
- 'What are the follow-up arrangements?'

Conditions that may recur

These include peptic ulcer, tuberculosis, especially if previously inadequately treated, asthma and allergic reactions. Drugs can be covered later in the history but it is important not to forget reactions to intravenous contrast agents, bee stings, elastoplast and such like.

Conditions that may give rise to long-term complications

One example is the importance of enquiring about a past history of jaundice or hepatitis, if only because of the potential risk to clinical and laboratory staff. The carrier state for hepatitis B is very common with a worldwide reservoir of about 200 million people. The virus can be transmitted by accidental inoculation from a needle used to take blood from a carrier or infected patient. Likewise, knowledge of HIV antibody status may be highly relevant in many clinical conditions. Tact and understanding are required in obtaining the information, and the patient's informed consent is normally necessary before testing HIV status. One approach is to ask if the patient has had the test previously. If the response is negative, the clinician can continue by explaining that for completeness sake it is desirable to exclude various viral infections, including HIV. Such questioning is also appropriate in a patient in a high-risk group. These include male homosexuals, bisexuals, intravenous drug abusers and haemophiliacs or others who have previously received blood products.

Surgical history

This involves recording

- the nature and date of any surgical procedure
- any surgical complications
- follow-up arrangements. These may be very relevant; for example, patients with colonic polypi are at increased risk of developing carcinoma of the colon.

Residence or travel abroad

Any illness which was acquired abroad may be relevant. With air travel even illnesses with very short incubation periods, including tropical or subtropical infections, may present in areas where they are not normally encountered. Amoebiasis can be misdiagnosed as ulcerative colitis, or malaria as influenza with potentially catastrophic results. The onus is on the doctor to make the relevant enquiry and to ask details about immunisation and prophylactic medication for malaria.

Obstetric and gynaecological history

This should include details of the following:

- number of pregnancies (full-term or premature delivery)
- complications of pregnancies (e.g. hypertension)
- miscarriages
- terminations
- menstrual history.

Other sources of information

If previous medical records and radiographs are available these should be consulted. A medical examination for insurance purposes may also provide valuable findings. Family planning clinics often record the blood pressure. These previous measurements may assist in the investigation and management of a woman presenting with hypertension.

Illustrative case

Past history
Thus in Mr A.P.T, our patient with chest pain, the past history (PH) was:
Six years ago (February 1988)
While residing in another city, myocardial infarction. Admitted to coronary care unit at hospital X for 5 days.
   After discharge severe angina for 6 months. Admitted for further investigation.
October 1988
Coronary artery bypass graft (CABG). Reviewed for 12 months and then discharged from follow-up.
   No other operations. No other chronic illnesses.

Family history

Many diseases have a significant genetic basis. With certain conditions there may be a well-defined mode of inheritance. For example, cystic fibrosis is inherited as Mendelian recessive. The diagnosis implies that both parents are asymptomatic heterozygotes and that any sibling of the patient has a one-in-four chance of being affected. In other diseases such as hypertension and coronary artery disease, the mode of inheritance is more complex and environmental factors such as diet and smoking play a role. Environmental factors may cause illness within a family, for example use of an infected water supply or exposure to industrial hazards, including asbestos. Likewise, faulty hygiene or close proximity may result in infections such as dysentery or tuberculosis being spread within the family. Thus information about the age and health or cause of death of a patient's relatives is often valuable:

- 'How many siblings and children are in the family?'
- 'Are your close relatives (parents, sibs and children) still alive?'
- If not, 'What was the cause of death and the age at death?'. If alive, 'Do they have any significant illness or are they on known medication?'.
- 'Is there a family history of any relevant specific conditions such as diabetes, hypertension or thyroid disease?'

The symbols used in the construction of a family tree (pedigree chart) are illustrated in Figure 1.4.

A family history has to be elicited with tact and care. Patients may have unwarranted fears that they have inherited a severe disease. Conversely, patients may fail to appreciate or deliberately not wish to know that they might have an inherited condition such as Huntington's disease.

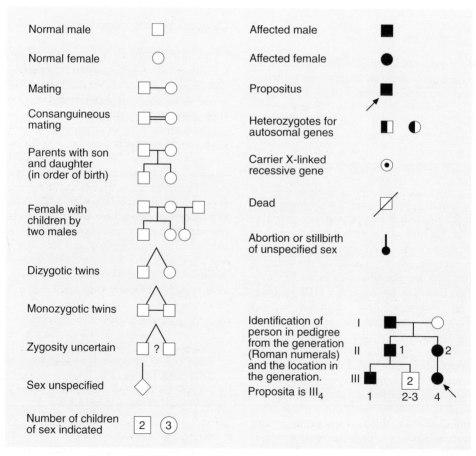

Fig. 1.4 Symbols used in pedigree charts. Drawing up a family tree begins with the affected person first found to have the trait (propositus if male, proposita if female). Thereafter relevant information regarding siblings and all maternal and paternal relatives is included. (Reproduced with permission from Emery A E H Mueller R F 1992 Elements of medical genetics, 8th edn. Churchill Livingstone, Edinburgh.)

Illustrative case

Family history
The family history (FH) of Mr A.P.T. was particularly revealing:

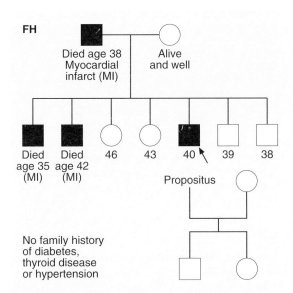

FH

Died age 38
Myocardial
infarct (MI)

Alive
and well

Died
age 35
(MI)

Died
age 42
(MI)

46

43

40

Propositus

39

38

No family history
of diabetes,
thyroid disease
or hypertension

Fig. 1.5   Mr A.P.T.'s family history.

The strong family history of ischaemic heart disease with early death suggests an inherited condition such as familial hypercholesterolaemia. This has an autosomal dominant mode of inheritance. The heterozygote defect affects about one person in every 400–500 in the UK and USA. About half of male heterozygotes develop ischaemic heart disease by the age of 50. As a result of the history the clinician will look for those physical signs which may be associated with accelerated atherosclerosis, corneal arcus, xanthelasma and tendon xanthomata (p. 94). The history also suggests that specific biochemical investigations should be performed to determine the value of low-density lipoprotein–cholesterol (LDL–cholesterol) and high-density lipoprotein–cholesterol (HDL–cholesterol) and raises the possible need for family screening.

Social history

Hospital doctors usually see the patient away from the home environment. Often the general practitioner will have a much better appreciation of this and can be an important source of help in assessing domestic problems.

Discussion about the home circumstances often provides a clearer impression of patients and their personal relationships. It may allow the patient an opportunity to raise issues such as sexual difficulties, marital or financial problems, or problems with children or elderly relatives. These may require advice, support or counselling in their own right and may also affect an individual's well-being. It is also important to know about the family as a source of strength and support to a patient trying to cope, or come to terms, with a particular illness.

When taking a history it is useful to enquire about the home, occupation, personal interests and habits. This factual information can be obtained by asking a fairly standard set of questions (see Appendix, p. 365). However, there is a continuing need to be aware of the potential significance of connections between the patient's past and present lifestyle and the current problem. At times, much more detailed questioning is necessary.

The home

It may be helpful to know about the details of patients' homes, such as other occupants, the number of rooms, the toilet and bathroom arrangements, the heating or lack of it. For patients with conditions such as angina, chronic bronchitis or rheumatoid arthritis, it is useful to ascertain the number of steps leading up to the home or bedroom and whether it is possible for the patient to sleep on the ground floor. More detailed information about the home situation may be obtained from the general practitioner or by a domiciliary visit by a social worker or occupational therapist. This also offers an opportunity to assess how the patient copes at home with such things as cooking and toileting.

Occupation

An occupational history is a useful part of any history. It may help to establish a rapport with the patient and may also provide important diagnostic clues. The classic observation by Percivall Pott in 1775 of the high incidence of scrotal cancer in chimney sweeps led to the realisation that soot contains a carcinogen. Exposure of a shipfitter or pipe lagger to asbestos may lead years later to the development of a malignant pleural tumour – a mesothelioma. Prior exposure to asbestos also markedly increases the risk of lung cancer in cigarette smokers.

Unemployment may also be associated with a variety of mental and physical problems. An occupational history may also provide insight into the patient's financial situation. Relevant aspects include compensation for an occupationally related illness or accident, or the receipt of a pension or invalidity benefit.

Personal interests

The doctor needs to be aware of a patient's leisure pursuits. This allows a better appreciation of the patient's lifestyle and may be diagnostically relevant. For example, amenorrhoea is common in young women who take a lot of physical activity.

Habits

Certain habits such as alcohol, tobacco or drug abuse can have serious consequences for health.

Some patients will deny drug abuse. Others will grossly underestimate their tobacco or alcohol intake. It may be useful to ask the patient to give an account of their normal working and leisure days. This may enable the physician to get a more accurate picture of smoking and drinking habits. If examination reveals features suggesting an alcohol-related problem, or if investigations show a raised mean corpuscular volume and an elevated gamma-glutamyltransferase it is important to retake the history and to ask a close relative or friend for their assessment of the patient's drinking habit.

If heavy drinking is suspected the doctor should try to assess the quantity of alcohol consumed per day or per week. This is usually expressed in terms of units. One unit of alcohol comprises 10 g, equivalent to half a pint of beer, one glass of wine or one measure of spirit. The regular consumption of more than 21 units of alcohol per week in males, or 14 units in females, confers a significant risk of developing an alcohol-related disorder. These include chronic liver disease (Fig. 6.10), peripheral neuropathy (p. 249), cerebral atrophy (Table 7.20), pancreatitis and alcoholic cardiomyopathy. There is also a liability to develop hypertension. If an alcohol problem is suspected, information should be obtained regarding:

- the nature and quantity of alcohol presently consumed per week
- the amount of money spent on alcohol per week, as sometimes this reveals a striking discrepancy
- the age of onset of drinking
- previous drinking habit, including maximum weekly intake and presence or absence of bout drinking
- previous episodes of 'the shakes', delirium tremens and admission to hospital
- time of taking the first drink in the day (regular morning drinking is strongly suggestive of dependence)

- with whom and where drinking occurs, at home or in a 'pub'.

Illustrative case

Social history
In Mr A.P.T. the social history was important.
Home
Lives in third floor flat with no lift.
Occupation
Carpet salesman for last 12 years. Very stressful job involving extensive travelling and entertaining of clients. No financial problems.
Personal interests
Takes no form of regular exercise.
Habits
Previously smoked 30 cigarettes per day until the heart attack. Then stopped for 3 years but restarted and presently smoking 20 per day. Average alcohol intake 5 units per day for 12 years. No problem with alcohol withdrawal but avoids breakfast and usually has 1 or 2 pints of beer with his lunch.

Systemic history

It is important to enquire about other symptoms which might indicate the presence of unsuspected disease; A list of standard questions is given in Table 1.1. It is not necessary to ask every patient all these questions. However, while learning to take a history it is useful to go through a full 'checklist'. If a positive response is elicited then more detailed questions may be required.

Illustrative case

Systemic history
In Mr A.P.T. systemic enquiry revealed that 4 months ago he experienced pain in his left calf on walking more than 800 yards. This pain was relieved by rest but had not occurred recently and his present exercise tolerance was limited by chest pain.

Drug history

It is essential to obtain full details of all the drugs and medications taken by the patient. Not infrequently patients forget to mention, or forget the name of, drugs they take. Some may be over-the-counter prescriptions unknown to the general practitioner. The significance of others, such as herbal remedies or laxatives, may not be appreciated by the patient.

In patients receiving medication it is necessary to determine the precise identity of the drug, the dose used, the frequency of administration and the patient's compliance or lack of it.

It is important to ask about known drug allergies or suspected drug reactions and to record the information in such a way on the front of the notes that it is obvious to any doctor seeing the patient. *Failure to ask the question or to record the answer properly may be lethal.*

Illustrative case

Drug history
In Mr A.P.T. this revealed that he was taking glyceryl trinitrate 0.5 mg sublingually when required for chest pain. In the week prior to referral his dose had increased from about five tablets per week to five tablets per day. He was taking 150 mg of aspirin per day but no other medication.

Conclusions at the end of the history

The history is the first step towards making a diagnosis. At this stage, by analysing the available information, it should be possible to reach a provisional diagnosis. This will influence the emphasis placed on different components of the physical examination.

Illustrative case

Provisional diagnoses
In Mr A.P.T. these were:
1. Ischaemic heart disease: unstable angina.
2. Peripheral vascular disease: left intermittent claudication.
3. ? Familial hypercholesterolaemia.

KEY POINTS

- Encourage the patient to describe the presenting complaint in detail up to the time of taking the history.

- The onus is on the clinician to enquire about residence or travel abroad.

- Previous medical notes and films should be consulted, if available.

- The past history may be incomplete because the patient forgets, or fails to appreciate any possible relevance, or because of embarrassment.

- A detailed social history often provides insight into the patient's personality.

- The nature of patients' occupation, or lack of it, may have an important impact on their health.

- Alcohol-related problems are very common; the extent of the problem may require detailed enquiry not only from the patient but also from a third party.

- The drug history is often relevant and poor compliance is a common problem.

THE PHYSICAL EXAMINATION

There is no correct sequence of performing a physical examination. It is important for all doctors to develop their own approach. By so doing the clinician will reduce the risk of making mistakes. The time-honoured sequence of physical examination is:

1. inspection
2. palpation
3. percussion
4. auscultation.

These have to be integrated into the examination and can be altered as deemed necessary. For example, it may be advisable to listen to bowel sounds before palpating the abdomen.

Although the tendency is to teach the techniques of physical examination system by system, in practice these require to be integrated because this approach is less tiring to the patient.

Environment and equipment

It is essential that the physical examination is performed in privacy and with optimal conditions of lighting and heating. Privacy may be readily obtained in a patient's home. It may be more difficult to achieve in a hospital ward.

The examination couch should be of an adjustable height or a stool provided to facilitate access. It is useful if the couch has an adjustable back-rest. This is particularly valuable if the patient is unable to lie flat without becoming breathless.

The part of the body being examined needs to be properly exposed and illuminated. The rest of the patient should be covered with a blanket or sheet, and care should be taken to prevent the patient becoming cold.

Not uncommonly a patient's relatives attend a consultation. They should be tactfully asked to leave prior to the physical examination. However, sometimes it is helpful for one to remain behind, especially if the patient is a child or if there is language problem. If a rectal or vaginal examination is to be performed then the presence of a nurse or relative is essential.

The equipment that is required will depend upon the nature of the examination. In the outpatient department the clinician will usually have a stethoscope, pen–torch and measuring tape. Other equipment such as an ophthalmoscope, auroscope, sphygmomanometer, tendon hammer, tuning fork, cotton wool, pins, disposable wooden spatula to use as a tongue depressor, disposable gloves, lubricant jelly and proctoscope and facilities for testing urine should be readily available. An accurate weighing machine and height scales (preferably a Harpenden stadiometer) should be standard equipment. When visiting the patient's home the doctor will require a fairly wide range of similar equipment.

Although the examination is integrated, the results are conventionally recorded in terms of systems. One method is described in detail in the Appendix.

Illustrative case

Physical examination
In Mr A.P.T. this revealed the following:
General assessment
Overweight for height (95 kg, 160 cm). Non-cushingoid distribution of fat, i.e. no centripetal obesity. Sternotomy scar.
Corneal arcus.
Xanthelasma. Tendon xanthomas found on both tendon Achilles and on the tendons on the dorsum of R and L hands.
Cardiovascular system
Pulse 72 per minute, regular. Carotid pulses normal.
R carotid artery bruit.
Jugular venous pressure (JVP) not elevated.
Apex beat fifth intercostal space, mid-clavicular line.
Cardiac impulse normal. No thrills.
Heart sounds normal. No added sounds. No murmurs.
Peripheral pulses: no pulses palpable below the femoral in L leg.
L femoral artery bruit. L leg cooler than R.
Respiratory system
Nil abnormal detected (NAD).
Alimentary and genitourinary system
NAD (rectal examination not performed).
Nervous system
NAD.
Locomotor system
NAD.
Psychological examination
Anxious. Particularly concerned about the family history of early death from coronary heart disease.

Clinical diagnoses in Mr A.P.T.
1. Ischaemic heart disease: unstable angina.
2. Peripheral vascular disease: left femoropopliteal obstruction.
3. Familial hypercholesterolaemia.
4. Anxiety.

FURTHER INVESTIGATION

At the end of the clinical examination the features may be so clear-cut that a final diagnosis is apparent. Often this is not the case and further investigations have to be arranged to clarify the nature or the severity of the problem. The number of investigations different doctors perform varies greatly depending on such factors as knowledge, experience and philosophy. In different countries the approach may be influenced by the health care system, the patient's financial resources and the extent of malpractice litigation. However, unnecessary investigations can never be justified and will become increasingly unacceptable as medical audit is established. The critical question to ask is 'What is the benefit of this test to this patient?'.

In spite of the increasing sophistication of modern medical technology, the key to the correct diagnosis remains in the history and physical examination.

KEY POINTS

- There is no correct sequence of performing a physical examination.

- An integrated approach to physical examination is recommended because it is less tiring for the patient.

- Investigations which can bring no benefit to the patient cannot be justified.

THE EXPLANATION

The final component of the clinical interview is the explanation. This involves the clinician explaining the overall assessment of the problem to the patient, preferably accompanied by a close relative. From the point of view of the patient, it is the most important aspect of the consultation. As with the history and physical examination, the prerequisite is to adopt a flexible and integrated approach. Just as the examination starts at the beginning of the interview so the explanation, or at least part of it, may be given either during the interview or the clinical examination. The tearful patient requires immediate comfort and re-assurance, and this usually involves a discussion or explanation of the problem. During the examination a doctor may note a benign lesion, such as a lipoma. If the patient expresses relief that it has been detected and concern that it might be malignant, the reassurance is best provided immediately.

Specific time, however, requires to be set aside to discuss matters with the patient, and this is best done after the examination. In a hospital setting the same principles involving privacy apply. However, it is often useful to ask patients if they would like an accompanying relative to be present and also if they would agree to a nurse attending. This ensures that the nursing staff are involved and made fully aware of what has and what has not been discussed. The details of the discussion will depend upon many factors including the nature of the problem and the personality of the patient. The aspects that should be discussed include:

- An explanation of the diagnosis or, if this is uncertain, the differential diagnosis or nature of the problem.
- A description of the immediate management plan. This includes the purpose and nature of any necessary investigations and also a discussion of the treatment.
- General advice about any change in lifestyle that may be appropriate, including such aspects as occupation, exercise, smoking and alcohol.
- The prognosis, though it must be emphasised that clinicians are not clairvoyant and the best that can be preferred is no more than an informed guess.
- Question time; patients should be given the opportunity of asking questions regarding their illness.

Illustrative case

Explanation
In Mr A.P.T. the initial explanation given to him and his wife covered the following issues:
Diagnosis
He was told that his own diagnosis of angina was correct and that, in addition, there was evidence of narrowing of a blood vessel to his left leg.
Management
Because his pain had occurred at rest, he was offered immediate admission to a coronary care unit so that treatment could be started without delay and under close medical supervision. He was told that his drug treatment would be altered and that a repeat angiogram might be arranged in the near future.
General advice
He was advised to use his admission to try to stop smoking and it was also suggested that he should reduce his alcohol intake.
Prognosis
He was told that the future was uncertain but that he should be optimistic. The anticipation was that treatment would considerably improve his pain and might resolve it completely.

The question of screening his two children and the surviving sibs was discussed. He was told that a final decision would be made depending upon the results of blood tests and once the previous case notes had been obtained and reviewed.
Questions
Mr A.P.T. asked about his leg. He was told that this was not the immediate priority but that before discharge arrangements would probably be made for him to obtain a specialist opinion.

His wife asked about the duration of his stay in hospital and was told that this would be for at least 5 days but depended on his progress and

the result of the possible angiogram. At this stage a further decision would be made and one option might be to consider surgery or angioplasty.

They were told that at present any discussion about the timing of his return to work was premature.

Breaking bad news

Many people find it difficult to break bad news, not because they lack compassion but because they feel inadequate in coping with the distress that the news will cause. Clinicians are no exception. However, breaking bad news is an inevitable component of caring for patients. There is no right way to undertake this responsibility – the most important thing is that the clinician behaves naturally. The circumstances have a profound effect. The way of breaking the news that a child or young adult has been killed following a road traffic accident differs from the approach adopted when explaining to a patient that they are suffering from an inoperable malignancy. This section attempts to provide a few general principles concerning breaking bad news to patients.

1. Give warning

It is best to warn patients about possible bad news. This can be achieved by first asking if they are the kind of person who wishes to be kept informed or if they would prefer not to be told of the final diagnosis. If, like most patients, they wish to be informed, it may be best to then explain that the range of diagnostic options is considerable.

2. Choose an appropriate setting

Privacy is essential. Patients should be asked if they would like a close relative to attend, and this should be encouraged. The presence of a relative provides the patient with an additional source of comfort and support and ensures that the relative personally knows what has been discussed. In hospital it is often helpful to involve a senior nurse; nursing staff will be available to answer questions and provide continuing support in the clinician's absence.

3. Take time

Bad news is best broken in stages. This gives the patient and relative the chance to assimilate the news and the clinician the opportunity to defer mentioning some information if the patient becomes distressed.

4. Use appropriate language

News must be given in a way that makes it comprehensible. If medical terms are used, their implications must be explained. Some words, such as cancer, multiple sclerosis and dementia, are highly emotive. Once they are used the patient, and often the relative, may be so upset that they fail to take in any further information. There is a difference between telling a patient that they have cancer of the colon but that all the evidence would suggest that this can be successfully treated and telling them that they are suffering from a condition which has been detected at an early stage and that there is every reason to believe that it can be cured by surgery. Cancer may be mentioned later in the interview or during a subsequent interview.

5. Confirm that the patient understands

It is valuable to ask the patient if they have understood the explanation and to invite them to summarise what they have been told. This ensures that there is no misunderstanding. The patient and relative should then be invited to ask questions.

6. Emphasise the positive

Frequently patients misunderstand the implication of having an inoperable condition. The concept that 'nothing further can be done' must be avoided by emphasising the positive aspects of any situation. These might include the commitment to provide continuing support, an assurance that pain relief is available, if required, and that other complications will be treated if and as they arise.

7. Discuss the prognosis

The common response to bad news is that the patient wants to know 'how long?'. Before attempting to answer this question, it is helpful to ask patients why they wish to know. There may be a particular reason, for example a business to hand over or a relative to visit, or the patient may want to resolve some personal problem or assuage a feeling of guilt about a previous relationship. These issues can then be discussed.

In attempting to give a prognosis, the clinician must emphasise the remarkable uncertainty of medical practice and should try to avoid suggesting a finite life expectancy.

8. Supplement the verbal message

Even if the initial explanation is understood, many subjects will be left with a distorted or false impression of what they have been told. For this reason, it is desirable to supplement the conversation by writing down the most important information or even by providing patients and relatives with a tape recording of the interview which they can play back as required.

9. Arrange a follow-up session

The patient should be given the opportunity of asking for further clarification after a period of time. At this stage the patient will be starting to come to terms with the situation and is usually much more anxious to ask questions and obtain additional information.

Breaking good news

Patients are usually greatly relieved to be told that nothing is seriously amiss. Sometimes, however, even good news requires to be broken with tact. Some patients are anxiously looking for a diagnosis and are distressed that no explanation has been found for these symptoms. To such patients the use of terms like 'nothing is wrong' may appear confrontational and imply that the consultation has been a waste of time. Tact and honesty are required in offering reassurance to patients whose symptoms are 'psychosomatic'. One approach is to explain that medical knowledge is limited – but expanding all the time – and that the clinician's responsibilities are restricted to excluding those conditions which can be diagnosed. This having been done, the patient can be reassured that, whatever is responsible for the symptoms, they are not caused by a serious or progressive medically recognised condition. Such an approach then provides the opportunity for the doctor and patient to discuss coping strategies and the possible role of stress as an aetiological factor.

KEY POINTS

- The explanation is an intrinsic component of the clinical examination.

- Should the patient so wish, it is helpful if a close relative is present.

- Patients and relatives often have difficulty in grasping the implications of bad news. Some words in particular are highly emotive.

- It may help to break bad news in stages, and to supplement the verbal message with written information.

- In hospital, nurses play a critical role in providing support and it is often helpful for a nurse to be involved from the onset.

PATIENTS' RIGHT OF ACCESS

The Health Records Act of 1990 gives patients the right to see, or even to receive, a copy of their case notes. This emphasises the importance of never making comments which might be construed as being derogatory, condescending or facetious. This is particularly important in case notes which contain detailed descriptions of patients' behaviours and personalities, and of their relationships with other people. Patients can be denied access to any part of their case notes if it is considered that this would be 'likely to cause serious harm to the physical or mental health of the patient' (or of any other individual), or if it would result in disclosure of information relating to or provided by an identifiable person other than the patient. For this reason it is advisable to use separate sheets of paper to record sensitive information (such as sexual abuse).

It is also important that notes should be comprehensible to all others who have access to them. They should not contain obscure acronyms or abbreviations. Increasing use is being made of storing details of patients on computer. This information is kept confidential.

The Data Protection Act 1994 provides patients with the right of access to the information held on computer.

M. J. Ford • S. Nixon

2

The analysis of symptoms

Despite major advances in investigative techniques, an analysis of the history and the clinical examination remain the foundation on which correct diagnosis and sound treatment are based. Diagnosis is the balancing of probabilities, based on the presence or absence of specific symptoms and signs, and the application of scientific method. The accuracy of diagnosis improves with practice and clinical experience.

Some symptoms are of little value in precise diagnosis. For example, nausea is common in many different disorders, e.g. motion sickness, heart disease, brain tumours and gastrointestinal disorders. In contrast, the symptom of vomiting of blood is more specific as it suggests mucosal disease of the oesophagus, stomach or duodenum; it may however occur in severe nose bleeds or coagulation disorders.

Cardinal symptoms such as blood in the sputum, urine, faeces or vomit cannot be ignored because they are often associated with serious conditions; others such as transient loss of function in the arm or leg, or chest, pain on exertion are important because they may herald catastrophic events, e.g. a major stroke or myocardial infarction. A basic principle of medical diagnosis is that common diseases are common; when rare disorders are considered before common conditions have been excluded, the diagnosis is likely to be erroneous.

Probability mathematics and its application to medicine has become increasingly relevant and can be illustrated by the following example. Given a patient with unilateral lower abdominal pain, appendicitis should be suspected. The clinician knows that this disease is common and may know the local incidence of the disease (*probability analysis*). In addition, the doctor compares the patient's symptoms and signs with those of patients previously encountered, or with textbook descriptions. The clinician may also assess the pattern of symptoms, e.g. central pain moving into the right iliac fossa (*cluster analysis*) or use a 'flow chart' approach (*algorithm*), e.g. gynaecological diseases must be considered if the patient is female; torsion of a testicle if male and aged < 30 years.

Computer-assisted diagnosis has evolved with the availability of large patient databases and with the refinement of appropriate mathematical models. Most computer systems use one of the techniques illustrated above; however, the diagnostician uses them all, often in combination, and more. A brief description of probability theory is included in the Appendix.

APPROACH TO THE DIAGNOSIS

In establishing a medical diagnosis, the doctor considers a series of increasingly specific questions:

- Is the patient ill?
- Which organ system is principally affected?
- Are other organ systems also involved?
- What is the likely underlying pathological process?
- What is the precise diagnosis?

Running parallel with this process are secondary questions, the answers to which may become even more important that those listed above. These are:

- Why has the patient chosen to seek help now?
- What other problems may be present?
- What are the implications of the diagnosis for the patient?

One could argue that any patient attending a doctor with symptoms must be 'ill', but clearly there are grades of ill-health. The patient's perception of illness may be very different from the doctor's. Factors which appear to influence requests for medical consultation include employment status, female sex, chronic symptoms and psychological distress. The mere attendance of the patient indicates the concern that there may be a significant health problem, but perceptions vary widely. The anxious patient may consider minor complaints to be life-threatening, while the stoic may tolerate extreme pain without admitting ill-health. Furthermore, the presenting complaint may not be the only or the most important problem requiring the doctor's attention. A patient may have chosen the presenting symptom from a number of symptoms for several possible reasons; it may be the most severe, or the most familiar to the patient or even, from previous experience, the most 'medically acceptable'.

Severe symptoms are likely to present early; other modifying factors include speed of onset, chronicity and the distress and disruption associated with symptoms. Since a patient may experience mild symptoms for many months before seeking help, the clinician must also ask the question 'Why now?'. Either the symptoms have changed in frequency or severity or life events or other difficulties may have made the patient less able to cope with symptoms that were previously tolerable. The clinician must consider each of these possibilities and remain sympathetic, realising that a very few patients wilfully attempt to deceive, e.g. the drug addict trying to acquire drugs and the 'Munchausen' patient wanting to be admitted to hospital.

Differences between doctors' and patients' interpretations of common descriptive terms are universal. Nonetheless, the use of lay terms like 'wind', 'dizziness' or 'indigestion' is preferable to medical jargon such as 'borborygmi', 'vertigo' or 'dyspepsia' when asking patients to describe their symptoms. Such lay terms then need to be carefully analysed so that the clinician is in no doubt as to the nature of the symptom that is being experienced. The mode of onset, pattern of development and clustering of symptoms should be noted together with the time-scale in order to deduce the nature of the pathological process and the organ or systems involved. Alterations in lifestyle and daily activities should be sought to assess the social impact of the illness. Whilst the student is encouraged to take a complete history, the experienced doctor may require the answers to only a limited number of key questions to establish the correct diagnosis. In doing so, the doctor is employing a multivariate analytical approach, having recognised by experience the relevant symptoms which hold most of the predictive power. For example, in predicting the likely survival of women with breast cancer, there are over 50 known prognostic factors. However, 95% of the power of prediction comes from just four factors. Multivariate analysis is able to identify the most powerful predictors and generate a mathematical formula to allow a doctor to calculate the exact probability of diagnosis or outcome (see Appendix).

Most patients present with a constellation of symptoms, not just one complaint. This facilitates the diagnostic process because the presence of various symptoms alters the probabilities. However, some patients will be unaware of the importance of 'minor' complaints, and this emphasises the need to obtain as comprehensive a history as possible. This approach will be illustrated by analysis of a few common symptoms.

KEY POINTS

- Common diseases are common. Diagnostic problems are much more frequently due to unusual presentations of common disorders than to rare conditions.

- The presenting complaint may not be the only, or the most important, problem for which the patient is seeking help.

- It is often better to use lay terms rather than medical jargon when enquiring about symptoms, but a positive response requires further analysis.

- Most patients present with a number of symptoms, not just one complaint. This simplifies the diagnostic process as different constellations of symptoms suggest different pathological conditions.

SYMPTOM ANALYSIS

Tiredness, breathlessness, chest pain, abdominal pain and headache are common presenting symptoms. In most patients the diagnosis can be established or serious underlying disease excluded by a careful history and clinical examination without extensive further investigations. Some of these symptoms are therefore considered in detail to exemplify the importance of an analytical approach.

Tiredness

Tiredness is experienced by everybody and is the natural consequence of prolonged physical or mental activity often associated with sleep deprivation. The clinician must determine when physiological tiredness is compounded by the pathological tiredness associated with disease. Chronic tiredness is a common symptom and is experienced by approximately 25% of patients attending their general practitioner. Patients may complain of 'being tired all the time' yet there may be little evidence of incapacity or alteration in daily activity.

States of chronic fatigue may be described as being *peripheral* in origin when tiredness is predominantly perceived as weakness of the limbs with limitation of exercise tolerance, *central* in origin when loss of energy is expressed as a loss of drive and motivation or as a combination of both. Chronic tiredness is often associated with significant psychiatric illness and stressful life events but may occur with physical illness. It may be the main presenting complaint in anaemia, sleep apnoea syndrome and thyroid, cardiac, connective tissue and infectious disorders. Before embarking on investigations, the physician should consider whether the results might alter patient management, influence the prognosis or simply provide reassurance (see Tables 2.1 to 2.3).

Few patients however are prepared to attribute chronic tiredness to emotional or social factors; many demand extensive investigation. It is a strange paradox that many patients with vague symptoms such as tired-

Table 2.1 Checklist for the history of tiredness

Tiredness at rest	*Tiredness on exertion*
Onset – acute, recurrent or chronic	Anaemia
Variability day to day	Claudication or angina
Degree of social disability	Cardiac failure
Associated psychological symptoms	Respiratory failure
Associated physical symptoms	
Past medical and drug history	

Table 2.2 Psychological correlates in tiredness

- Absence of weight loss, fever or systemic illness
- Previous similar episodes of tiredness
- Symptoms of hyperventilation syndrome
- Symptoms of anxiety or depressive disorders
- History of stressful life events or difficulties

Table 2.3 Differential diagnosis in chronic tiredness

Psychiatric	Anxiety and depressive disorders
Infection	Glandular fever-like illnesses
Anaemia	Chronic bleeding, marrow disorders
Malignancy	Haematological, gastrointestinal
Drugs	Iatrogenic
	Self-administered
Alcohol abuse	
Endocrine disease	Thyroid, adrenal and pituitary
Connective tissues	Rheumatoid arthritis, systemic lupus erythematosus, polymyalgia
Cardiac	Ischaemic heart disease
	Cardiac failure
Respiratory	Chronic respiratory failure

ness would rather be given an unpleasant diagnosis than be told 'there is nothing wrong with you'. Such a statement usually provokes an unhelpful conflict between the clinician and patient.

It is often better to accept that the cause of tiredness may remain unknown and that the purpose of investigation is to exclude underlying disease. In this way, patients may be helped to recognise that somatic, emotional and situational factors may all have a part to play and to adopt a behavioural and cognitive approach necessary for effective management.

The *chronic fatigue syndrome*, previously termed post-viral fatigue syndrome or myalgic encephalomyelitis (ME), is a disorder characterised by extreme chronic tiredness. Explicit stringent criteria for its diagnosis have been suggested by the Center for Disease Control (CDC), Atlanta, USA. The major criterion is recent-onset severe fatigue unrelieved by rest which persists for at least 6 months in the absence of otherwise diagnosable physical or psychiatric illness.

KEY POINTS

- Tiredness is a natural consequence of sleep deprivation and of prolonged physical or mental activity.

- Chronic tiredness is more often psychological than physical in origin. The cause may remain unknown and the purpose of investigation is to reassure the patient by excluding those conditions that can be diagnosed.

Breathlessness

Contributory factors

The complaint of shortness of breath (*dyspnoea*) indicates a conscious appreciation of increased work done during breathing and is a natural consequence of strenuous physical exercise. Rapid, shallow breathing (*tachypnoea*) is less energy consuming than an increase in both ventilatory depth and rate (*hyperpnoea*).

The principal factors contributing to the production of breathlessness include an increase in the work of breathing, increased ventilatory drive and impaired respiratory muscle function. Each has a variety of causes and a number of factors may operate, either singly or in combination, in an individual patient to produce dyspnoea. The clinical analysis of the breathless patient comprises both an assessment of the severity of breathlessness and identification of its cause.

In general, there is little correlation between the respiratory rate and the sensation of breathlessness until ventilation has at least trebled. While some patients with severely impaired respiratory function may complain of minimal breathlessness, others with minor respiratory dysfunction may experience severe dyspnoea. Only when hypoxaemia is severe does it contribute significantly to the sensation of breathlessness. Similarly, there is little correlation between the symptom of breathlessness and the severity of hypercapnia. Though a rise in arterial $PaCO_2$ rapidly induces hyperventilation and breathlessness in healthy subjects, it may fail to do so in patients with chronic ventilatory failure in whom the respiratory centre is less responsive to arterial $PaCO_2$. Stimulation of pulmonary stretch receptors in the alveolar capillary walls (*J receptors*) may mediate the sensation of dyspnoea in pulmonary thromboembolism and congestive cardiac failure.

Breathlessness associated with increased work of breathing. The work of breathing is increased by airflow obstruction in either the small or large airways, reduction of pulmonary compliance ('stiff lungs') and restriction of chest expansion (Table 2.4).

Breathlessness associated with increased ventilatory drive. An increase in the physiological dead space (ventilation–perfusion mismatch) and stimulation of the respiratory centre (hyperventilation) may each contribute to an increase in ventilatory drive either singly or in combination, to produce dyspnoea.

Increased physiological dead space occurs when ventilation and perfusion are mismatched. The net result is often tachypnoea, hyperpnoea or both. Examples of abnormalities in ventilation include consolidation or collapse, obesity and pleuritic chest pain limiting chest

Table 2.4 Increased work of breathing

Airflow obstruction
Bronchial asthma
Chronic bronchitis and emphysema
Tracheal obstruction

Decreased pulmonary compliance
Pulmonary oedema
Pulmonary fibrosis
Extrinsic allergic alveolitis

Restricted chest expansion
Ankylosing spondylitis
Respiratory muscle paralysis
Kyphoscoliosis

wall expansion. Abnormalities in perfusion occur in pulmonary thromboembolism and congestive cardiac failure.

Hyperventilation resulting from stimulation of the respiratory centre may occur in response to chemical or neural stimuli (see Table 2.5). Hyperventilation associated with emotional distress may produce a respiratory alkalosis with decreased intracellular potassium, magnesium and alkali reserves and decreased ionisation of extracellular calcium. Breathing is often deep, irregular and sighing; patients may describe needing to take an extra breath or to breathe more deeply or the inability to fill the lungs completely. When hyperventilation is acute and sustained, tetany and even epilepsy may occur.

In the chronic hyperventilation syndrome (*effort syndrome*), the metabolic effects on neural and myoneural junctions may explain the spectrum of symptoms observed (see Table 2.6).

Breathlessness associated with impaired respiratory muscle function. Neuromuscular disorders may impair the function of the intercostal muscles and diaphragm to produce partial or complete respiratory paralysis. Examples include poliomyelitis, Guillain–Barré polyneuropathy, cervical cord transection, muscular dystrophies and myasthenia gravis.

Table 2.5 Chemical and neural stimulation of respiration

Increased arterial hydrogen ion concentration, e.g. metabolic acidosis producing 'air hunger' (*Kussmaul respiration*)

Increased arterial $Pa{CO}_2$, e.g. respiratory acidosis

Decreased arterial $Pa{CO}_2$ via aortic, carotid and brainstem chemoreceptors, e.g. pneumonia; impaired oxygen delivery due to anaemia, shock and stroke also stimulates the chemoreceptors

Increased central arousal, e.g. exertion, anxiety, thyrotoxicosis and phaeochromocytoma

Pulmonary J receptor discharge, e.g. pulmonary oedema

Table 2.6 Symptoms in chronic hyperventilation syndrome

- Lightheadedness, faintness and dizziness
- Dullness of hearing and tinnitus
- Peripheral and circumoral paraesthesiae
- Cold hands and feet and cold sweats
- Muscle cramps, muscle aches, trembling, shivering
- Constant tiredness and generalised weakness
- Breathlessness at rest with sighing and yawning
- Chest tightness, heaviness and palpitation
- Abdominal 'butterflies', cramps and bloating
- Urgency and frequency of defecation and micturition
- Restlessness, anxiety and panic attacks

Breathlessness associated with multiple factors. The pathophysiological mechanisms responsible for the production of dyspnoea in individual disease states are often complex and multifactorial (see Table 2.7).

Although pathophysiological considerations may help to explain the mechanisms of breathlessness, the cause of dyspnoea can often be assessed by obtaining a detailed history (see Tables 2.8 and 2.9).

Table 2.7 Specific factors producing breathlessness

Disorder	Factors
Pneumonia	Pyrexia stimulating respiratory centre
	Pleuritic pain limiting chest expansion
	Increased work – 'stiff lungs'
	Ventilation – perfusion mismatch
	Stimulation of pulmonary J receptors
	Hypoxaemia
	Low $Pa{CO}_2$
	Septic shock
Pulmonary oedema	Ventilation – perfusion mismatch
	Increased work – 'stiff lungs'
	Hypoxaemia
	Low $Pa{CO}_2$
	Cardiogenic shock
	Increased work – bronchiolar obstruction
	Hyperventilation – fear and anxiety

Table 2.8 Checklist for the history of breathlessness

- Mode of onset – acute or chronic
- Exercise tolerance – daily activities
- Associated symptoms
  Cough, sputum, haemoptysis
  Wheeze, chest pain
- Past history of allergic, cardiac or respiratory disorder
- Occupation – exposure to dust, pollens, animals, chemicals
- Tobacco consumption – past and present
- Recent travel abroad

Table 2.9 Causes of breathlessness

Physiological	*Pathological*
Exercise	Obesity
High altitude	Anaemia
	Respiratory disorders
Psychological	Cardiac disorders
Hyperventilation	
Pharmacological	
Drug-induced respiratory disorders	
Drug-induced cardiac disorders	

Table 2.11 Acute breathlessness: diagnostic value of associated symptoms

With chest pain	*Without chest pain, cough or wheeze*
If lateralised and pleuritic consider	*consider*
Pneumonia	Pulmonary embolism
Pulmonary infarction	Tension pneumothorax
Rib fracture	Hypovolaemic shock
Pneumothorax	Metabolic acidosis
If central and non-pleuritic consider	
Myocardial infarction	
Massive pulmonary embolism	
With cough and wheeze but without chest pain consider	
Asthma	
Pulmonary oedema	
Pneumothorax	

Clinical patterns

The cause of breathlessness is often indicated by the clinical pattern of its onset, duration and progression, variability, aggravating factors, relieving factors and associated symptomatology.

Mode of onset, duration and progression. The principal patterns of breathlessness may occur either independently or in combination and include rapid onset and progression over minutes, gradual onset and slow progression over days and slow onset and progression over months (see Table 2.10).

Variability, aggravating and relieving factors. Diurnal and day-to-day variability may be characteristic. Breathlessness which improves at the weekend or on holiday suggests extrinsic allergic alveolitis. In asthma, symptoms may be particularly striking after coughing or laughing or following exertion or exposure to smoke, dust, animal or plant allergens. Asthmatics usually complain of cough and wheeze with difficulty in exhaling. In children nocturnal coughing is often more obvious; the response to bronchodilator therapy may be of diagnostic value.

Breathlessness which wakes the patient from sleep is a typical feature of asthma because of diurnal variation in the calibre of the small airways. It also occurs in pulmonary oedema (*paroxysmal nocturnal dyspnoea*) (see p. 86) and in severe chronic obstructive airways disease. The patient often finds that sleeping upright, supported by several pillows, is more comfortable than lying flat. In cardiac failure, breathlessness which occurs on lying flat (*orthopnoea*) is the result of the postural increase in venous return further compromising cardiac output; in emphysema, orthopnoea is the result of reduced diaphragmatic movement which, in the upright position, is gravity assisted. Similarly, a postural increase in dyspnoea is a notable feature in patients with bilateral diaphragmatic paralysis.

Associated symptomatology. The common symptoms associated with breathlessness include cough, wheeze, sputum, haemoptysis and chest pain. Their presence associated with the acute onset of breathlessness may determine the likely diagnosis (see Table 2.11 and illustrative case study).

Severity

It is important to assess the severity of breathlessness in terms of daily activities. If these are impaired, the precise limiting factor should be identified. For example, the exercise tolerance of an elderly patient may be more limited by intermittent claudication, angina pectoris or osteoarthritic hips than by breathlessness attributable to chronic bronchitis. Though grading systems exist to assess cardiac and respiratory disabilities, simple questions about daily activity provide an effective functional assessment of the severity of dyspnoea (see Tables 2.12 and 2.13).

Table 2.10 Modes of onset, duration and progression

Minutes to hours	Hours to days	Months to years
Pneumothorax	Pneumonia	Pulmonary TB
Acute asthma	Pleural effusion	Chronic bronchitis
Pulmonary oedema	Anaemia	Bronchial carcinoma
Pulmonary embolism	Guillain–Barré Syndrome	Spondyloarthritis

Table 2.12 Functional assessment of breathlessness

- Is sleep disturbed by breathlessness?
- Does breathlessness occur at rest?
- Does breathlessness interfere with normal conversation?
- Does dressing or washing produce breathlessness?
- How far can the patient walk on the flat without stopping?
- How many stairs can the patient climb without stopping?
- What does breathlessness prevent the patient from doing?

Table 2.13 New York Heart Association classification: severity of heart failure

Grade I	No dyspnoea at rest or on moderate exertion
Grade II	Dyspnoea on moderate exertion No symptoms at rest or on mild exertion
Grade III	Dyspnoea on mild exertion but minimal at rest
Grade IV	Significant dyspnoea at rest and often bed bound Severe dyspnoea on minimal exertion

Note: Patients with major heart disease may have no, or only minor, symptoms, while patients with only minor heart disease may have major symptoms especially if they are anaemic, pregnant or anxious.

Illustrative case

A 60-year-old male was awakened by severe breathlessness causing him to get out of bed and open his bedroom window. The breathlessness settled after 20 minutes and there was no associated chest pain, cough or wheeze, reducing the possibilities of myocardial infarction, pneumothorax or asthma. He revealed that he had also noticed increasing central chest tightness on exertion over the previous 3 weeks. His younger brother, who had angina, had offered him one of his glyceryl trinitrate tablets, and this had rapidly relieved the chest tightness. The patient's age, family history, relationship of symptoms to exertion and the response to drug therapy strongly suggested ischaemic heart disease complicated by left ventricular failure; a subsequent electrocardiogram revealed an acute myocardial infarction.

KEY POINTS

- The assessment of the breathless patient involves considering the diagnostic possibilities and also assessing the functional severity of the dyspnoea.

- The rate of onset of breathlessness is often of diagnostic importance.

- Paroxysmal nocturnal dyspnoea is a feature of pulmonary oedema but also occurs in asthma.

Pain

The diagnostic importance of pain cannot be over-estimated; a meticulous analysis of pain will often reveal its cause. A careful clinical history should always be obtained because the experience gained from a thorough assessment of each and every variation of a painful disorder will greatly improve the diagnostic accuracy in typical cases.

The patient should be encouraged to describe the features of pain in detail and without interruption. Thereafter, further information should be sought by systematic analysis based upon the following characteristics:

- Main site
- Radiation
- Character
- Severity
- Duration
- Frequency and periodicity
- Special times of occurrence
- Aggravating factors
- Relieving factors
- Associated phenomena

Main site

The site at which pain is felt depends upon whether the innervation of the diseased organ is somatic or autonomic. Somatic pain is usually accurately localised, e.g. the sprained ankle, broken bone, skin abscess. Visceral pain derived from organs deeply placed in the body is less well localised. When single (unpaired) organs are the source, e.g. heart, gut and uterus, the pain is usually perceived in the midline. Pain arising from a paired organ, e.g. lungs, kidneys and ovaries, is felt to one or other side and rarely midline. Visceral pain may be distinguishable from somatic pain by its character, radiation and associated phenomena.

It is important to observe any gesture or body language the patient makes when localising a pain. For example, patients with a peptic ulcer may localise the pain to the midline of the upper abdomen with a finger, while in biliary disorders upper abdominal pain may be localised by rubbing the palm of the hand over the right upper quadrant, midline or lower chest. In angina pectoris, central chest pain is usually localised with a clenched fist or by gripping the chest between both hands.

Radiation

Pain may spread from the initial site of disease to other sites as a result of extension of the disease process or may be referred to anatomical sites remote from the site of disease.

Referred pain is the perception of sensory stimuli at any site along the distribution of a peripheral nerve or autonomic plexus. Diaphragmatic pain, due to pleurisy or peritonitis, may be experienced either over the back and lower abdomen via intercostal nerves (thoracic dermatomes T10–T12) or over the tip of the shoulder via the phrenic nerve (cervical dermatomes C3, C4, C5). Similarly, the pain of biliary tract disease may be felt over the shoulder blade or shoulder tip.

Pain may be experienced exclusively as referred pain without any pain at the site of the disease process. Thus, pain in the left forearm or shoulder could be due to angina pectoris, oesophagitis, cervical spondylosis or carpal tunnel syndrome. Similarly, pain due to lumbar disc compression of the lumbar nerve root (L5) may be felt as pain which radiates from the low back to the buttock, posterior thigh, calf or dorsum of the foot or in any single site or combination of sites along the distribution of the nerve root, even with a pain-free gap.

Spread of pain due to extension of disease is a characteristic feature of intra-abdominal diseases. In acute appendicitis, for example, pain is usually first felt around the umbilicus; after several hours, extension of the inflammatory response through to the serosal surface of the appendix and the overlying parietal peritoneum results in the pain moving to the right lower quadrant of the abdomen. Sometimes, pain due to disease extension may be the first indication of disease, e.g. duodenal ulceration may be asymptomatic until the acute onset of pain due to perforation.

Character

Superficial pain, e.g. a cut or burn, can be accurately identified by its pricking or burning character. Deep pain has a uniquely different character akin to the diffuse aching sensation reproduced by squeezing the Achilles tendon.

The behaviour of patients in pain may be helpful. In biliary or renal colic, restlessness is often marked as patients try many different positions in futile attempts to seek relief. In peritonitis, however, patients lie still to avoid aggravating abdominal pain. In acute conversion hysterical disorders, restlessness, groaning and weeping are prominent yet may abate temporarily when the patient is distracted by conversation. Characteristic descriptions of pain are shown in Table 2.14.

Table 2.14 Characteristic pain descriptions

Peptic ulcer pain	Gnawing, boring, hunger-like pain
Renal/Biliary colic	Severe gripping, cramp-like pain
Myocardial pain	Heavy, crushing, squeezing, vice-like, like a weight or a tight band on chest
Dissecting aneurysm	Tearing, searing, crushing pain
Pleurisy	Sharp, stabbing, knife-like pain
Tension headache	Like a tight band around the head
Migraine headache	Blinding, throbbing, sickening pain
Trigeminal neuralgia	Sharp, stabbing, knife-like pains like red-hot needles through the face

Severity

Patients differ widely in their pain thresholds and tolerances; the subjective intensity of pain is also dependent upon their state of mind and concentration. A remarkable indifference to pain may be observed in states of religious fervour, hypnosis, mania or during life-threatening events. In contrast, depression, anxiety, loneliness and introspection tend to aggravate pain severity.

In practice, an accurate assessment can usually be made of the intensity of pain, particularly if the patient is witnessed during its occurrence. Pain may be so severe in certain disorders, e.g. acute pancreatitis, peritonitis, biliary and renal colic and dissecting aortic aneurysm, that it is unusual to obtain an articulate description of its quality.

Duration

Pain may last for less than a second, as in trigeminal neuralgia, or days or weeks, as in osteomyelitis. Intestinal colic is felt in waves, each lasting less than a minute, while the pain of an uncomplicated duodenal ulcer rarely lasts longer than 2 hours. Exertional angina ceases within minutes of rest, whereas the pain of myocardial infarction may continue for several hours. The subjective assessment of the duration of pain can be very inaccurate and is best assessed in conjunction with its frequency and periodicity.

Frequency, periodicity and onset

Some pains occur intermittently in waves with a characteristic frequency, e.g. uterine contractions in labour and intestinal colic in obstruction occur every few minutes. In biliary 'colic', bouts of severe and sustained abdominal pain occur unpredictably with days, weeks or months between episodes; they are, however, so memorable that patients can often recall the exact number of painful episodes. In peptic ulceration, episodes of pain tend to occur over several days with pain-free intervals lasting weeks or months; during painful bouts, pain recurs predictably, often more than once a day, especially in the early hours of the morning. Information about the severity, duration and frequency of pain can be usefully summarised in the form of time–intensity graphs (see Fig. 2.1).

The speed of onset may give a valuable clue as to the pathological process. A sudden onset suggests a vascular cause. This may be produced by arterial occlusion with thrombus or an embolus, e.g. myocardial infarction, bowel infarction and acute ischaemia of the leg.

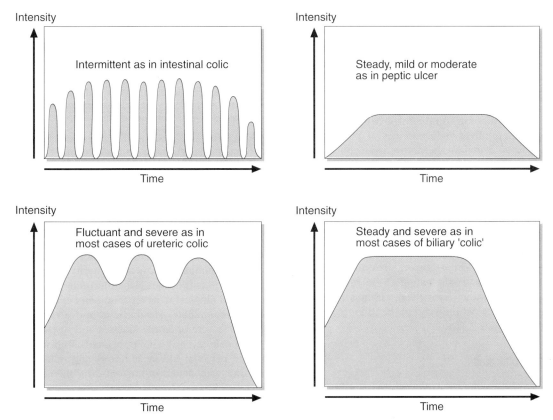

Fig. 2.1 Time–intensity graphs in pain syndromes.

Release of blood clot from venous thrombosis in the pelvis or lower limb leads to pulmonary embolism and infarction with sudden onset of pleuritic pain. Rupture of the abdominal aorta may cause sudden, acute back pain, and rupture of an intracerebral vessel produces sudden, severe headache. Perforation of the bowel also leads to rapid pain, as in perforated peptic ulceration of stomach or duodenum. Pain arising from an inflammatory process is usually progressive rather than sudden, e.g. appendicitis, pneumonia. An exception is acute pancreatitis, which can present as sudden severe pain, indistinguishable from perforated ulcer. Obstruction of the bowel may occur suddenly but results in slowly progressive pain as the intensity of smooth muscle contractions increases over time.

Special times of occurrence

It is important to establish the predictability of pain by careful questioning about special times of occurrence. For example, bone pain and neural pain are characteristically more troublesome when resting in bed.

Questions to ask might include:

- Has the patient ever experienced this pain before?
- Does pain wake the patient up during a sound sleep?
- Is pain present immediately on awakening?
- Is pain more likely to occur in the forenoon, afternoon, evening or at night?

Aggravating factors

The patient should first be asked if any aggravating factors are known before more specific questions are asked to determine if the pain is related to specific activities or postures, such as resting, exertion, sleeping, eating, defecation, micturition or sexual intercourse. Positive responses should be carefully assessed for reliability and reproducibility. For example, if bending apparently induces pain, is the patient able to tie shoelaces and, if so, how? Questions should be framed to avoid the expectation of a direct association: 'Does exercise make any difference to the pain?' is preferable to 'Does exercise aggravate the pain?'. Corroboration of a positive association should be sought

Table 2.15 Typical relieving factors in painful syndromes

- Resting in a darkened room in migraine
- Lowering the arm in carpal tunnel compression
- 'Walking off' the discomfort of restless legs syndrome
- Sitting upright and bending forward in pancreatitis or pericarditis

by further questioning to establish whether or not the patient purposefully avoids activities or postures that induce pain and makes alternative arrangements, e.g. by asking a neighbour to help carry heavy shopping.

Relieving factors

Similar caution should be exercised before accepting statements about relieving factors. Many pains resolve spontaneously and the apparent remedy may be just a placebo response. For example, abdominal pain in peptic ulceration is usually relieved 5–15 minutes after the ingestion of an antacid; relief within a minute or after 30 minutes is unlikely to be due to antacid therapy (see Table 2.15).

Associated phenomena

Pallor, sweating, nausea, vomiting and a sensation of impending death (*angor animi*) are common associated features of pain in myocardial infarction. In migraine, premonitory symptoms such as hunger, depression or an unusual feeling of well-being may herald an attack and give way to the typical visual disturbances experienced before the onset of headache and vomiting. Other examples include rigors prior to the onset of pleuritic chest pain in pneumonia or the loin pain of acute pyelonephritis, haematuria accompanying renal colic and the dark-brown urine associated with biliary colic.

These features should help characterise most pain syndromes. Examples are given of the application of the method in the assessment of chest pain (p. 87 and p. 138), abdominal pain (p. 163) and headache (see below).

KEY POINTS

- Detailed analysis of pain should provide the clinician with the likely site of origin and underlying pathological process.

- Precipitating, relieving, aggravating and associated factors often provide the best clues.

- Pain with no accompanying features should raise the possibility of a psychological rather than physical basis.

- Visceral pain is often less accurately localised than somatic pain. When arising from a single organ, such as the heart or gut, visceral pain is usually perceived in the midline.

- The subjective assessment of the duration of pain is often very inaccurate, unlike the speed of initial onset.

- A remarkable 'tolerance' of pain may occur in situations which are life-threatening.

Headache

Headache is one of the commonest and most demanding of symptoms to assess. A detailed history is frequently more important and more helpful than the physical examination. In the majority of patients, the diagnosis is tension headache; no underlying disease or abnormal physical signs are found and emotional factors often predominate. Headache is also a common non-specific feature of febrile illnesses and systemic diseases (see Table 2.16). The past medical history, family history, personal and social history and systemic enquiry together with details of current drug therapy are often relevant. The assessment of headache should include its characterisation using the method described for pain.

Main site

Whether headache affects the entire head, half the head or a smaller area in one part of the head, neck or face is often of paramount diagnostic significance. Typical examples of headaches and their relationship to the site are shown in Table 2.17.

Table 2.16 Common causes of headache

Extracranial disorders	*Example*
Temporomandibular joint	Osteoarthritis
Cervical spine	Cervical spondylosis
Ophthalmological	Glaucoma
Teeth	Dental sepsis
Middle ear	Earache
Paranasal sinuses	Sinusitis
Arteries	Cranial arteritis
Intracranial disorders	
Migraine	
Meningitis	
Intracranial hypertension	
Tumour	
Subarachnoid bleed	
Psychosomatic disorders	
Tension headache	

Table 2.17 Relationship between the cause and site of headache

Disorder	Site
Tension headache	Bilateral, generalised or nuchal
Migraine	Unilateral; different sides on separate occasions
Cluster headache	Unilateral; eye, nose, cheek
Cranial arteritis	Unilateral with scalp tenderness
Trigeminal neuralgia	Unilateral; maxillary or mandibular branches of the trigeminal nerve
Post-herpetic neuralgia	Unilateral; ophthalmic branch of the trigeminal nerve

Radiation

Unilateral pain radiating to the throat, ear, eye, nose, cheek or face is typical of the neuralgias. Facial pain extending beyond the territory of the trigeminal nerve and which may be bilateral or involve the tongue or mouth suggests a psychogenic cause. Pain radiating to the neck with tenderness of the neck muscles is typical of tension headache.

Character

Pain likened to a tight band around the head or like a pressure over the head is characteristic of tension headache; in contrast, headaches that are described as sickening, dull aching or throbbing are usually migrainous in origin. Lancinating, paroxysmal pain like red-hot needles thrust through the face suggests trigeminal neuralgia.

Severity

The explosive onset of severe headache associated with neck stiffness is a common feature of subarachnoid haemorrhage, while a slowly progressive headache increasing in duration and severity is typical of raised intracranial pressure from a cerebral tumour. Severity is often also marked in migraine, cluster headache and trigeminal neuralgia; in the last, paroxysms of severe pain may cause the patient to wince and cry out momentarily.

Duration

It is important to establish whether headache lasts seconds, minutes, hours, days or weeks; whether pain is intermittent or constant and if there is more than one type of headache. The longer the history without progression, the more likely its cause is benign. Migraine attacks often last longer than 24 hours but occasionally last less than six hours. Episodes of cluster headache typically last less than an hour. In trigeminal neuralgia, each paroxysm lasts only seconds recurring over several minutes. In contrast, tension headache may last several days without disrupting sleep.

Frequency and periodicity

Attacks with a sudden onset occurring in repeated short bursts with pain-free intervals lasting weeks or months are characteristic of migraine, trigeminal neuralgia and cluster headache. Post-herpetic neuralgia and cranial arteritis have an acute onset but are continuous, and meningitis and subarachnoid haemorrhage have an acute onset with rapid progression and are continuous.

Special times of occurrence

Severe pain waking a patient from sleep in the early hours of the morning is typical of cluster headaches and raised intracranial pressure. Pain precipitated by facial movement such as eating, drinking, shaving or brushing the teeth suggests trigeminal or glosso-pharyngeal neuralgia. Jaw pain during chewing is typical of cranial arteritis. Headaches occurring at the onset of menarche and premenstrually suggest migraine.

Aggravating factors

Headache that is increased by bending, straining and coughing suggests raised intracranial pressure. Migraine may be aggravated post-partum, by hunger, intake of chocolate, cheese, alcohol and citrus fruits and by the contraceptive pill. The headache of benign intracranial hypertension is associated with weight gain and with the use of corticosteroids, tetracycline and contraceptive drug therapy.

Relieving factors

Migrainous attacks are characteristically less frequent and less severe during pregnancy. Headaches usually respond well to analgesic therapy; those that are poorly responsive are usually tension headaches. In contrast, migraine responds rapidly to sumatriptan, a $5-HT_1$ agonist. A rapid and dramatic response of cranial arteritis to corticosteroid therapy is similarly characteristic.

Associated phenomena

Nausea and vomiting are typical of migraine and raised intracranial pressure but unusual in other causes of headache, including tension headache. Diarrhoea, polyuria and syncope are also occasionally experienced in migraine. Intolerance to light (photophobia) or noise (phonophobia), irritability, food cravings and hunger, visual disturbances (teichopsia), peripheral and circumoral paraesthesiae are all common premonitory features of migraine. Patients with cluster headaches may experience watering of the eye or nose or even ptosis of an eyelid.

KEY POINTS

- The site of headache is often diagnostically significant.
- Tension headache is very common. It may last for several days without disturbing sleep patterns.
- Unlike tension headache, headaches caused by organic disease are often progressive in nature.

Fits, faints and funny turns

The terms 'blackout', 'dizziness' and 'funny turn' are commonly used to describe the sudden onset of an altered state of consciousness. Such episodes may denote any of the following syndromes:

- *Vertigo*: a sensation of unsteadiness and loss of balance associated with a feeling of rotational movement due to impaired vestibular function of either a central or peripheral origin.
- *Syncope*: lightheadedness or faintness associated with the feeling of impending and/or actual loss of consciousness due to a reduction in cerebral blood flow.
- *Epilepsy*: loss of consciousness associated with generalised seizures due to paroxysmal, neuronal discharges.
- *Drop attack*: falls occurring without warning or loss of consciousness associated with sudden weakness of the legs.

Vertigo

The vestibular system includes the peripheral vestibular apparatus of the inner ear and vestibular nerve and the central connections of the vestibular nuclei within the brain stem.

Any disorder which disrupts the balance of the two vestibular inputs may produce vertigo of varying severity from a 'swimming sensation' in the head to severe unsteadiness of gait with nausea and vomiting. A *peripheral disorder* producing vertigo is suggested by the association with cochlear symptoms, e.g. unilateral

Table 2.18 Patterns of vertigo and their causes

Without deafness and tinnitus	With deafness and tinnitus
Acute	
Viral vestibular neuronitis	Skull fracture
Multiple sclerosis	Meniere's disease
Acute and recurrent	
Benign positional vertigo	Meniere's disease
Migraine	Chronic otitis media
Multiple sclerosis	Acoustic neuroma
Chronic and persistent	
Multiple sclerosis	Ototoxic drugs
Vertebrobasilar ischaemia	Acoustic neuroma

or bilateral *deafness* and *tinnitus* (abnormal noises in the ear). A *central disorder* producing vertigo is suggested by the association with neurological symptoms. It is important to establish the mode of onset: brief, acute episodes are usually due to a peripheral labyrinthine disorder, although acute brainstem ischaemia, temporal lobe epilepsy and Meniere's disease may also present in this way; chronic vertigo of gradual onset not associated with cochlear symptoms suggests a central lesion (see Table 2.18).

Syncope

Transient reductions in cerebral blood flow may result from a reduction in cardiac output, increased peripheral vasodilation or a combination of the two (see Table 2.19).

Vasovagal syncope or simple faints usually occur in the standing position and rarely during lying or on exertion. Prodromal features include nausea, weakness and sensations of heat, tinnitus and dimming of vision. Bradycardia, peripheral vasodilatation and hypotension produce the transient loss of consciousness, which may be averted by lying down or putting the head well

Table 2.19 Causes of syncope

Vasovagal syncope
Postural syncope
Cough or micturition syncope
Vertebrobasilar arterial insufficiency
Carotid sinus hypersensitivity
Cardiogenic syncope
   Arrhythmias
      bradyarrhythmias (Stokes–Adams)
      tachyarrhythmias
   Outflow obstruction
      aortic, pulmonary or mitral stenosis
      hypertrophic cardiomyopathy
      atrial myxoma, constrictive pericarditis

down. Sweating and skin pallor are often observed, and episodes commonly follow prolonged standing or intense emotional stimuli.

Postural syncope occurs soon after standing upright or on prolonged standing and is common after prolonged bed rest. Its occurrence suggests impaired vasomotor reflexes due to autonomic neuropathy or vasodepressor drug treatment, or sodium and water depletion due to adrenal or renal insufficiency, excessive intestinal or cutaneous losses or following intense exertion.

Exertional syncope occurs during rather than following exertion and suggests impaired cardiac output due to pericardial, myocardial or valvular heart disease.

Syncope due to cardiac arrhythmias characteristically occurs suddenly and without warning; the patient may appear dead and be pale and pulseless as a result of either ventricular tachycardia or asystole. Recovery is often rapid and accompanied by facial flushing.

Syncope associated with head movements suggests either carotid sinus hypersensitivity or vertebrobasilar arterial insufficiency; carotid sinus massage or extension of the cervical spine during upward gaze may precipitate further episodes.

Syncope on coughing characteristically follows a prolonged, purple-faced paroxysm of coughing in a chronic bronchitic.

Syncope on micturition is uncommon and occurs in elderly males with prostatism who strain to empty their bladder in the upright position after rising from sleep.

Epilepsy

Epileptic discharges may arise from one small area of the cortex and remain localised (*partial or focal seizures*) or may arise from structures deep within the central brain and spread rapidly to both hemispheres (*generalised seizures*). Partial seizures may be *simple* and not impair consciousness or *complex* and impair consciousness; both simple partial and complex partial seizures may progress to become generalised seizures (see Tables 2.20 and 2.21).

The cause of epilepsy. Recognition that a patient's blackouts are epileptic in origin is only the first stage in the diagnostic process as the cause must then be established. Epilepsy may be familial, congenital or acquired (see Table 2.21).

Differential diagnosis of syncope and epilepsy

Most blackouts are due to either syncope or epilepsy. Patients who fall to the ground may attribute the episode to a trip; those who are unable to recall hitting the ground have usually lost consciousness before

Table 2.20 Classification of seizures

Generalised seizures
Absence attacks – petit mal (3 Hz spike and wave)
Myoclonic seizures – myoclonic jerks
Tonic clonic seizures (grand mal or major fits)
Tonic seizures
Atonic or akinetic seizures

Partial seizures (minor fits)
Simple partial seizures – no loss of consciousness
Complex partial seizures – loss of consciousness
Partial seizures evolving into generalised seizures
Generalised seizures with only EEG evidence of focal onset

Pseudo-seizures (hysterical conversion disorder)

Table 2.21 Aetiological clues in the history of epilepsy

Feature	Possible cause
Childhood onset	Idiopathic
Headaches	Intracerebral bleed or tumour
Focal symptoms	Intracerebral tumour
Nocturnal fits	Idiopathic Hypoglycaemia
Alcohol abuse	Alcohol withdrawal Subdural haematoma Hypoglycaemia
Sexual promiscuity or drug abuse	HIV infection
Drug therapy	Iatrogenic
Pregnancy	Eclampsia
Hypertension/CVA	Cerebrovascular disease

falling. The differential diagnosis of blackouts is entirely clinical and is best diagnosed by a trained observer who has witnessed an episode. As this is not often possible, every effort must be made to interview any available eyewitness. Without an eyewitness the diagnosis can only be inferred from the patient's account of antecedent and postcedent events.

Prodromal features. Nausea, visual dimming and a sense of impending loss of consciousness precipitated by prolonged standing or intense emotional excitement favour syncope. Hyperventilation may be a prodromal feature but may also produce epilepsy in susceptible patients. Episodes of unconsciousness occurring while sleeping or watching television or stroboscopic discotheque lights suggests epilepsy.

Eyewitness account. A history of tonic or convulsive movements, facial grimacing, grunting, jaw clenching, tongue biting or irregular noisy breathing clearly suggests seizures. However, syncope may result in urinary incontinence, and patients with seizures may appear syncopal with pallor, sweating and limpness. Cardiac arrhythmias may result in a seizure due to cerebral hypoxia.

Falls and drop attacks

Changes in the erect posture and balance are normally monitored by visual, proprioceptive and vestibular receptors. Disorders of these systems may impair balance and are often first manifested by increased sway. Severe disorders of balance usually only ensue when more than one of the sensory systems are impaired. Proprioception is particularly important in maintaining static balance, while the vestibular system is more important in dynamic balance, e.g. walking on uneven pavements. In normal healthy elderly subjects, shorter step length and increased sway alter both the gait and the balance. The increased risk of falls in the elderly is particularly marked in those with dementia or cerebrovascular or locomotor disorders.

Accidental falls (trips or slips) should be distinguished from *spontaneous falls*. A careful history will often reveal that patients feel unsteady or frightened that they are going to fall when standing or walking without any associated dizziness or impairment of consciousness. Less commonly, patients may experience *drop attacks*, a sudden, unpredictable loss of power in the lower limbs causing the patient to crumple to the ground without dizziness or loss of consciousness.

Table 2.22 Checklist for the history of falls

Was it an accidental fall?
Recall of event
Trip or slip
Walking surface
Footware
Illumination
Visual acuity

Was it a spontaneous fall?
Preceding symptoms
Onset with head movement or standing upright
Associated symptoms of vertigo, deafness or tinnitus
Associated chest pain or palpitation
Awareness of hitting the ground
Eyewitness account
Resulting injuries or incontinence
Recall of events at the time
Ability to regain erect posture
Previous confusion, dementia or parkinsonism
Previous hypertension, blackouts or epilepsy
Previous drug therapy – antidepressants, hypnotics
Alcohol consumption

KEY POINTS

- Any eyewitness account of a 'blackout' is often the most critical part of the clinical examination.

- Patients who fall may attribute the episode to a trip. Those who lose consciousness before falling cannot recall hitting the ground.

- Epilepsy is not a diagnosis; it is always important to establish the underlying cause of the convulsion.

Characteristically, even with help, patients with drop attacks are unable to stand upright for several minutes afterwards (see Table 2.22).

Weight loss

Body weight is best assessed using the *body mass index* [weight (kg)/height^2 (m); normal = 19–25]. In health, body weight fluctuates by several kilograms from year to year. In menstruating females, there is often a marked fluctuation in weight due to premenstrual fluid retention. Loss of body fluid for any reason, e.g. diuretic therapy, can produce rapid and dramatic weight loss (1 litre of water = 1 kilogram). In most patients with weight loss, however, there is a reduction in both adipose and fat-free mass. Weight loss of this nature is either produced by reduced energy intake or increased energy expenditure. Significant weight loss occurring as an isolated symptom is rarely associated with serious disease. In most instances, a careful history will elicit other symptoms and alert the clinician to the underlying cause (see Table 2.23 and illustrative case study).

Table 2.23 Aetiological clues in the history of weight loss

Symptom	Possible cause
Feeling low	Grief, depression
Absence of anorexia	Thyrotoxicosis, diabetes mellitus
Polyuria	Diabetes mellitus, Addison's disease
TB contact	Tuberculosis
Sexual promiscuity or drug abuse	HIV infection
Alcohol abuse	Malnutrition, TB, pancreatic disease
Haemoptysis	Bronchial carcinoma
Haematuria	Renal carcinoma
Breathlessness	Cardiac failure, chronic bronchitis
Pruritus	Haematological malignancy
Altered bowel habit	Colonic carcinoma
Vomiting	Anorexia nervosa, gastric carcinoma
Diarrhoea	HIV, malabsorption syndromes
Travel abroad	Tropical sprue

Weight loss is usually the result of reduced calorie intake rather than increased energy consumption. While some patients can accurately quantify their weight loss, many cannot. The patient may assess the rate and severity of weight loss from ill-fitting clothes. Whenever possible such subjective assessment should be confirmed objectively. Review of previously documented weights from case records may avoid needless investigation in patients who mistakenly believe they are losing weight. Weight loss may result from physical, psychological or social factors. In addition to a search for serious underlying disease, the physician should enquire of changes in the social well-being and lifestyle of the patient. Grief, depression and chronic alcohol abuse are commonly associated with weight loss. Weight loss with amenorrhoea in an adolescent female suggests the possibility of anorexia nervosa.

Illustrative case

A 14-year-old girl presented with a history of weight loss of 14 lb over the previous year. Though menarche had occurred at the age of 12, menstruation had stopped 6 months previously, raising the possibility of anorexia nervosa. On further questioning, however, it emerged that 1 year ago she had developed generalised aches and pains with arthralgia associated with a painful skin rash over the lower limbs. She remembered the date of onset as her grandfather had returned to Jamaica following his visit to the UK. For 3 months prior to the consultation, she had complained of night sweats and a dry cough. The probability of pulmonary tuberculosis was suggested by a family history of TB, presumed erythema nodosum, persistent febrile symptoms and the absence of BCG inoculation. The diagnosis was rapidly confirmed by chest radiograph and sputum microscopy.

KEY POINTS

- Weight loss, as an isolated symptom, is infrequently associated with serious underlying organic disease.

- Many people respond to stress or depression by changing eating habits, and depression in particular may present as weight loss.

REFERENCES

Knill-Jones R P 1987 Logic in medicine: diagnostic systems as an aid to clinical decision making. British Medical Journal 295: 1392–1396.

Macartney F J 1987 Logic in medicine: diagnostic logic. British Medical Journal 1987 295: 1325–1331.

3

J. A. A. Hunter • J. F. Munro

General examination and the external features of disease

The physical examination starts as soon as the clinician meets the patient and includes an assessment of general appearance, dress, demeanour and personal hygiene. A remarkable number of conditions can be identified at first glance. Some are very obvious, such as gross obesity; others less so, such as the increased arterial neck pulsation in aortic incompetence or the blue sclera of severe iron deficiency anaemia and osteogenesis imperfecta (Fig. 3.1A). The student can test the skill of making these observations on the general public! First impressions are often invaluable. For example, hypothyroidism may be identified on first sight but overlooked by somebody in regular contact with the patient who has failed to appreciate the onset of the insidious changes in voice and facial appearance.

The converse, however, is equally important. Physical signs may be easily missed during a routine examination unless the clinician looks specifically for them. The very concept of performing a complete physical examination is misleading and should be avoided

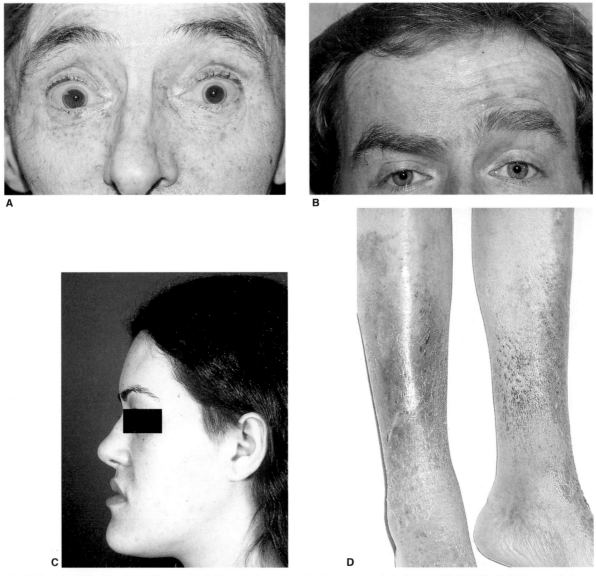

Fig. 3.1 Examples of the value of 'spot diagnoses'. **A.** Blue sclera in a patient with osteogenesis imperfecta (Courtesy of Dr D.H.A. Boyd). **B.** VII nerve palsy in a patient with sarcoidosis (Courtesy of Dr D.H.A. Boyd). **C.** The facies in acromegaly. **D.** Legs of an elderly patient showing dry, cracked skin, pigmentation and purpura. The features suggest severe malnutrition with scurvy.

except as an exercise in practising examination techniques. It is time-consuming and inappropriate to test every patient's sense of smell and colour vision and to always examine the abdomen for shifting dullness. But it is essential to perform these tests in certain circumstances. It follows that, once the history has been obtained, the clinician should consciously, or with experience subconsciously, consider what physical features may be present and to then examine the patient accordingly. A useful maxim is 'You only find what you look for'.

There is no one correct way or correct sequence of performing the physical examination. Some clinicians may start by examining that system which appears to be most affected; others may first examine the hands and others examine the patient from the feet upwards. Students should be encouraged to develop their own sequence and 'style' of examination rather than to follow uncritically a rigid regime. This book does not attempt to describe *the* method of physical examination but rather to provide a satisfactory and effective method of examination. The purpose of this chapter is to describe the following:

- the significance of those general observations that can be made before formally examining the patient
- the examination of the hands and head, which can be performed without asking the patient to undress
- the examination of the skin
- those other components of the examination which cannot be assigned to any single system. This includes examination of the lymphatic system and the breasts. It also includes an assessment of the endocrine disorders, which may be diagnosed by the alert clinician but, if the diagnosis is not considered at an early stage, may not be made at all.

GENERAL OBSERVATIONS

DEMEANOUR

Early impressions of the patient's condition are influenced by many factors including the greeting, mobility and facial expression.

The handshake

This usually provides the first opportunity for the clinician to make physical contact with the patient, and is a useful prelude to the more intimate aspects of examination. A friendly handshake at the onset will offer the patient reassurance. Strength of handshake may provide an index of the patient's personality and may also give diagnostic clues. It is abnormal in many neurological or locomotor disorders, such as spastic hemiparesis or severe Dupuytren's contracture. Indeed, it is advisable to always check surreptitiously that the patient's right hand is present and reasonably functional. If this is not the case, it is best to avoid shaking hands or to proffer the left hand. Much information may be available from a 'normal' handshake (see Table 3.1.).

Posture and gait

Useful information can be obtained by observing a normal gait, which ranges from the brisk and erect to the slouched and shuffling. Abnormalities in gait should be carefully analysed as they may indicate a neurological (p. 203) or a locomotor disturbance (p. 281). Similar observations should be made about the posture of the patient sitting or lying in bed. Much information may also be available by observing the bed itself and the surrounds, for example,

- Is the bed level or tilted?
- Has the bed got 'cot sides'?
- Is there a bed cage, ripple mattress, monkey rail or other apparatus?
- How many pillows are in use?
- Is there a sputum mug?
- Is oxygen in use or available for use?
- Has the patient been catheterised?

Facial expression

Facial expression, including the presence or lack of eye-to-eye contact, is a useful index of physical and psychological well-being (see Table 3.2).

The recognition of the looks of pain, fear, anxiety, anger or grief does not require medical training but should alert the clinician to explore the underlying emotional issues. Without intending to deceive, some patients may manage to conceal their apprehension or cloak their feelings in an air of feigned cheerfulness.

Table 3.1 Some information available from a normal handshake

Features	Diagnosis
Large hands with excessive sweating	Acromegaly
Hot and sweaty hands	Thyrotoxicosis
Cold and sweaty hands	Anxious
Dry and coarse skin	Hypothyroidism
Delayed relaxation of grip	Dystrophia myotonica

Table 3.2 Examples of abnormal facial expressions

Features	Diagnosis
Poverty of expression	Parkinsonism
Startled	Hyperthyroidism
Apathy and poverty of expression	Depression
Agitation	Hypomania
Peering	Myopia
Apparent indifference	Hysterical conversion

The doctor should avoid adopting, or being misled by, such a patient's apparently lighthearted attitude. The experienced clinician behaves naturally and thereby reduces risks of misunderstanding.

COMPLEXION

Abnormalities of complexion may be noticed by patients or by their friends or relations. With careful observation, complexion may provide a sensitive index of disease. The appearance of skin complexion may be influenced by artificial lighting.

The colour of the face depends upon variations in oxyhaemoglobin, reduced haemoglobin, melanin and, to a lesser extent, carotene. Unusual skin colours, excluding those which have been applied externally, are due to abnormal pigments such as the sallow brownish tinge seen in uraemia. The bluish tinge of 'enterogenous' cyanosis, produced by abnormal haemoglobins such as sulphaemoglobin and methaemoglobin, may be caused by drugs such as dapsone and some sulphonamides. The pink colour characteristic of carbon monoxide poisoning from coal gas is due to excessive carboxy-haemoglobin in the blood. Metabolites of drugs may themselves, or in combination with melanin, cause striking abnormal coloration of the skin, for example mepacrine (yellow), clofazamine (red) and phenothiazines (slate grey on exposed areas) (Fig. 3.2B).

Haemoglobin

Untanned Caucasoid skin is pink owing to the red pigment oxyhaemoglobin in the capillary-venous plexuses of the superficial dermis. The contribution of haemoglobin to the complexion is influenced by the proportion which is oxygenated or reduced.

Pallor may be due to anaemia or to vasoconstriction, which may occur when subjects are frightened or faint. The observation by relatives or friends of increasing pallor may be an early feature of progressive anaemia. Examination of the mucous membranes may help to distinguish the pallor of anaemia from that of other causes.

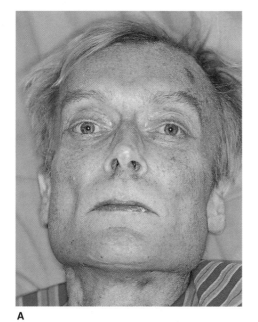

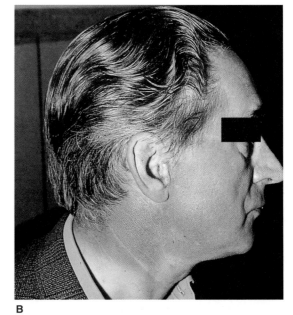

A

B

Fig. 3.2 Abnormal coloration of the skin. **A**. Jaundice (Courtesy of Dr M.A. Eastwood). **B**. Phenothiazine-induced pigmentation.

Vasodilation may produce a deceptive pink complexion even in the presence of anaemia. An unduly plethoric complexion may be seen in polycythaemia, some alcohol abusers with a pseudo-Cushing's syndrome and in Cushing's syndrome itself (see Fig. 3.4B, p. 47). The plethora of Cushing's syndrome is due to thinning of the skin with enhanced visibility of superficial blood vessels.

Cyanosis

This is discussed on page 94.

Melanin

This pigment is normally formed in the deepest layer of the epidermis and colours the skin brown or even black. The amount present is largely determined by hereditary influences. The pigment increases or diminishes in amount with exposure to, or withdrawal from, ultraviolet light. The amount and distribution of melanin is modified in a number of situations (see Table 3.3).

Vitiligo and albinism may affect any race, whereas the characteristic pallor of hypopituitarism is only apparent in white races.

The overproduction of melanin in adrenal insufficiency results in the development of brown pigmentation of the skin, particularly in creases, in scars, overlying bony prominences and on areas exposed to pressure from belts, braces and tight clothing. Melanin may also be deposited in the mucous membranes of the lips and of the mouth, where it results in patches of a slatey grey–brown pigmentation (Fig. 3.20, p. 62). Pregnancy is commonly associated with a blotchy pigmentation of the face, 'melasma' or 'chloasma', and increased pigmentation of the areolae, the linea alba and around the genitalia.

Table 3.3 Local and generalised causes of abnormal melanin production

Underproduction	
Patchy (vitiligo)	Autoimmune loss of melanocytes
Total absence (albinism)	Genetic failure to form tyrosinase
Partial absence (hypopituitarism)	Diminished pituitary formation of melanotrophic peptides
Overproduction	
Adrenal insufficiency (Addison's disease)	Excessive pituitary formation of melanotrophic peptides
Pregnancy	Owing to oestrogen, progesterone and pituitary melanotrophic peptides
Heavy metals including iron	As in haemochromatosis
Freckles, lentigines and pigmented naevi	Local overproduction

In both Addison's disease and hypopituitarism vasoconstriction occurs in the skin, so that pigmentation and pallor respectively are accentuated.

Carotene

Hypercarotenaemia occasionally occurs in vegetarians or in subjects who eat a lot of raw carrots and tomatoes. The orange–yellow pigment carotene is unevenly distributed in the subcutaneous fat and epidermis. It is seen particularly on the face, palms and soles but not in the sclerae. A yellowish discoloration of the face may appear in hypothyroidism because of impaired hepatic metabolism of carotene.

Bilirubin

In jaundice, the sclerae, mucous membranes and skin are lemon–yellow in colour (Fig. 3.2A). A useful site to look for jaundice is the sublingual mucosa. Jaundice that is obvious in daylight may be undetected in artificial light.

In haemolytic jaundice there is an increase in circulating unconjugated bilirubin, which is not excreted in the urine. The stools are dark and the urine looks normal but contains an excess of urobilinogen.

In hepatocellular and obstructive jaundice bilirubin has been dissociated from plasma albumin and conjugated with glucuronic acid by the liver. Conjugated bilirubin is water soluble and readily passes through the renal glomeruli. The urine is brown like beer and the stools tend to be pale in colour like putty, because of the reduction in the amount of bile in the faeces. If jaundice is deep and long-standing a distinct greenish colour develops in the sclerae and in the skin due to the presence of biliverdin. Scratch marks may be prominent in obstructive jaundice; the precise cause of the associated pruritus is unknown but may be attributed to the retention of bile acids. The causes of hepatocellular and obstructive jaundice are discussed on page 167.

Haemosiderin

This is another haemoglobin breakdown product. It may be difficult to distinguish from melanin though it has a more gingery hue. It occurs frequently in the wake of purpura (Fig. 3.10, p. 40) and is seen most commonly on the lower legs, like a sprinkling of pepper, where blood under the influence of gravity is most likely to leak from small capillaries.

ABNORMAL MOVEMENTS

Involuntary movements may be due to organic disease of the central nervous system, particularly when the extrapyramidal system is involved. Disorders of movement may also result from primary disease elsewhere (see Table 3.4).

The 'flapping tremor' of encephalopathy due to hepatic failure may not be apparent except by inspecting the outstretched arms with the hands dorsiflexed. The sign consists of irregular jerky movements of the hands due to flexion and extension of the wrists and fingers.

ABNORMAL SOUNDS

Normal speech depends upon the tongue, lips, palate and nose, the integrity of the mucosa, muscles and nerve supply of the larynx and the ability to expel sufficient air from the lungs.

The neurological abnormalities which cause disturbances of voice and speech are described on page 204. Many of the other causes can be recognised by inspection, for example a cleft palate, nasal obstruction, loose dentures or a dry mouth. Hoarseness of the voice may be neurological in origin, due to laryngitis or the result of excessive smoking. The voice in myxoedema may be so characteristic that the diagnosis can be made over the telephone without seeing the patient. The normal inflections of tone disappear, speech is low-pitched, slow and deliberate, and seems to require more effort than normal; it sounds 'thick'. Many of these changes are due to myxoedematous infiltration of the tissues concerned in voice production.

Several other types of abnormal sound may be heard. Wheezing, rattling or stridor (p. 139) may help in the differentiation of dyspnoea. The character of a cough may be revealing (p. 137). Witnesses may give an account of a whoop suggestive of pertussis or the cry of an epileptic fit. Audible noises of cardiovascular and alimentary origin are described in the appropriate chapters.

ABNORMAL ODOURS

The body normally produces an odour. This largely arises from apocrine sweat contaminated by diphtheroid bacteria and may be reduced by the use of deodorants or concealed with perfume. Excessive sweating causes an increase in body odour which becomes pungent. Poor personal hygiene results in an exaggeration of this smell, which may be compounded by the odour of dirty and soiled clothing and the smell of dried-out urine. Where washing and toilet facilities are available, malodour usually only occurs in:

- the very elderly and infirm
- those with a physical disability that prevents normal toileting
- subjects with severe learning difficulties or personality disorders
- those with dementia and other causes of progressive brain damage.

Some abnormal odours are sufficiently characteristic as to be diagnostic:

- the sickly 'fetor hepaticus' of liver failure
- the sweetness of the breath in diabetic or starvation ketoacidosis, which is obvious to some observers but is not appreciated at all by others
- the smell of wounds or ulcers infected by *Pseudomonas aeruginosa*
- the characteristic smell of wet gangrene, chronic suppuration, necrotic tumours or some skin disorders.

Halitosis or malodorous breath is often unrecognised by the patient but offensive to others. Sometimes halitosis occurs without any obvious explanation. It may be caused by decomposing food wedged between the teeth, gingivitis, stomatitis, atrophic rhinitis and tumours of the nasal passages, as well as pulmonary suppuration. Bronchiectasis may be associated with offensive breath, and in some cases the patient may notice that expectorated sputum tastes foul. In patients with gastric outlet obstruction from scarring or carcinoma of the stomach, foul-smelling eructations may occur, but probably the most offensive odour of this type is associated with a gastrocolic fistula caused by the faecal contents of the stomach.

Tobacco has a characteristic lingering smell which pervades clothing. Marijuana can also be identified by smell. Its presence and that of alcohol should prompt the doctor to ask appropriate questions from the patient and, if necessary, from others about the subject's habits. If alcohol can be detected in the breath before midday, there is a high probability that the patient has a significant drink problem.

Table 3.4 Some abnormal movements

Nature	Condition
Increase in physiological tremor	Anxiety Thyrotoxicosis Beta agonists (e.g. salbutamol)
Twitching and myoclonic jerks	Chronic renal failure with uraemia Respiratory failure with carbon monoxide retention
Flapping tremor	Hepatic encephalopathy

ANTHROPOMETRY

A routine examination should include the measurement of weight and height, both for their immediate value and for future reference. Other measurements, such as span, sitting height and pubis to ground height are made only when a more precise evaluation of growth and development is required, especially in infants and young children (p. 328).

Increase in height

Gigantism is very uncommon as a feature of hyper-pituitarism. Some patients with hypogonadism may give the impression that they are disproportionately tall because the limbs continue to grow for longer than usual in the absence of sex hormones, which normally serve to close the epiphyses after puberty. Thus the sitting height of the patient (head, neck and trunk) will be considerably less than half the height of the patient measured standing. Likewise the span of the fully extended arms will exceed the height standing or, more significantly, twice the sitting height.

In Marfan's syndrome the appearances are rather similar, the limbs being longer than appropriate to the length of the trunk. Additional features distinguish the patient with Marfan's syndrome, in particular long slender fingers and narrow feet, a high arched palate, dislocation of the lens and sometimes dilatation of the aorta, causing aortic regurgitation.

Decrease in height

Short stature is normally familial. Adult height is influenced by polygenic inheritance and has a normal distribution. Any significant illness in childhood will have an impact on the rate of growth. Most conditions that result in short stature can usually be identified from coexistent features (see Table 3.5). Possible exceptions include selective failure of growth hormone secretion, chronic renal disease, intestinal mal-absorption and, in girls, Turner's syndrome if the neck webbing is overlooked.

NUTRITIONAL STATUS

In adults it is becoming increasingly common to express nutritional status in terms of the body mass index (BMI), which is derived from the formula Wt/Ht^2, measured in kg/m^2. The normal range is 19–25. Weight loss, as a symptom, has been discussed in Chapter 2 (p. 36–7). Adults are significantly under-weight if the BMI is 18 or less. They are overweight when the BMI is between 25 and 30 and obese if it is in excess if 30. BMI can be calculated from the formula or derived from the nomogram (Fig. 11.1).

Table 3.5 Some causes of short stature

Hereditary	Constitutionally small
Genetic	Down's syndrome Turner's syndrome Achondroplasia
Nutritional	Intrauterine growth retardation Protein and energy deprivation Rickets
Systemic disease	Chronic wasting diseases including renal failure and biliary disease
Endocrine	Juvenile hypothyroidism (cretinism) Hypopituitarism, craniopharyngioma
Alimentary	Malabsorption including gluten enteropathy, Crohn's disease, cystic fibrosis
Cardiorespiratory	Congenital heart disease Suppurative lung disease
Locomotor	Severe scoliosis

Obesity

Life expectancy is shortened by obesity. Obesity will only develop when dietary intake exceeds energy expenditure. The causes are probably multifactorial, but in many subjects, particularly females, a vicious circle situation may develop whereby weight gain results in 'comfort eating' and further weight gain. Obesity is associated with hypertension, hyperlipidaemia and diabetes mellitus. Its presence should alert the clinician to consider these possibilities and various other compli-cations (see Fig. 3.3).

The amount of subcutaneous fat can be estimated by measuring the skinfold thickness over the triceps or below the scapula by means of a special pair of calipers or more simply by picking up the skinfolds between the finger and thumb. Recent evidence suggests that regional distribution of fat may be of greater prognostic significance than the absolute degree of obesity. Waist–hip ratio provides a simple assessment of visceral adipose fat. Subjects with a 'pear-shaped' configur-ation and a waist–hip ratio of 0.8 or less have a good prognosis; 'apple-shaped' subjects with a waist–hip ratio of 0.9 or greater carry a greater risk of developing the complications of obesity whether or not they are significantly overweight.

Ask about:

Family history
Obstetric history
Psychological stress
Anxiety and depression
Binge eating
Alcohol and other fluid
intake
Symptoms of diabetes

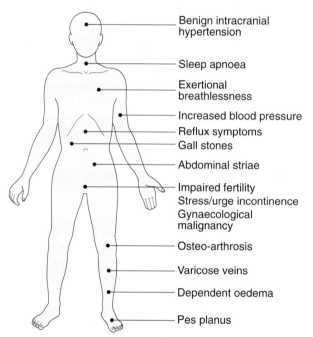

Benign intracranial
hypertension

Sleep apnoea

Exertional
breathlessness

Increased blood pressure

Reflux symptoms

Gall stones

Abdominal striae

Impaired fertility
Stress/urge incontinence
Gynaecological
malignancy

Osteo-arthrosis

Varicose veins

Dependent oedema

Pes planus

Fig. 3.3 Complications of obesity.

Subnutrition

Malnutrition and even starvation remain major problems in many parts of the world. In developed countries malnutrition due to poverty is rare. It occurs in the psychological disorder anorexia nervosa. It may be associated with chronic abuse of alcohol and other addictive drugs and is a feature of HIV infection.

Scurvy affecting elderly people living alone is almost the only vitamin deficiency disease of dietetic origin seen in British adults (Fig. 3.1D). In its most florid form it may present with extensive ecchymosis. In Asian immigrants vitamin D deficiency used to be quite common and probably resulted from differences in dietary intake and absorption of the vitamin and from its decreased formation in the skin.

Specific abnormalities of fat distribution

- *Localised deposits.* Lipomas are commonly found around the trunk and are soft, circumscribed, lobulated swellings.
- *Progressive lipodystrophy* is a rare condition in which subcutaneous fat is reduced in the face, neck, arms, chest and trunk but may be deposited in excess on the lower trunk and thighs, the line of demarcation varying from patient to patient. Diabetes mellitus is common and mesangiocapillary glomerulonephritis may also occur.
- *Localised atrophy of subcutaneous fat* occasionally may develop in diabetics at the site of injection of some insulin preparations.
- In *Cushing's syndrome* the distribution of fat is abnormal. This syndrome can result from excessive endogenous secretion of cortisol or as a result of administration of supraphysiological amounts of glucocorticoids such as cortisone or prednisolone or from injections of adrenocorticotrophic hormone (ACTH). Fat deposition tends to be restricted to the trunk, neck and face, when it causes mooning (Fig. 3.4A and B), together with an increase of the normal pad of fat over the lower cervical and upper thoracic vertebrae. The limbs remain relatively thin or are actually wasted, the whole impression giving rise to the term 'buffalo obesity'. Other features that may may alert the clinician to the possibility of Cushing's syndrome are shown in Table 3.6.

Table 3.6 Other features of Cushing's syndrome

Features	Comment
Facial mooning	Face round and plethoric (see Fig. 3.4)
Plethoric appearance	Caused by thinning of dermis
Purple striae	Noticeable on trunk and limbs
Bruising	Increased capillary fragility
Diabetes	Glucocorticoid effect
Hypertension	Mineralocorticoid effect
Vertebral collapse	Osteoporosis may lead to shortening of stature
Personality change	May progress to psychosis

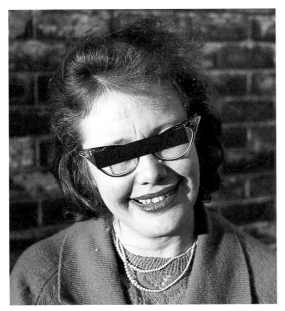

A

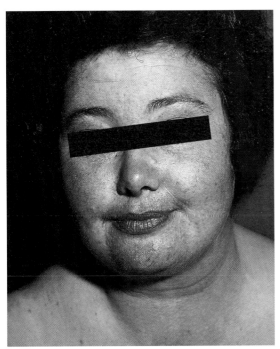

B

Fig. 3.4 Patient with Cushing's syndrome showing facial appearance.
A. 3 years before and **B.** at time of diagnosis.

THE STATE OF HYDRATION

Dehydration

The state of hydration should be assessed in all cases of fluid loss, notably from vomiting, diarrhoea, sweating or polyuria. Unless the possibility of dehydration is considered, its existence may be overlooked or its severity underestimated. A detailed history of the nature and quantity of fluid loss is important but, if the patient's usual weight is known, the most satisfactory assessment is obtained by weighing. A dry tongue is apt to be deceptive as it may be due to mouth breathing. In an adult, a total of 4–6 litres has to be lost before the skin becomes dry, loose and wrinkled. Loss of skin elasticity is a poor index relating more to collagen damage than to water loss. It can be demonstrated by pinching up a fold, which then remains as a ridge and subsides abnormally slowly. The eyeballs are soft, due to lowering of the intraocular tension (Fig. 8.6, p. 262). The change in elasticity of the skin with age and the difficulty in manually assessing intraocular pressure make these unsatisfactory physical signs. The blood pressure may be low and the presence of a postural drop in blood pressure may be a useful index of intravascular volume depletion. Elevation in the haemoglobin concentration, packed cell volume and plasma osmolality provide evidence of the severity of dehydration, and serial readings will indicate when treatment has been adequate.

Oedema

Oedema means swelling of the tissues due to an increase in interstitial fluid.

- *Generalised oedema* may be dietary in origin or due to a disorder of the heart, kidneys, liver or gut. Occasionally the cause is idiopathic.
- *Localised oedema* may arise from venous or lymphatic obstruction, allergy or inflammation.
- *Postural oedema* is relatively common but unimportant.

Clinical manifestations

When oedema is due to generalised fluid retention its distribution is determined by gravity. It is usually observed in the legs, back of the thighs and the lumbosacral area in the semirecumbent patient. If the patient lies flat, it may involve the face and hands, as in children with acute glomerulonephritis. Regional rises in venous pressure also influence the distribution of oedema as exemplified by pulmonary oedema in left heart failure and by ascites in portal hypertension.

The cardinal sign of subcutaneous oedema is the pitting of the skin, made by applying firm pressure with the examiner's finger or thumb for a few seconds. The pitting may persist for several minutes until it is obliterated by the slow redistribution of the displaced fluid. However, pitting on pressure may not be demonstrable until body weight has increased by as much as 10% to 15%. Day-to-day alterations in weight usually provide the most reliable index of progress or response to treatment.

Myxoedema is due to infiltration of the tissues by a firm mucinous material. In contrast to oedema it does not pit on pressure. Chronic lymphoedema may also fail to pit.

Genesis

Increase in interstitial fluid will occur if fluid intake exceeds fluid loss from the urine, skin, breath and other sources. The renal excretory capacity may be reduced by disease of the kidneys or by extrarenal factors. For example, in the early stages of cardiac failure, a fall in renal blood flow leads to a reduction in glomerular filtration rate and an increase in obligatory water absorption by the proximal tubule. Renal tubular reabsorption of water may be enhanced when a rise in circulating aldosterone increases the reabsorption of sodium and chloride, as occurs in some patients with hepatic cirrhosis, the nephrotic syndrome or cardiac failure.

The traditional concept that the accumulation of interstitial fluid is caused by a change in the balance between hydrostatic pressure within the vessels and the osmotic pressure of the proteins in the interstitial fluid fails to take into consideration the importance of the pulsatile nature of capillary flow. Although the mean capillary pressure is equal and opposite to the osmotic gradient, it is the capillary pulsation which is responsible for fluid exchange between plasma and interstitial space.

The mean capillary pressure varies widely at different sites. For example, in the pulmonary capillaries during recumbency it is less than 10 mmHg, while in the glomerular capillaries it is about 75 mmHg and the theoretical mean capillary pressure in the feet of a person of average height during quiet standing is at least 110 mmHg. It is not surprising that some swelling of the feet at the end of the day may be normal.

The types and causes of oedema

Oedema may be generalised or localised and it results from factors disturbing the physiological control of body fluid.

Generalised oedema (Fig. 3.5). There are two principal causes of generalised oedema, hypoproteinaemia and fluid overload. Clinically, these two causes can be distinguished because fluid overload results in a rise in

Ask about:

    Cardiac causes
    (e.g. past history
    or rheumatic fever,
    breathlessness,
    palpitations)
    Malabsorption
    (e.g. stool odour,
    bulk and colour)
    Malnuitrition
    Liver disease
    Renal disease
    (e.g. diabetes, sore
    throat, colour of urine,
    frothing of urine)
    Fundal haemorrhage
    Periorbital oedema

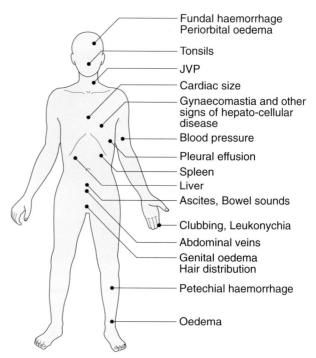

Fundal haemorrhage
Periorbital oedema

Tonsils

JVP

Cardiac size

Gynaecomastia and other
signs of hepato-cellular
disease

Blood pressure

Pleural effusion

Spleen

Liver

Ascites, Bowel sounds

Clubbing, Leukonychia

Abdominal veins

Genital oedema
Hair distribution

Petechial haemorrhage

Oedema

Fig. 3.5 Generalised oedema checklist.

JVP (p. 99), whereas the JVP is not elevated in hypo-proteinaemia.

Hypoproteinaemia.. The osmotic pressure is mostly due to the serum albumin so that a fall in the concentration of this protein in particular predisposes to oedema. Hypoproteinaemia may arise for a variety of reasons:

- Inadequate intake of protein may be responsible, as in kwashiorkor, the most important nutritional disorder in the world. Famine conditions, self-imposed dietary restrictions or pyloric obstruction with vomiting may also impair the protein intake.
- Failure of digestion of dietary protein results from impairment of the exocrine secretion of the pancreas, as in chronic pancreatitis.
- Failure of absorption of the products of digestion may occur after resection of considerable lengths of small intestine or in conditions such as Crohn's disease or gluten enteropathy.
- Reduced synthesis of albumin is found in hepatocellular disease, including cirrhosis. When the portal venous pressure is high, ascites is a more prominent feature than dependent oedema.
- Excessive loss of protein may occur in the urine in the nephrotic syndrome. Uncommonly protein may be lost into the gut in protein-losing enteropathy, which occurs in a variety of gastrointestinal disorders. The repeated removal of body fluids, especially ascites, will also aggravate depletion of protein.

In one patient several of these reasons may coexist. In addition a low intravascular volume may cause secondary hyperaldosteronism via the renin–angiotensin system, promoting sodium retention and an increase in the oedema.

The cause of hypoproteinaemia can usually be identified from the history. The nephrotic syndrome can be excluded in the absence of heavy proteinuria and most patients with a hepatic cause will show the features of hepatocellular failure (Fig. 6.10, p. 178) and/or of cirrhosis, which is associated with ascites, splenomegaly and venous changes (p. 174).

Fluid overload. This may have a number of causes:

1. Cardiac causes. The causes of oedema in cardiac failure are multiple and are not fully understood. Significant factors are:
   - Impairment of renal blood flow. The reduction in renal blood flow, alteration in the pulsatile pattern of renal perfusion, and possibly alteration in the distribution of blood flow within the kidney promote excessive reabsorption of salt and water – this is the main cause of 'cardiac' oedema.
   - Increased venous pressure. There is a rise in venous pressure proximal to the failing chamber. In right-sided failure this can be detected by inspection of the neck (p. 78). In left-sided failure, pulmonary venous congestion is manifested by the development of dyspnoea and cough and the auscultatory finding of crepitations in the lungs. However, the heights of the rises in venous pressure do not correlate with the degrees of oedema and it is clear that the hydrostatic effect alone does not account for the fluid retention.
   - The effect of aldosterone. In some cases secondary hyperaldosteronism occurs and contributes to the oedema.
   - Antidiuretic hormone. There is evidence of increase in antidiuretic substances in the urine of some patients.
   - Lymphatic factors. Lymphangiectasis, incompetent valves and poor lymph drainage have been demonstrated.
   - Osmotic pressures. A combination of chronic passive congestion of the liver reducing albumin synthesis, a poor appetite and loss of protein into the oedema fluid and the urine may sometimes account for a significant drop in the concentration of the serum albumin. The protein content of the interstitial fluid may rise to as much as 1g% compared with 0.02g% in normal interstitial fluid. This change has sometimes been interpreted as evidence for an increase in capillary permeability supposedly due to ischaemia, but it is likely to be mainly due to lymphatic failure.

2. Renal causes. In acute glomerulonephritis the cause of the fluid retention is not fully understood. There is an expansion of the circulating fluid volume as well as the extracellular space due at least in part to increased tubular reabsorption of sodium and consequent reduction in urine volume. Should normal fluid intake be maintained, oedema results.

3. Iatrogenic. Excessive fluid replacement, especially if given intravenously, will result in fluid overload. The danger is greatest in infants and young children. The same mechanism can operate if oral intake is unrestricted when urine production is diminished or absent in renal failure.

Localised oedema. This may be due to venous, lymphatic, inflammatory or allergic causes.

Venous causes. External pressure upon a vein, venous thrombosis or incompetence of the valves due to previous thrombosis may each contribute to a rise in capillary pressure in the areas of drainage. A common example is deep thrombosis in a leg vein. Venous return will also be impaired if the normal pumping action of the muscles is diminished or absent, and accordingly oedema (with or without thrombosis) may occur in an immobile bedridden patient, in a paralysed limb or even in a normal person sitting still for long periods as, for example, during air travel.

Lymphatic causes. The small quantity of albumin filtered at the capillary is normally removed through the lymphatics. In the presence of lymphatic obstruction, the water and solutes are reabsorbed into the capillaries as the tissue pressure rises, but the protein remains until its concentration approaches that in the blood. Ultimately, fibrous tissues proliferate in the interstitial spaces and the whole part becomes hard and no longer pits on pressure.

Lymphatic oedema (lymphoedema) is common in some tropical countries due to lymphatic obstruction by filarial worms. One or both legs, the female breast, or the external genitalia in either sex, are the parts most frequently involved. The skin of the affected area may eventually become very thick and rough – elephantiasis. Lymphoedema is comparatively rare in Britain. It may be due to congenital lymphangiectasis or hypoplasia of the lymph vessels of the legs (Milroy's disease), recurrent lymphangitis (resulting in fibrosis of lymphatics) or may affect an arm after radical mastectomy and irradiation for carcinoma of the breast.

Inflammatory causes. Damage to tissues by injury, infection, ischaemia or chemicals such as uric acid results in liberation of histamine, bradykinin and other factors which cause vasodilation and an increase in capillary permeability. The inflammatory exudate, therefore, has a high protein content. The resulting oedema is accompanied by the classical signs of inflammation, namely redness, heat and pain. Testing for pitting on pressure in inflammatory oedema causes pain and should be avoided.

Allergic causes. Increased capillary permeability also occurs in allergic conditions but, in contrast to inflammation, there is no pain, there is less redness and the exudate, which has a high protein content, contains eosinophils rather than polymorphs and red cells. Angio-oedema is a specific example of allergic oedema; it is particularly prone to affect the face and lips. The swelling develops rapidly, and it is pale or faintly pink in colour. The condition may be life-threatening if the tongue and glottis are affected.

Temperature

The normal oral temperature is 37°C. Circadian variations of about 0.5°C occur, the lowest temperature being in the early morning. Rectal temperature is usually about 0.5°C higher than the mouth, which in turn is 0.5°C higher than the axilla. It is normal practice to record body temperature either beneath the tongue, which is the most convenient, or in the rectum, which is the most reliable. If possible, alternative sites, the axilla, groin or natal cleft, should be avoided.

The warmth of the skin to the touch usually provides a remarkably good indication of fever, but the skin of a patient with a normal temperature may feel cold, and an apparently normal skin temperature does not exclude hypothermia.

Fever is usually due to organic disease. An otherwise inexplicable transient rise may be due to a recent hot drink or a hot bath. Malingerers sometimes falsify their temperatures by a variety of tricks, including the use of hot-water bottles, in order to feign illness.

Hypothermia may be overlooked, particularly if the ordinary clinical thermometer, which reads from 35°C, is not shaken down below this level before the temperature is measured. Low-reading clinical thermometers are readily available and should be used when hypothermia is suspected. Temperatures as low as 27°C are not uncommon and core body temperatures below 20°C have been recorded in patients who subsequently survived.

Hypothermia is associated with various situations:

- elderly patients living alone who have fallen down and are unable to rise
- near-drowning
- prolonged unconsciousness in low environmental temperatures, especially when the result of alcohol intoxication, other drug overdosage or head injury
- severe hypopituitarism and hypothyroidism.

Because many of the features of severe hypothyroidism and near-drowning mimic death, such subjects may require to be fully resuscitated and rewarmed before assessing viability.

Examination

❑ Greet the patient with a handshake and note its characteristics.
❑ Observe and define any abnormality of gait or posture.
❑ Inspect the patient's dress.
❑ Note any features beside the bedside.
❑ Identify any abnormalities in movement, smell or voice and complexion.
❑ Assess any abnormalities in stature.

⌐ Record the weight of outpatients in indoor clothing without shoes, and of inpatients wearing pyjamas and dressing gown.

⌐ Record height using a rigid arm sliding on a vertical scale with the patient standing erect and without shoes.

⌐ Determine the BMI.

⌐ Determine waist–hip ratio in the erect patient by measuring the girth at the level equidistant between costal margin and iliac crest and at the level of the greater trochanters.

⌐ Look for any evidence of malnutrition or abnormal fat distribution.

⌐ Assess the state of hydration by testing skin elasticity and intraocular pressure, recording the blood pressure and looking for a postural drop.

⌐ Check for dependent oedema by firm pressure at the ankle behind the medial malleolus and, when present, assess its extent elsewhere by pressing over the tibia, in the medial thigh and in the sacral area.

⌐ Examine the JVP (p. 99).

⌐ Record the temperature either beneath the tongue or in the rectum. Use a low-reading thermometer if there is a possibility of hypothermia.

KEY POINTS

- First impressions are often invaluable.

- The concept of performing a complete physical examination is inappropriate. As a general rule 'you only find what you look for'.

- Check to make sure that the patient's right hand is functional before shaking hands.

- Skin complexion is influenced by artificial lighting.

- A liver 'flap' may only become apparent when the outstretched hand is dorsiflexed.

- Regional fat distribution can be roughly assessed from the waist–hip ratio and is probably as useful a prognostic index as overall degree of obesity.

- Dehydration in an adult only becomes clinically apparent after substantial fluid loss.

- The JVP is useful in distinguishing between the oedema of fluid overload and that of hypoproteinaemia.

- Hypothermia can be missed if a clinical thermometer is not shaken down to below 35ºC.

THE PHYSICAL ASSESSMENT

After completing the initial appraisal of the patient, the more formal physical assessment usually begins with examination of the hands and pulse.

THE HANDS

The hand is a highly developed structure and its area of representation in the cerebral cortex is appropriately extensive. While the palmist may claim to read more from the hand than is justified, critical examination can indeed provide much reliable information. Attention should be paid first to general features and then to detailed consideration of individual structures on an anatomical basis. The examination of the function of the hand is described on page 290–94, and the significance of right or left handedness on page 205.

General features

Movements. Some people, including those of Mediterranean origin, 'speak' with their hands. For example, the hand pressed flat on top of the head accompanying a complaint of headache suggests a psychogenic symptom 'something weighing on the mind'.

Tremors are studied with the hands at rest and then outstretched. Characteristic tremors are described in Table 3.4 (p. 44).

Tetany may be recognised by the presence of carpal spasm. Latent tetany may be detected by Trousseau's sign. This is positive if the characterised position of the hand, opposition of the thumb, extension of the interphalangeal flexion of the metacarpophalangeal joints is induced within four minutes when a sphygmomanometer cuff is inflated to a level above the systolic blood pressure.

Posture. This may be almost diagnostic. Examples include the flexed hand and arm of hemiplegia, wrist drop or radial nerve palsy and ulnar deviation in long-standing rheumatoid arthritis.

Shape. Trauma is the commonest cause of deformity of the hand. Other unusual shapes include the long thin fingers of arachnodactyly, while a short fourth metacarpal, best seen when making a fist, strongly supports a diagnosis of Turner's syndrome in a girl with primary amenorrhoea. Short metacarpals, especially the fourth and fifth, are found in patients with pseudohypoparathyroidism.

Size. In acromegaly the hands are large and broad. Rings may be difficult to remove or may have been cut off or enlarged. The increase in bulk consists largely of soft tissues. These are also thickened in myxoedema. Oedema may be part of a generalised process or be local from venous or lymphatic obstruction or disuse, as with a hemiplegia.

Colour. By and large changes in the colour of the hands are similar to those of the skin in general (p. 42). The purported cigarette consumption should be reconciled with a degree of nicotine staining of the fingers. Coal miners may have small blue tattoo marks in the skin of their hands and in other sites where particles of coal dust have been embedded in the scars of minor injuries. Professional tattoos may provide information about the subject's personality (Fig. 3.7) and also act as a source of hepatitis B viral infection. In both miners and those with professional tattoos the

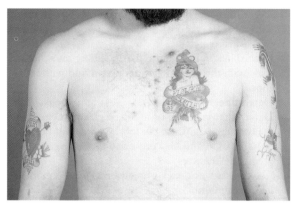

Fig. 3.7 Professional tattooing as a guide to personality.

blue colour is due to black particles (carbon or Indian ink) changed in appearance by the scatter of light as it passes through and is reflected back from the skin. This explains why veins normally look blue, while in the elderly, with very thin skin, the true red colour of the blood may be seen.

Temperature. In a cold or cool climate the temperature of the patient's hand is a good guide to the blood flow. If the hand is warm and cyanosed it can be deduced that arterial oxygen saturation is reduced. In most patients with heart failure the hands tend to be cold and cyanosed due to vasoconstriction in response to a low cardiac output. The combination of central cyanosis and finger clubbing suggests congenital cyanotic heart disease (Fig. 3.6A). If they are warm the cause of the heart failure may be hyperthyroidism or cor pulmonale.

Detailed features

Skin

The smooth, hairless hands of a child become lined and hairy in the adult male unless hypogonadism is present. Manual work may produce specific callosities due to pressure at characteristic sites. In contrast, disuse results in a soft, smooth palmar skin and prolonged recumbency affects the soles likewise.

The skin may feature a wide variety of specific skin disorders or dermatological manifestation of systemic disease. An example of the former is contact dermatitis due to a rubber glove (see Fig. 3.27D), whereas in progressive systemic sclerosis the skin may have a shiny, glazed appearance and be tightly stretched over the underlying tissues, limiting the movement of the fingers, which are held in a semiflexed position.

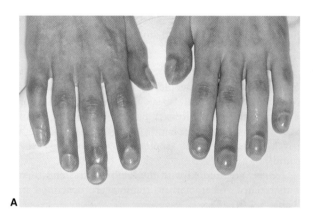

A

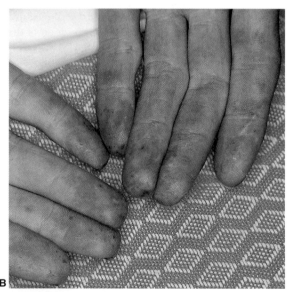

B

Fig. 3.6 The fingers as a diagnostic aid.   A. Cyanosis and finger clubbing in a patient with congenital heart disease. **B.** Acute vasculitic lesions in a boy with systemic lupus erythematosus.

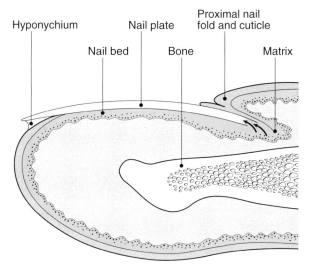

Hyponychium Nail plate Proximal nail fold and cuticle

Nail bed Bone Matrix

Fig. 3.8 Anatomy of the nail.

Nails

The keratinous nail plate is produced mainly in the nail matrix, which lies in an invagination of the epidermis, the nailfold, on the back of the terminal phalanx of each digit. The matrix runs from the end of the floor of the nailfold to the distal margin of the lunula ('half-moon'), and from it the nail plate grows forward covering the nail bed (Fig. 3.8). A small part of the nail, the undersurface, is formed from cells in the nail bed. Fingernails grow more quickly than toenails.

Nails grow throughout life, the growth in fingernails being approximately 1 cm in 3 months. Growth is slowed by acute illness and ischaemia. It is increased in psoriasis. Injury to the nail matrix is by far the most

Table 3.7 Important signs in the nails

Feature	Association
Bitten nails	Anxious personality
Finger clubbing	(see p. 141)
Splinter haemorrhages	Minor trauma, systemic vasculitis
Koilonychia	Chronic iron deficiency anaemia
Pitting	Psoriasis
Onycholysis	Trauma, psoriasis
Striate leuconychia	A 'normal' finding, ? minor trauma
Severe leuconychia (white nails or Terry's nails)	Hypoalbuminaemia, chronic liver disease, other wasting diseases
Transverse ridging (Beau's line)	Recent acute illness
Fungal infection	Thickening, crumbling and discoloration
Red half-moons	Congestive cardiac failure
Blue half-moons	Hepatolenticular degeneration; Wilson's disease
'Half and half' nails	Chronic renal failure

common cause of changes in the nails and may permanently impair their growth.

Some important changes in the nails are indicated in Table 3.7.

Longitudinal ridging and beading of the nail plate is not abnormal and increases with age. Similarly, occasional white transverse flecks (striate leuconychia) are seen frequently in normal nails; they are probably caused by minor and repeated trauma to the nail matrix and, contrary to the popular lay belief, are not due to insufficient calcium. Excessively shiny or polished nails are striking proof of frequent rubbing of the skin by the nails.

Systemic vasculitis producing splinter haemorrhages (Fig. 3.9A) may also cause haemorrhages in the skin and retina and, occasionally, tender nodules in the fingertips (Osler's nodes). Although one or two are commonly seen under the nails of manual workers, multiple splinter haemorrhages raise the possibility of infective endocarditis.

Onycholysis, separation of the nail plate from the nail bed, may be due to minor trauma (especially if the nails are left long) and psoriasis. It is also reported to be a feature of thyroid disease. Nail pitting (Fig. 3.9B) is seen commonly in psoriasis though rarely in other conditions, such as alopecia areata and when eczema affects the proximal nailfold. In koilonychia (Fig. 3.9C) the nails become brittle and flat, and ultimately spoon-shaped. It is a sign of iron deficiency and is seen most often in countries where malnutrition is prevalent. Beau's lines, due to temporary arrest of nail growth (Fig. 3.9D), are transverse grooves which appear at the same time on all nails a few weeks after an acute illness and which move out to the free margins as the nail grows. Colour changes are sometimes seen in nails. Whitening of the nails is a rare sign of hypoalbuminaemia, as in cirrhosis of the liver. Occasionally 'half and half' nails (white proximally and red–brown distally) are seen in patients with chronic renal failure. Rarely, drugs (e.g. antimalarials and phenothiazines) discolour nails.

The nailfolds

Examination of the nailfolds should accompany examination of the nails. Paronychia is the term used to describe inflamed, bolstered and swollen nailfolds. Chronic paronychia is seen most commonly in those with a poor peripheral circulation, in those involved in wet work, in diabetes and those who are overenthusiastic when manicuring their cuticles. Ragged cuticles and dilated or thrombosed capillaries in the proximal nailfold are an important pointer to connective tissue disease (Fig. 3.9E).

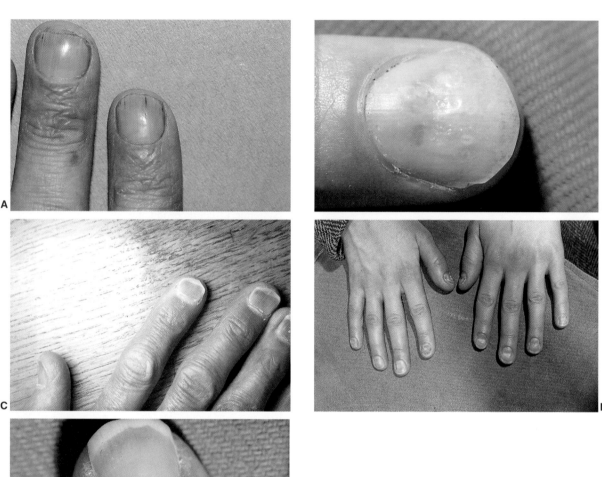

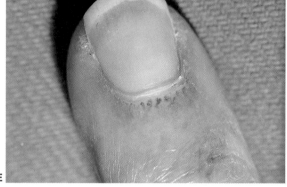

Fig. 3.9 The nail as a diagnostic aid. **A.** Splinter haemorrhages. **B.** Onycholysis with pitting in psoriasis. **C.** Koilonychia. **D.** Beau's lines. **E.** Dilated capillaries in the proximal nailfold in systemic lupus erythematosus.

Subcutaneous tissues

In Dupuytren's contracture there is thickening and shortening of the palmar fascia, resulting in flexion deformities, particularly of the fifth and ring fingers. Firm, painless subcutaneous nodules occur in rheumatoid disease; these occur more frequently over the upper end of the ulna than on the hands. Finger clubbing is discussed on page 141.

Joints

Arthritis frequently involves the small joints of the hands (p. 291–296).

Rheumatoid arthritis (Fig. 9.25) affects the proximal interphalangeal, metacarpophalangeal and carpal joints and causes pain, stiffness, swelling, restriction of movement and, ultimately, often gross deformity.

Osteoarthrosis affects mainly the terminal interphalangeal joints where it causes little or no disability. The characteristic changes are Heberden's nodes, which are visible and palpable osteophytes projecting from the dorsal surface of the base of the terminal phalanx.

In *psoriatic arthropathy* the terminal interphalangeal

joints are affected by a diffuse swelling with rheumatoid-like changes in other joints.

Muscles

Wasting is common in rheumatoid arthritis. It also occurs in lesions of the lower motor neurone. Causes include syringomyelia, poliomyelitis, lesions of the first thoracic nerve root, the peripheral neuropathies and motor neurone disease, in which fasciculation is often present. Lesions of the ulnar and median nerves will affect specific muscle groups, e.g. in leprosy. In the carpal tunnel syndrome median nerve compression may result in selective wasting of the thenar muscles. This may occur in rheumatoid arthritis, autoimmune hypothyroidism and acromegaly, or may be associated with premenstrual fluid retention or pregnancy.

Tendons

Excessive use of a tendon may result in tenosynovitis. This commonly produces a sensation of local crepitus and swelling over the tendon sheath. A common site is the extensor pollicis longus tendon at the wrist where it crosses the radial styloid (de Quervain's tenosynovitis) (p. 296). Thickening of a flexor tendon may result in a trigger finger or thumb (p. 292). A tendon may be ruptured from its involvement in hypertrophied synovial membrane on the dorsum of the hand in rheumatoid arthritis.

Bones

In fractures of the scaphoid the only finding may be tenderness localised in the anatomical snuffbox. Occasionally the bones of the hand, particularly the phalanges, may be involved in granulomatous or other generalised disorders such as sarcoidosis, Paget's disease or hyperparathyroidism. Acute dactylitis is characteristic of sickle cell disease in children. Graves' disease, autoimmune hyperthyroidism, may be associated with finger clubbing and periosteal new bone formation in the phalanges.

Nerves

In sensory polyneuropathy there is a characteristic impairment of a glove distribution affecting both hands; the feet are usually also involved. An example, common in the tropics, is the late result of dimorphous or lepromatous leprosy. Secondary infection through abrasions leads to deformities from absorption of the phalanges or from loss of fingers by ulceration. In tuberculoid leprosy the lesions are likely to be asymmetrical or unilateral.

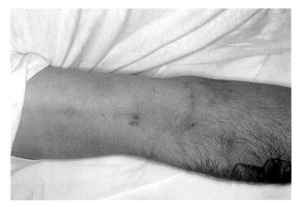

Fig. 3.10 The linear marks of intravenous injection at the right elbow.

Blood vessels

Palmar erythema is a mottled, bright-red cutaneous vasodilation seen mainly over the thenar and hypothenar eminences. Though found in normal persons, it is suggestive of liver dysfunction. Arteritis may occur in infective endocarditis and in connective tissue disorders; it may cause small necrotic lesions around the base of the nail and on the pulps, most commonly in systemic lupus erythematosus (Fig. 3.6B). Raynaud's phenomenon is described on page 127. Venous abnormalities are seldom seen, but the linear marks following the intravenous injection of drugs of addicts ('mainliners') are characteristic (Fig. 3.10).

Examination

- ❑ Inspect the general features of the dorsal and then the palmar aspects of both hands.
- ❑ Note specific changes in the skin, nails, tendons and joints.
- ❑ Look for evidence of muscle wasting.
- ❑ Assess the temperature, degree of sweating and skin texture.
- ❑ Test the power of the intrinsic hand muscles (p. 292) and look for any sensory disturbance (p. 240–44).
- ❑ Assess the range of joint movements (p. 292).

KEY POINTS

- The importance of the hand is indicated by its area of representation in the cerebral cortex.
- Some people 'speak' with their hands.
- The skin is smooth and soft with disuse, whereas manual work produces distinctive callosities in the hands.
- Trauma is a common cause of changes in the nails.

THE HEAD

The examination of the various components of the head is described in topographical sequence – the cranium, hair, face, eyes, ears, nose and mouth. In practice this routine is rarely followed.

The cranium

The examination of the cranium in infancy and child-hood can be very valuable. In the adult inspection may reveal generalised enlargement in Paget's disease or localised bony bossing overlying a meningioma. The supraorbital ridges often enlarge in acromegaly as a result of increase in the size of the frontal sinuses. In cranial arteritis the temporal arteries may be visibly or palpably enlarged and tender (Fig. 3.11). On auscultation a bruit may occasionally be detected in the presence of an intracranial arteriovenous malformation (p. 207).

The hair

The hair follicle is the sac-like housing of the hair shaft. The germinative part of the hair shaft is the hair matrix (see Fig. 3.23). Melanocytes migrate into the matrix and the melanins that they produce are responsible for the different colours of hair. Each follicle

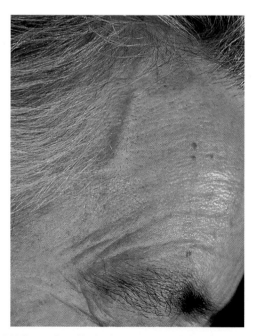

Fig. 3.11 Temporal arteritis showing an enlarged palpable artery.

passes, independently of its neighbours, through regular cycles of growth (anagen) and resting/shedding (telogen), the duration of these stages varying in different regions of the body. The anagen phase of scalp hair may last for up to 5 years, accounting for its length. This phase is shorter and the telogen phase longer in eyebrow and sexually determined hair. Moulting does not normally occur in humans unless the hair cycles in neighbouring follicles become synchronised, as sometimes occurs after childbirth and various pyrexic illnesses (telogen effluvium).

There are three main types of hair. Fine long *lanugo* hairs cover the fetus but are shed about 1 month before birth. They are replaced by fine short *vellus* hairs, which cover much of the body surface. *Terminal* hairs then replace vellus hairs on the scalp. At puberty the vellus hair of the pubic region is replaced by darker, coarser and curlier hair. This begins earlier in girls (average age 11.5 years) than in boys (average age 13.5 years). The early development of pubic hair is related to adrenal androgen production (adrenarche). This occurs in the absence of gonadotrophin secretion. Thus patients with isolated gonadotrophin deficiency may have early pubic hair but no other signs of pubertal development. Axillary hair appears about 2 years after the start of pubic hair growth and, in boys, coincides with the development of facial hair. Last of all body hair develops, and its extent increases throughout the years of sexual maturity though there is a wide variation in its pattern.

There are striking racial differences in hair. Asians tend to have straight hair, Negroids to have curly hair and Europeans to have wavy hair. Mongoloids have sparse facial and body hair. Mediterranean people have more hair than northern Europeans.

Scalp hair

Certain follicles of the scalp regress with age to produce fine vellus instead of coarse terminal hairs. This patterned baldness often starts as temporal recession progressing to thinning of hair over the crown. It is common in males and is androgen dependent, prevented by prepubertal castration but not reversed by castration in maturity. Temporal recession is less common in women and may suggest virilisation. Loss or thinning of hair over the frontal region is an almost constant finding in the rare condition myotonic dystrophy, and is also seen in systemic lupus erythematosus.

Alopecia is the term used to describe hair loss. It has many causes and patterns. Complete hair loss may occur following the administration of some cytotoxic

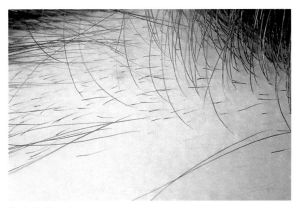

Fig. 3.12 Alopecia areata.

drugs. The most common local disease of the hair of the scalp is alopecia areata, in which the hair falls out in patches. In active spreading alopecia areata, hairs shaped like exclamation marks (Fig. 3.12) are found at the periphery of the bald area, which is clean and smooth. Alopecia areata may rarely cause total scalp baldness (alopecia totalis) or loss of all body hair (alopecia universalis), both distressing conditions. Alopecia may also be caused by a fungal infection. In this condition the affected area contains hairs broken off close to the skin. In assessing alopecia it is helpful to distinguish if the hair loss is due to an abnormality of the hair shaft (as in some inherited disorders of sparse hair) or of the scalp and, if the latter, whether or not there is evidence of scarring. A search for nits (Fig. 3.13) and lice is essential when faced with an itchy

scalp and posterior cervical lymphodenopathy. Nits (the ova of lice) are firmly adherent to the hair shaft, whereas dandruff (desquamating scalp scales) is easily shed.

Facial and body hair

Hirsutism is an excessive growth of coarse hair in the female on the face, trunk and limbs in the pattern normally seen in males. The pubic hair spreads from its normal flat-topped distribution up towards the umbilicus, this being described as a male escutcheon. Mild hirsutism is a common complaint. Many hirsute subjects have higher than average levels of circulating testosterone, but the amount of hair varies considerably in normal subjects and is influenced by racial and familial factors. Some increase in facial hair is common after the menopause. Hirsutism associated with other signs of virilisation (the development of masculine physical features in a female), including enlargement of the clitoris and menstrual irregularity or cessation, may be a sign of an androgen-secreting or pituitary tumour.

Hypertrichosis is an excessive growth of coarse hair but one which does not follow an androgen-induced pattern. It may be due to many different causes including drugs (e.g. minoxidil and cyclosporin), trauma and cutaneous porphyria. It is also a feature of primary hypothyroidism (Fig. 3.14A and B).

Secondary sexual hair on the face in the male, and in the axillae and on the pubis of both sexes, may fail to develop normally in hypogonadism; it may diminish in quantity in old age or be lost in hypopituitarism or as a result of hepatic cirrhosis. In severe hypopituitarism (Fig. 3.15) the loss is ultimately complete, including the hair follicles, so that the axillae and pubis return to the smooth appearance seen in childhood.

Eyebrows. The amount of hair in the eyebrows varies very widely. Thinning of the outer third of the eyebrows is so common in normal people as to be of little value in the diagnosis of hypothyroidism.

Examination

❏ Inspect the scalp hair for its lustre, calibre, structure, tensile strength and density.
❏ If alopecia is present, determine if the abnormality affects the hair shaft or the scalp itself.
❏ Inspect for evidence of fungal infection, nits and lice.
❏ Examine the body and secondary sexual hair for its nature and distribution.

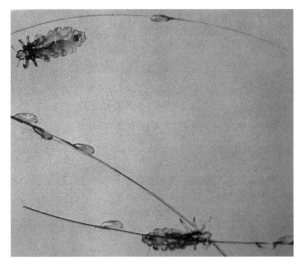

Fig. 3.13 Nits and head lice.

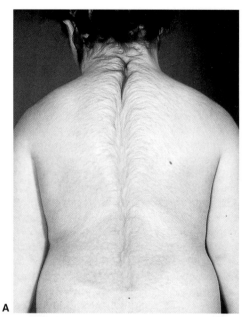

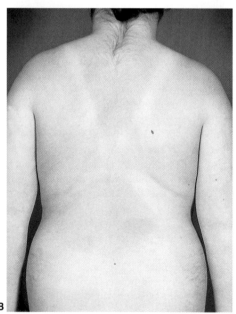

Fig. 3.14 Hypertrichosis as the presenting sign in a young girl with hypothyroidism. A. before and B. 1 year after the introduction of thyroxine replacement therapy.

Ask about:

Obstetric history	Cold intolerance
Menstrual pattern	Thirst
Sexuality	Visual problems
Previous trauma	Headache
Fatigue	

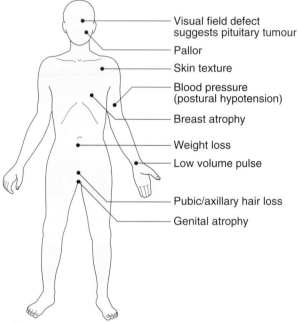

- Visual field defect suggests pituitary tumour
- Pallor
- Skin texture
- Blood pressure (postural hypotension)
- Breast atrophy
- Weight loss
- Low volume pulse
- Pubic/axillary hair loss
- Genital atrophy

Fig. 3.15 Panhypopituitarism in a woman.

Table 3.8 Examples of facial appearance characteristic of specific diseases

Endocrine	Hyperthyroidism
	Hypothyroidism
	Cushing's syndrome
Genetic	Down's syndrome
Renal	Nephrotic syndrome
Cardiovascular	Superior vena caval obstruction
Infective	Risus sardonicus in tetany
Neuromuscular	Myasthenia gravis
	VII nerve palsy

The face and eyes

The face may provide important diagnostic information (Fig. 3.16). Some facial appearances are characteristic of specific diseases (Table 3.8). In children, study of the face is particularly rewarding (Figs 10.4 and 10.5).

Some examples of the more common and more significant findings in the eyes, ears, nose and mouth are provided.

Examination of the eyes is very important. It is considered separately in Chapter 9.

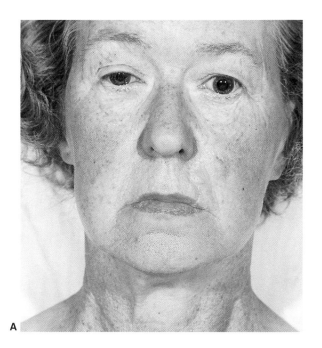

syndrome the auricles are usually small and the lobule may be rudimentary or absent. The helix of the ear is a recognised site of gouty tophi – white chalky nodules consisting of sodium biurate crystals deposited in the cartilage. Local trauma to the ear may cause haemorrhage. When frequent, partial organisation can lead to permanent deformity and the features of 'cauliflower ear'.

Acute otitis media usually causes earache, which may be severe, but in infants it may present as an acute febrile illness without local pain.

The normal drum appears pearly grey, with the handle of the malleus visible and lying almost vertically near the centre of the tympanic membrane. A cone of light is reflected from its lower end downwards and forwards to the periphery of the drum (Fig. 3.17).

The common abnormalities on inspection of the drum are acute inflammation and perforation.

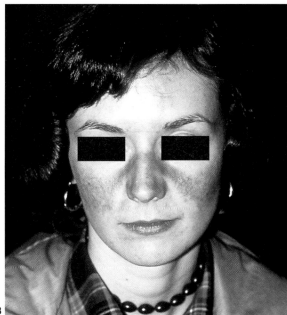

A

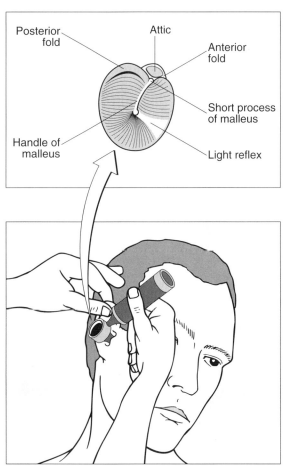

B

Fig. 3.16 The face as a diagnostic aid.   A. Right Horner's syndrome in a patient with bronchogenic carcinoma. Note the ptosis and enophthalmos. (Courtesy of Dr D.H.A Boyd) **B.** The characteristic rash of systemic lupus erythematosus.

The ears

Normal ears vary widely in size, shape and form. There are some genetic deformities. For example, in Down's

Fig. 3.17 Auroscopic examination.

Auriscopic examination

Indications include adults with a hearing difficulty or headache and infants with any febrile illness (p. 349).

Examination

- ❏ Confirm that the light of the auriscope is working.
- ❏ Select a speculum of appropriate length and with the largest diameter that will fit the meatus in comfort.
- ❏ Gently retract the pinna upwards and backwards to straighten the external meatus (Fig. 3.17), thereby facilitating insertion of the speculum.
- ❏ Examine the external meatus, then identify and examine the ear drum.
- ❏ If the vision is obscured by wax, remove this using a wax hook or by gentle syringing with warm water.

Wax commonly obscures the view and may need to be removed. Hard wax may need to be softened by the application of a few drops of olive oil or an appropriate preparation for two or three days before removal. Syringing should not be undertaken except by an expert if there is a history of middle ear disease or in the presence of perforation.

Foreign bodies in the external meatus are not uncommon in children.

The nose and sinuses

The nose may be deformed as a result of an old fracture, or enlarged, red and bulbous (rhinophyma) in the late stages of rosacea (Fig. 3.18).

Destruction of the nasal septum may produce flattening of the bridge and a 'saddle-nose' appearance. This is frequently the result of local trauma. Other causes include Wegener's granulomatosis, congenital syphilis or nasal sniffing of cocaine. This may also produce ulceration of the nasal mucosa. Other common mucosal abnormalities include:

- narrowing of the nose when there is chronic obstruction of the airway in childhood. When associated with mouth breathing this produces the 'adenoidal facies'
- widening of the nose, one of the early features of acromegaly
- nasal polyps; these are pearly grey in colour and bleeding points can be readily identified on the nasal septum.

Infection of the frontal air sinuses may cause a headache, which characteristically reaches a peak

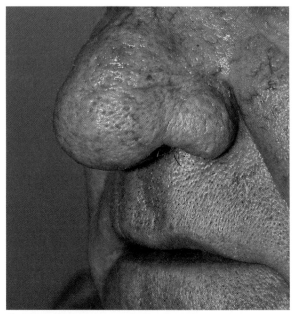

Fig. 3.18 Rhinophyma as a complication of rosacea.

within 2 or 3 hours of rising and then spontaneously subsides as the day proceeds. Involvement of the maxillary sinuses may simulate toothache. A purulent nasal or post-nasal discharge is often present and there may be tenderness on pressure over the affected sinus.

Examination

- ❏ Test the patency of the nasal airways by asking the patient to sniff as each nostril is occluded in turn by finger pressure.
- ❏ Using a nasal speculum, examine the state of the mucosa of the nose and identify the anterior ends of the inferior terbinates.
- ❏ If sinusitis is suspected, apply firm finger pressure over the frontal and maxillary areas to identify any localised tenderness.

The mouth

The examination of the mouth involves the inspection of the lips, teeth, gums, tongue, floor of the mouth, mucosa of the cheeks, palate, tonsils and the oropharynx. These may be involved by local disease or may show lesions which are part of a systemic disorder.

The lips

Exposure to cold commonly causes dryness followed by desquamation and cracking of the lips. Somewhat resembling this is the much rarer cheilosis of ribo-flavine deficiency causing red, denuded epithelium at the line of closure of the lips, peeling towards the mucocutaneous junction. A similar appearance may result from the use of lipstick to which the patient is hypersensitive.

Angular stomatitis, consisting of painful inflamed cracks at the corners of the mouth, is often caused by ill-fitting dentures allowing saliva to dribble out of the mouth, followed by infection with *Candida albicans*. Angular stomatitis may also be due to deficiency of iron or riboflavine.

A fissure of the lip in an elderly patient, which fails to heal in spite of treatment, should be regarded as a possible epithelioma and requires biopsy.

The teeth

Inspection of the 32 so-called 'permanent teeth' may give some indication of the patient's attitude towards health issues. There are three common findings:

- *Discoloration* is usually due to staining from tobacco or from poor hygiene, but devitalised teeth also gradually become grey. The teeth may be pitted and mottled yellow in fluorosis.
- *Caries* is related to lack of fluoride and can be kept in check by regular dental care. Extensive caries may be an index of self-neglect.
- *Missing teeth* are most commonly the molars; as these are used for grinding rather than biting, their absence is important in connection with alimentary symptoms.

Notched, separated and peg-shaped upper incisors occur in congenital syphilis (Hutchinson's teeth), and poorly developed teeth are a feature of juvenile hypo-parathyroidism. Eruption of the teeth may be retarded as part of any disorder responsible for delayed develop-ment, especially rickets.

The gums

Gingivitis is very common. At first bleeding is apt to occur, and a narrow line of inflammation can be seen at the free border of the gum, and the interdental papillae are swollen. If the condition progresses, food debris, bacteria and pus tend to accumulate between the teeth and the gum margin (pyorrhoea alveolaris). Halitosis may be apparent and the teeth may become loose. Pus or even a tooth may be aspirated into the bronchial tree and initiate pneumonia. Badly affected gums are associated with frequent transient bacter-aemia, the usual organism being *Streptococcus viridans*. This may cause infective endocarditis, especially in

Table 3.9 The gums in systemic conditions

Phenytoin treatment	Firm and hypertrophied
Scurvy	Soft, haemorrhagic
Acute leukaemia	Hypertrophied and haemorrhagic
Cyanotic congenital heart disease	Spongy and haemorrhagic
Chronic lead poisoning	Punctate blue line

patients with valvular heart disease. Painful ulcero-membranous gingivitis may be due to Vincent's infection (p. 63).

Changes in the gum may also be a feature of systemic disease (Table 3.9). If phenytoin causes distressing hyperplasia, it is advisable to change to another anticonvulsant.

The tongue

The surface of the tongue. This normally varies greatly in regard to both colour and appearance. Shades of pink and red or even yellow, brown or almost black may be of no medical significance though they are a potential cause of anxiety to the subject. Variations in colour may be caused by foods, particularly coloured sweets, or they may be due to quantitative or qualita-tive changes in the haemoglobin. Central cyanosis can best be assessed clinically by inspection of the tongue (p. 94). A clean tongue, often red with prominent papillae, can result from antibiotic treatment. Iron or vitamin B_{12} deficiency cause a smooth clean-looking tongue from diffuse atrophy of the papillae.

The fungiform papillae are small, red, flat elevations on the surface, especially at the tip and edges; the filiform papillae are more numerous at the centre and give rise to the fur. Transient denuded islands (geographical tongue) constitute a symptomless change of no known significance. Excessive furring occurs in healthy people and in fever or dehydration.

Separating the anterior two-thirds from the posterior third of the tongue are the circumvallate papillae set in a wide V with its apex pointing backwards. Patients who discover these may be alarmed by the thought that they might be cancerous.

Congenital fissuring of the tongue has no pathological significance. In contrast, leukoplakia is a precancerous condition. It is characterised by grey opaque areas interspersed with a few red inflamed patches. Ulcers of the tongue may be caused by sharp, damaged teeth, but malignancy must always be considered.

Movement and size of the tongue. The request 'please put out your tongue' may provide general information. For example, a stuporous patient who responds obviously hears and understands. Neurological disease, a tight frenulum, a painful condition of the mouth or modesty may restrict the protrusion. Fasciculation (p. 228), with the tongue at rest, is a feature of motor neurone disease. Lesions of the hypoglossal nerve cause wasting of half the tongue (p. 225), which protrudes toward the affected side. The tongue is enlarged in Down's syndrome, acromegaly, myxoedema and in some patients with amyloidosis.

The palate

The hard palate comprises the anterior two-thirds, and the soft palate with the uvula lies posteriorly. Abnormalities include cleft palate and a narrow high arched palate. This is of little importance by itself, but may be associated with other congenital conditions. The uvula varies greatly in size and shape; it seldom presents clinical problems except to some patients with obsessional anxiety. The examination of movement of the soft palate is described on page 223.

The tonsils

The tonsils are masses of lymphoid tissue that lie beneath the mucous membrane between the pillars of the fauces. In common with lymphoid tissue elsewhere, the tonsils enlarge to reach a maximum between the ages of 8 and 12 years, after which involution takes place. Failure to recognise this normal phase of lymphoid hyperplasia has led to erroneous recommendations for tonsillectomy. In streptococcal tonsillitis the tonsils are swollen and inflamed, often with pus exuding from the tonsillar crypts. Less common causes of sore throat include infectious mononucleosis, Vincent's infection and diphtheria (p. 63).

Tumours of the tonsils may also occur either in isolation or as part of lymphatic leukaemia or lymphoma.

The pharynx and buccal mucosa

Small lymphatic nodules can normally be observed on the posterior wall. With infection in the nose or sinuses, mucus or pus may be visible trickling down the back of the throat.

Koplik's spots. In measles small white spots on an erythematosus background are distributed over the mucosa of the cheeks opposite the molar teeth and sometimes throughout the mouth. These Koplik's spots are of diagnostic value as they appear before the rash.

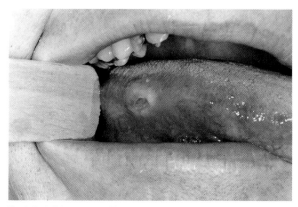

Fig. 3.19 Aphthous stomatitis causing a deep ulcer in a young patient with inflammatory bowel disease.

Pigmentation in the mouth. Melanin deposition in the buccal mucosa is normal in black people and is proportionally reduced as the skin becomes lighter. Pathological pigmentation in the mouth occurs in Addison's disease (Fig. 3.20). Other causes are chronic cachexia, the malabsorption syndrome, haemochromatosis or the rare Peutz–Jeghers syndrome. This comprises polyposis of the small intestine with pigmentation around and in the mouth and on the lips and fingers. If there are no other suggestive features of these disorders, the pigmentation is likely to be congenital in patients with black hair and brown eyes.

The salivary glands

While examining the mouth, the opening of the parotid duct may be seen on the buccal mucosa as a small papilla opposite the second upper molar tooth. The openings of the submandibular salivary gland

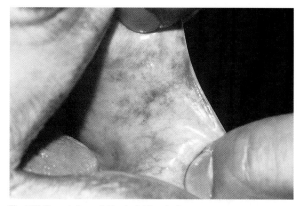

Fig. 3.20 Buccal pigmentation in Addison's disease.

ducts seldom require identification, but may be found near the midline in the sublingual papilla, adjoining the root of the frenulum of the tongue. Each of these openings is more readily seen if a free flow of saliva is provoked by something tasty. Purulent infections of the salivary glands may be investigated by culturing pus expressed through these orifices.

Causes of enlargement of the parotid gland include mumps, sarcoidosis (Fig. 3.21) and tumour. Obstruction of the duct may produce intermittent swelling with pain while eating, or may lead to infection of the gland. Obstruction due to salivary calculi is very much more frequent in the submandibular ducts. The submandibular glands may sometimes be affected by mumps in the absence of parotid swelling.

Some disorders of the mouth

Aphthous stomatitis. This is characterised by ulcers on the inner sides of the lips, the edges of the tongue, the insides of the cheek or on the palate. Initially small vesicles form, which quickly burst, leaving shallow ulcers usually surrounded by a red margin. Such ulcers can cause intense discomfort. They may heal quickly in a day or two, or they may progress into deep indurated ulcers which heal slowly (Fig. 3.19) and may leave a small scar. The lesions tend to occur in crops; a

patient may be free from ulcers for months only to suffer a relapse. The cause is obscure. They are often seen in patients with ulcerative colitis.

Ulcerative stomatitis. This is commonly due to the combination of a spirochaete and a fusiform bacillus which can be seen in a smear taken from one of the ulcers (Vincent's infection). The condition is painful and foul smelling.

Ulcerative stomatitis may complicate acute leukaemia or agranulocytosis and immunosuppression. In acute leukaemia the gums often bleed and may be so swollen that the teeth may be largely obscured. Agranulocytosis may present as a sore throat, which may progress to an ulcerative stomatitis.

Thrush. This may occur in the infants of mothers who carry infection with Candida albicans in the vagina. It also occurs, particularly in the elderly, in association with febrile or debilitating diseases. It is common in patients being treated with antibiotics, corticosteroids or immunosuppressive drugs (Fig. 3.22). The fungus may be seen as individual or coalescent white deposits adhering to the mucous membrane of any part of the mouth. There is very little evidence of inflammation.

Diphtheria. In this condition an adherent membrane forms on the tonsils or less commonly in the nose or larynx. The affected area bleeds if attempts are made to remove the membrane. The smell is characteristic. The causative organism can be identified on a direct smear and its pathogenicity determined by bacteriological examination. Infectious mononucleosis may also produce a membrane on the tonsils.

Syphilis. In the secondary stage syphilis causes highly infective mucous patches consisting of shallow ulcers with a narrow red margin and a surface covered by a thin white membrane; they resemble snail tracks. The primary ulcer or chancre of syphilis may also

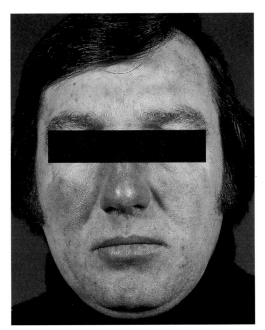

Fig. 3.21 Sarcoidosis associated with bilateral parotid swelling. The skin of the nose and right cheek is also involved ('lupus pemio')

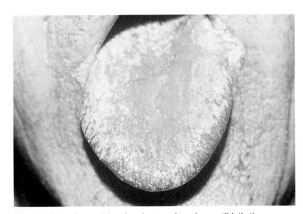

Fig. 3.22 Extensive oral thrush; a feature of previous antibiotic therapy.

occur on the lips and sometimes in other parts of the mouth.

Carcinoma. Carcinoma may be found on the lips, the tongue, the fauces, or the floor of the mouth, usually in the form of an ulcer. Any indolent ulcer requires a biopsy. Only in the later stages of disease may other signs of malignant disease appear, such as enlargement of the regional lymph nodes and fixation of the mass.

Examination

❏ Remove any dentures before examining the mouth.

❏ Use a pocket torch or other light source with a wooden tongue depressor or similar instrument.

❏ Note the symmetry, size and shape of the tongue and look for fasciculation.

❏ Carefully inspect the lips, teeth, gums, cheeks, floor of the mouth; use the spatula to separate the cheeks and tongue from the teeth and gums.

❏ Inspect the soft palate, tonsils and oropharynx; if a clear view cannot be obtained by asking the patient to say 'Ah', depress the tongue with the spatula.

❏ Use a suitable mirror to inspect the nasopharynx.

KEY POINTS

- Hirsutism is common, but is rarely associated with underlying disease.

- Thinning of the outer third of the eyebrow is a common feature in normal subjects.

- Removal of wax by syringing should only be performed by an expert if there is disease of the middle ear or perforation of the ear drum.

- Angular stomatitis is often caused by ill-fitting dentures.

- Dental disease may provide an index of self-neglect.

- The colour of the healthy tongue is extremely variable.

- Physiological enlargement of the tonsils occurs during childhood.

- Any dentures must be removed before examining the mouth.

THE SKIN

Anatomy and function of the skin

The skin of an adult weighs an average of 4 kg and covers an area of 2 m². It has three layers (Fig. 3.23). The outer avascular epithelium, the epidermis is firmly attached to, and supported by, a tough fibroelastic dermis. The dermis contains blood vessels, nerves, sweat and sebaceous glands and hair follicles. The third layer, the hypodermis, is of loose connective tissue, often containing abundant fat, which underlies the dermis.

Keratinocytes make up 90% of the epidermal cells. Their main function is to synthesise insoluble proteins, keratins, which are the main component of the impervious surface of the epidermis, the horny layer. Keratinocytes are generated by division of cells in the basal layers of the epidermis and move outwards, dying in the granular cell layer before being shed at the surface as anucleated horny squames (a significant proportion of common dust). The journey from the basal layer to the surface (epidermal turnover or transit time) takes about 60 days but is greatly accelerated in some skin conditions, for example psoriasis.

Two types of dendritic cell make up most of the remaining epidermal cells. Melanocytes are found mainly in the basal cell layer and are the only epidermal cells to contain tyrosinase, the enzyme essential for the synthesis of melanin from phenylalanine. Synthesised melanin is transferred to surrounding keratinocytes in the form of melanosomes. Langerhans cells form a network within the epidermis and are specialised macrophages which circulate between local lymph nodes and the skin. They are capable of presenting antigen to T lymphocytes (e.g. in allergic contact dermatitis), and play a part in immuno-surveillance of viral and tumour antigens.

The dermis supports the epidermis both structurally and nutritionally. It is separated from the epidermis by a basement membrane and has three principal components: cells (mainly fibroblasts and a few mononuclear phagocytes, lymphocytes, mast cells and Langerhans cells), fibres (collagen, reticulin and elastin) and an amorphous ground substance (mostly the glycosaminoglycans hyaluronic acid and dermatan sulphate). The functions of skin are listed in Table 3.10.

Ageing of skin

Ultraviolet radiation is the main factor speeding the ageing process in skin. This may be very obvious when the wrinkled and inelastic exposed skin of an elderly person who has spent a lot of time out of doors is compared with covered skin (e.g. buttock) of that same person. Ultraviolet rays, especially those of longer wavelength (UVA), damage and destroy the collagen and elastin in the dermis, causing the skin to lose its

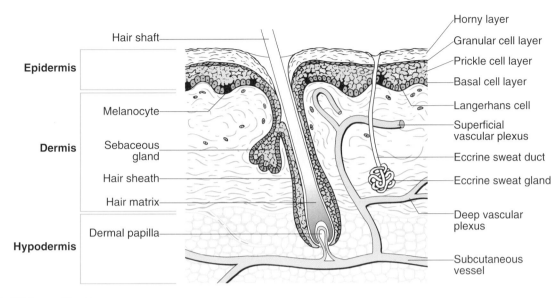

Epidermis

Dermis

Hypodermis

Hair shaft

Melanocyte

Sebaceous gland

Hair sheath

Hair matrix

Dermal papilla

Horny layer

Granular cell layer

Prickle cell layer

Basal cell layer

Langerhans cell

Superficial vascular plexus

Eccrine sweat duct

Eccrine sweat gland

Deep vascular plexus

Subcutaneous vessel

Fig. 3.23 Layers of the skin.

Table 3.10 Functions of the skin

Function	Structure/cell involved
Protection against	
Chemicals, particles	Horny layer
Ultraviolet radiation	Melanocytes
Antigens, haptens	Langerhans cells, lymphocytes, mononuclear phagocytes, mast cells
Microbes	Horny layer, Langerhans cells, mononuclear phagocytes, mast cells
Preservation of a balanced internal environment	Horny layer
Provontion of loss of water electrolytes and macromolecules	
Shock absorption	Dermis and subcutaneous fat
Strong, yet elastic and compliant covering	
Sensation	Specialist nerve endings
Calorie reserve	Subcutaneous fat
Vitamin D synthesis	Keratinocytes
Temperature regulation	Blood vessels Eccrine sweat glands
Lubrication and waterproofing	Sebaceous glands
Protection and prising	Nails
Body odour	Apocrine sweat glands
Psychosocial display	Skin, lips, hair and nails

tensile strength and elasticity. The wrinkled, prune-like faces of elderly Caucasoids living in sunny climates (Fig. 3.24) fuel a substantial business in cosmetic surgery; however, prevention of photoageing by reducing excessive exposure to ultraviolet radiation is better than any cure.

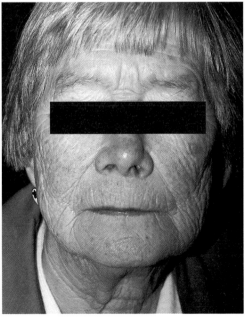

Fig. 3.24 Old face. Note the marked wrinkling and the lentigo on the left cheek.

The history

The ready accessibility of the skin makes it tempting to examine patients with skin disorders without the benefit of a good history. However, the principles of a general medical history should be followed with emphasis on the events surrounding the onset of skin lesions and the progression of the disease. A careful enquiry into drugs (both systemic and topical), a past or family history of skin disease and details of the occupation and any hobbies are especially important. As in other systems, the more difficult the diagnosis proves to be on examination, the more important the history. Although skin lesions may be caused by an exclusively dermatological problem, sometimes the history, or the lesion itself, may suggest that they are cutaneous manifestations of a more widespread condition (see Table 3.11 and Fig. 3.25).

Examination

Dermatology is primarily a visual specialty, and anything that impairs careful inspection will reduce the chance of making the correct diagnosis. Special consideration requires to be shown to the shy or embarrassed patient, but obtaining optimal views is an essential component of the clinical examination. A chaperone is often desirable.

Skin lesions often evolve over a short time span. Several examinations over the period of evolution may enable the diagnosis to be made more easily than a single snapshot of the appearance (Fig. 3.26).

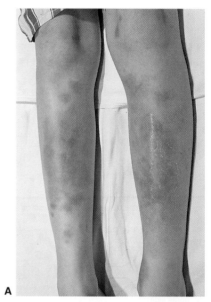

A

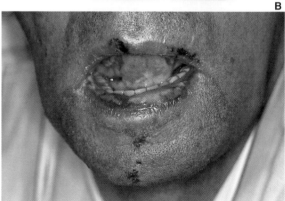

B

Fig. 3.25 The skin manifestations of systemic disease. **A.** Erythema nodosum. **B.** Steven–Johnston syndrome. This was a manifestation of a drug-induced widespread hypersensitivity reaction.

Table 3.11 Some examples of skin lesions and systemic diseases

Skin lesions	Associations	Ask about
Erythema nodosum	Sarcoid, tuberculosis post-streptococcal infection, connective tissue diseases, drugs, etc.	Cough and sputum, breathlessness, sore throat, drugs, etc.
Pyoderma gangrenosum	Ulcerative colitis, rheumatoid arthritis	Rectal bleeding, joint symptoms
Dermatitis herpetiformis	Gluten enteropathy	Family history, change in bowel habit
Generalised purpura	Idiopathic thrombo-cytopenic purpura and other haematological disorders	Family history, haematuria, fever and weight loss
Dermatitis artefacta	Personality disorders	Stresses or anxieties

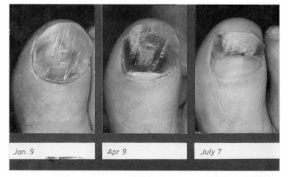

Jan. 9   Apr 9   July 7

Fig. 3.26 The patient, an ardent hill walker, had no recollection of injury of the left big toe and the initial diagnosis included a number of possibilities. The evolution of the disease was consistent only with trauma and a diagnosis of subungual haematoma.

The diagnosis of skin disorders is based on the distribution, morphology and configuration of the skin lesions.

Distribution. The temptation to look at skin lesions at nose length should be resisted until the distribution of the rash has been noted at arm's length. This may be the most valuable clue to the diagnosis. For example, it is not easy to diagnose herpes zoster by the appearance of the individual lesions, but it becomes simple once the dermatomal distribution is appreciated (Fig. 3.27A). Similarly, a photosensitive basis for a rash becomes obvious only after it is noted that exposed areas are involved and shielded areas spared (Fig 3.27B). Some skin conditions may affect certain areas (sites of

predilection) more than others. Whereas psoriasis preferentially involves the scalp, elbows, knees, natal cleft and nails, atopic dermatitis frequently picks out the antecubital and popliteal fossae in children (Fig. 3.27C) and seborrhoeic dermatitis is seen most often on the scalp, forehead, eyebrows, nasolabial folds and presternal area. The distribution of an eczematous rash may be the main pointer that the problem is due to a reaction from an external contactant (Fig. 3.27D).

Universal and symmetrical eruptions favour systemic or constitutional causes, whereas asymmetrical rashes which spread from a single focus are most often due to fungal, bacterial and some viral infections. Frequently, changes on the soles are mirrored by a similar appear-

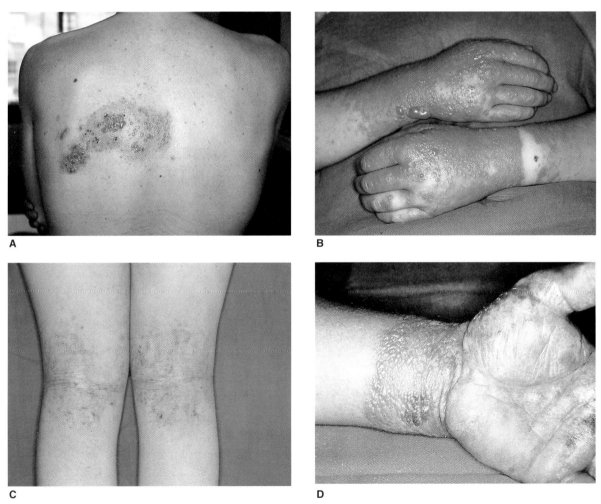

Fig. 3.27 Distribution of rashes as a key to diagnosis. **A.** Herpes zoster. **B.** Griseofulvin photosensitivity eruption. **C.** Atopic dermatitis. **D.** Allergic dermatitis from contact with rubber gloves.

ance on the palms. Sometimes clues as to the diagnosis may be found at sites distant to the presenting problem, for example a patient may consult the doctor about a solitary peri-ungual fibroma although the diagnosis of tuberous sclerosis becomes evident only after ash-leaf depigmented macules on the trunk and adenoma sebaceum on the face are noted. In summary, before looking at the detail of individual lesions, stand back from the patient and consider the following questions:

- Is the rash localised, universal or symmetrical?
- Does the rash follow any anatomical (e.g. derma-tomal) pattern?
- Does it affect special sites such as flexures?
- Are areas of predilection for some common disease involved?
- Are certain areas spared?
- Are there other clues to the diagnosis at sites distant to the presenting problem?
- Are there other incidental findings such as skin cancer which the patient has ignored?

Morphology.   After the distribution has been noted the morphology of the primary lesions should be defined. Unfortunately, scratch marks, crusting and ulceration may obscure the appearance of early lesions though these should be sought and, when found, inspected closely.

Most types of primary lesions have special names (Table 3.12), and these should be used if a skin disease is to be described properly. This encourages the clinician not only to look at the primary lesions carefully but also to record details concisely so that the description can be understood and the rash visualised by others.

With practice use of the terminology will save much time in describing the rash as well as point to the diagnosis. For example, 'violaceous, shiny, polygonal discrete and flat-topped papules on the fronts of the wrists' are probably due to lichen planus (Fig. 3.28A), but the diagnosis is clinched by recognition of the pathognomonic Wickham's striae on close inspection of the papules (Fig. 3.28B), and made indisputable by the observation of a white lacy network on the buccal mucosa (Fig. 3.28C); a biopsy for diagnostic purposes in this instance would be like checking the engine specifications of a car to determine its make rather than looking at the general shape of it and its name on the body!

Most skin lesions are pink; other colours may help in diagnosis, for example the yellow–orange hue of xanthomata, the violaceous tint of lichen planus, the slate-grey colour of drug-induced pigmentation (Fig.

Table 3.12 Terminology of skin lesions

Primary lesions	
Papule	Small solid elevation of skin, less than 0.5 cm in diameter
Plaque	Elevated area of skin greater than 2 cm in diameter but without substantial depth
Macule	Small flat area of altered colour or texture
Vesicle	Circumscribed elevation of skin, less than 0.5 cm in diameter, and containing fluid
Bulla	Circumscribed elevation of skin over 0.5 cm in diameter and containing fluid
Pustule	A visible accumulation of pus in the skin
Abscess	A localised collection of pus in a cavity, more than 1 cm in diameter
Wheal	An elevated white compressible, evanescent area produced by dermal oedema
Angioedema	A diffuse swelling of oedema that extends to the subcutaneous tissue
Nodule	A solid mass in the skin, usually greater than 0.5 cm in diameter
Papilloma	A nipple-like mass projecting from the skin
Petechiae	Pinhead-sized macules of blood in the skin
Purpura	A larger macule or papule of blood in the skin
Ecchymosis	A larger extravasation of blood into the skin
Haematoma	A swelling from gross bleeding
Burrow	A linear or curvilinear papule, caused by a burrowing scabies mite
Comedo	A plug of keratin and sebum wedged in a dilated pilosebaceous orifice
Telangiectasia	The visible dilation of small cutaneous blood vessels
Secondary lesions (which evolve from primary lesions)	
Scale	A flake arising from the horny layer
Crust	Looks like a scale, but is composed of dried blood or tissue fluid
Ulcer	An area of skin from which the whole of the epidermis and at least the upper part of the dermis has been lost
Excoriation	An ulcer or erosion produced by scratching
Erosion	An area of skin denuded by a complete or partial loss of the epidermis
Fissure	A slit in the skin
Sinus	A cavity or channel that permits the escape of pus or fluid
Scar	The result of healing, in which normal structures are permanently replaced by fibrous tissue
Atrophy	Thinning of skin due to diminution of the epidermis, dermis, subcutaneous fat
Stria	A streak-like linear, atrophic, pink, purple or white lesion of the skin caused by changes in the connective tissue

3.2B). Variation in colour, asymmetry and an irregular outline are key signs in distinguishing some malignant from benign lesions (Fig. 3.29). The surface charac-teristics of individual lesions may be equally important diagnostic pointers (Fig. 3.30). Finally, a tiny primary lesion, which might only be recognised with the help of

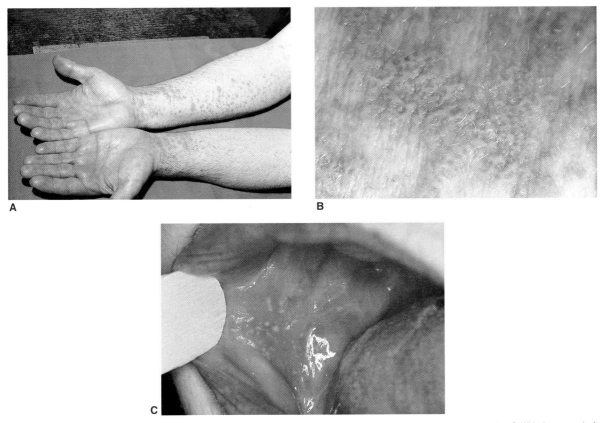

Fig. 3.28 Diagnostic sequence, lichen planus.   A. Discrete flat-topped papules at the wrist. **B.** Wickham's striae visible on close inspection. **C.** White lacy network of striae on buccal mucosa.

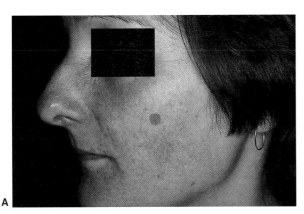

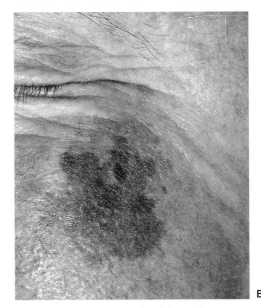

Fig. 3.29 Simple versus malignant lentigo.   A. Simple lesion with well-defined margin. **B.** Malignant lesion with irregular margin and pigmentation.

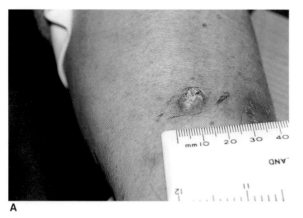

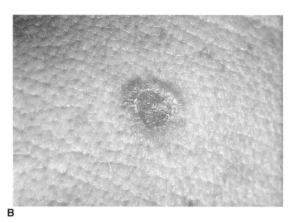

A

B

Fig. 3.30 Surface characteristics as a key to diagnosis.   **A.** Central keratin plug and fleshy shoulders of a Keratoacanthoma. **B.** Rolled margin around ulcer due to basal cell carcinoma.

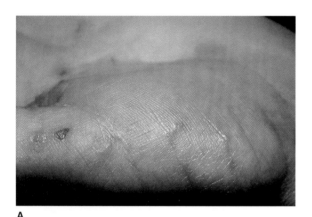

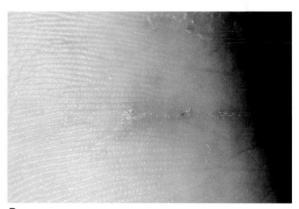

A

B

Fig. 3.31 Scabies burrow on the hand, A, and a close-up of a scabies burrow, B.

a lens, may provide the vital clue in diagnosing a widespread and non-specific rash. The best example of this must be the burrow caused by the scabies mite (Fig. 3.31).

Close to the patient, perhaps aided by a lens, the clinician should study individual lesions carefully and ask the following questions:

- What are their shape?
- What are their size?
- What are their colour?
- What are the characteristics of their margin and surfaces?

Configuration. Having studied the overall distribution of the rash and the morphology of individual lesions the examiner should note the arrangement or configuration of the lesion or groups of lesions. Dermatologists use a few special adjectives which help in this description; they help to describe both individual lesions and their groupings. Examples in which configuration of lesions aids diagnosis include the Köbner phenomenon in psoriasis and lichen planus, grouping of vesicles in herpes simplex (Fig. 3.32A), the patterning and peripheral spread of urticaria (Fig. 3.32B) and the linear appearance of insect bites (Fig. 3.32C).

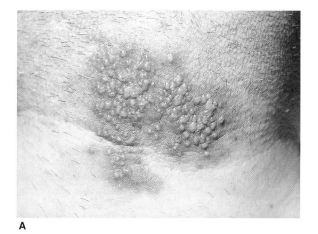

A

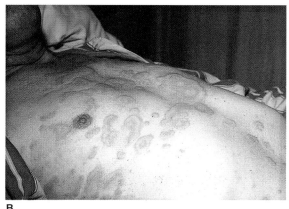

B

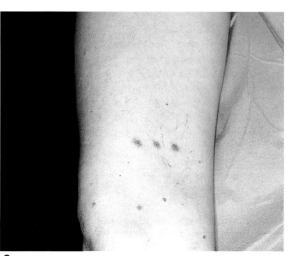

C

Fig. 3.32 Configuration of lesions as a key to diagnosis. **A.** Vesicles of herpes simplex under the chin. **B.** Extensive urticarial reaction. **C.** Insect bites.

Examination

☐ Ask the patient to remove any dressing, wigs and make-up (Fig. 3.33).

☐ Examine, using uniform and bright lighting, with the patient undressed if the skin lesions are widespread.

☐ First observe the overall distribution of the skin lesions.

☐ Then note the morphology of the lesion using a lens if necessary.

☐ Note the arrangement and configuration of the lesions.

KEY POINTS

- Ultraviolet radiation is the main factor speeding the ageing process in skin.

- Skin lesions often evolve over a period of time. Several examinations during the period of evolution often facilitate diagnosis.

- The overall distribution of a rash may be the most valuable clue to diagnosis.

- The morphology of the primary lesion may be obscured by secondary changes but whenever possible should be carefully defined.

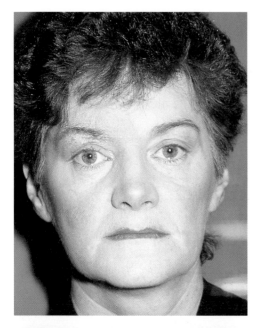

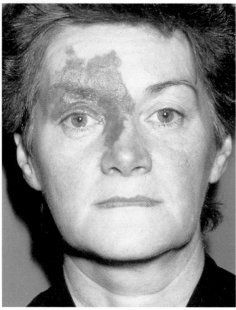

Fig. 3.33 The effect of camouflage make-up in a patient with an extensive port wine stain.

SWELLINGS

This section describes the common principles involved in the examination of any swelling.

The 'sudden' finding of a lump by a patient does not necessarily imply that it has only recently developed. It is important to ask if any change in size or other characteristics have been noted since it was first detected and whether there are any associated features such as pain, tenderness or colour changes. The history of preceding events may also be of diagnostic help. Sometimes physical examination will reveal a lump whose presence is unknown to the patient.

Inspection and palpation

Position. It is important to define the anatomical situation of any mass. The site of some swellings such as those in the breast, the thyroid or the parotid glands presents no difficulty. In others, the ease with which the lump can be localised will vary, especially in the abdomen. Other features such as shape or mobility will help to identify the anatomical origin.

Size. The size of any swelling requires to be accurately measured and documented. In this way significant changes can be recognised. Vague and misleading statements about size, such as large, medium or small, or comparisons with fruit, eggs or vegetables should be avoided.

Shape. The shape of a mass may be sufficiently characteristic to signify its origin. Examples in the abdomen include an enlarged spleen or liver, a distended bladder or the fundus of the uterus in later pregnancy.

Colour and temperature. The skin over acute inflammatory lesions is usually red and warm. There may also be a rise in skin temperature over a vascular tumour which ranges in colour from red to blue or purple according to the proportions of reduced haemoglobin present and the depth of the layer of skin through which it is seen. In haematomas the pigment from extravasated blood may produce the range of colours so familiar in a bruise. A brown or black colour is common in melanomas (Fig. 3.29), though some are not pigmented. A xanthoma is a small skin nodule which may be identified by its yellow colour because of the lipids it contains.

Pain and tenderness. Inflammatory swellings are characterised by tenderness. Some other swellings, such as large lipomas, may be entirely free from pain or tenderness, because they carry no nerve supply and have developed in an area where the mass can be accommodated without subjecting any structure to undue stretching. Tumours eroding bone or growing into nerve roots and plexuses cause severe persistent and intractable pain which is often worse at night.

Movement. A mass may be part of, attached to or free from adjacent structures, such as skin or bone. Fixation of the skin may be associated with a fine dimpling at the opening of the hair follicles resembling an orange skin when there is lymphatic obstruction ('peau d'orange'). Such a change is most commonly due to malignant disease.

Fixation to deeper structures may occur. For example, a breast tumour may become fixed to underlying muscle.

The presence or absence of movement on swallowing, respiration and coughing will produce information regarding the nature of a swelling in the neck (p. 78), abdomen (p. 178) and hernial orifices (p. 183) respectively.

Expansile pulsations arise from aneurysmal dilation of the aorta or other large arteries, or highly vascular tumours. In tricuspid incompetence, the liver is pulsatile and a transmitted pulsation may be detected if a mass is in contact with a major blood vessel.

Consistency. The consistency of a swelling may vary from soft and fluctuant through increasing degrees of firmness until this may be so striking as to merit the term 'stony hard'. Very hard swellings are usually malignant or calcified, or consist of dense fibrous tissue.

Fluctuation indicates a fluid-containing swelling, such as an abscess or a cyst. Soft encapsulated tumours such as lipomas may also show some degree of fluctuation.

Surface texture. The surface of a swelling may vary from the uniformly smooth to the grossly irregular. The texture often provides important evidence of the probable pathological process. For example, on palpation, the surface of the liver is smooth in acute right ventricular failure but is usually grossly nodular in metastatic malignancy.

Margin. The edge or margin may be well delineated or ill defined, regular or irregular, sharp or rounded. The margins of enlarged organs such as the thyroid gland, liver, spleen or kidney can usually be defined more clearly than those of inflammatory or malignant masses. An indefinite margin may suggest an infiltrating malignancy in contrast to the clearly defined edge of a benign tumour.

Associated swellings. Conditions in which multiple swellings occur include neurofibromatosis (Fig. 3.34), lipomatosis, metastases in the skin, lymph nodes in the lymphomas and fibrocystic changes in the breast. If there is suspicion that a tumour is malignant, the lymph nodes draining the area concerned should be thoroughly examined.

Percussion

This is of limited value but occasionally may be helpful in defining an abdominal mass (p. 180).

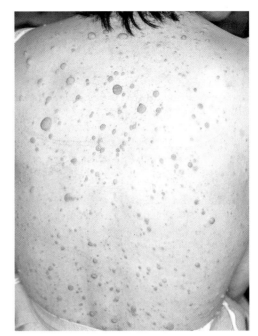

Fig. 3.34 Neurofibromatosis.

Auscultation

Vascular sounds. If the blood flow through a tumour is large, a systolic murmur (bruit) may be audible over the swelling and, if it is sufficiently marked, a thrill may be palpable. Systolic murmurs may also be heard over arterial aneurysms, while over the very rare swelling due to an arteriovenous fistula there is a continuous murmur, often accompanied by a thrill, similar to the bruit of a persistent ductus arteriosus (p. 111).

Fetal heart sounds. These may be audible over the pregnant uterus after 30 weeks. The noise of blood flowing through extensive vascular formation in the pregnant uterus may also be audible (uterine souffle).

Intestine and bowel sounds (p. 181). These may be heard over a hernia which contains intestine.

Friction. This may be sometimes heard over an enlarged spleen or liver when fibrinous perisplenitis or perihepatitis is present.

Transillumination

This may be useful in distinguishing between a swelling composed of solid tissue and one consisting of transparent or semitransparent liquid. For example, the sign may help to distinguish a hydrocele from other scrotal swellings. It must be borne in mind that a testicular tumour may lie within a hydrocele (p. 184).

Examination

❏ Inspect any mass carefully, noting change in the colour or texture of the overlying skin.

❏ Gently palpate to elicit any tenderness or change in skin temperature.

❏ Without causing undue tenderness define the site and shape of the mass by palpation. Measure its size and record the findings diagrammatically.

❏ Keep the hand still for a few moments on the mass to determine if it is pulsatile.

❏ Assess the consistency, surface texture and margins of the mass.

❏ Attempt to pick up a fold of skin over the swelling to assess skin fixation and contrast the mobility of the skin with the unaffected side.

❏ Determine fixation to deeper structures by attempting to move the swelling in different planes relative to the surrounding tissues.

❏ Look for fluctuation by compressing the swelling suddenly with one finger, using another finger to determine if a bulge is created.

❏ Confirm the presence of fluctuation in two planes.

❏ Auscultate for vascular bruits and other sounds.

❏ To elicit transillumination, the surroundings must be dark. Press the lighted end of an electric torch into one side of the swelling. A cystic swelling will light up if the fluid is translucent provided that the covering tissues are not too thick.

THE LYMPH GLANDS

The lymphoreticular system comprises the spleen, the lymph nodes and lymphatic ducts and lymphoid tissue elsewhere, including the tonsils, adenoids and the Peyer's patches of the ileum. It is important to distinguish between a normal lymph node which may be palpable and a pathological gland. Finding of pathological lymphadenopathy is frequently of considerable diagnostic or prognostic significance, for example in the staging of various lymphoproliferative and other malignancies. Pathological lymphadenopathy may be local or generalised.

Anatomy. The important groups of lymph glands available for clinical examination are shown in Figures 3.35 and 5.3 (p. 143). Other glands can only be assessed by investigation: for example, a chest radiograph may reveal hilar lymphadenopathy and CAT scan abodminal para-aortic nodes.

History

A patient's attention may be drawn to a lymphatic enlargement by the presence of pain. Sometimes pain-free glands are detected on inspection or by palpation, for example when taking a shower or a bath. Their finding may cause understandable but hopefully inappropriate concern. Frequently the dominant symptoms are those of the underlying pathological process and lymphadenopathy is only discovered during physical examination. This emphasises the need to be thorough. Where HIV infection is a possibility, the patient should be asked about possible drug abuse, sexual habits and other risk factors.

Examination

This involves not only detection but also an assessment of the various features of any swelling as previously described (p. 72).

Extent. In healthy subjects palpable glands can usually be detected, especially in the axilla and the groin. They are seldom greater than 0.5 cm in diameter and frequently smaller. They are usually described as soft, rubbery or shotty.

Generalised lymphadenopathy can occur in a number of conditions (see Table 3.13).

Localised lymphadenopathy is common and usually infective, as in acute tonsillitis. In many instances the precise aetiological factor remains obscure.

In the presence of pathological lymphadenopathy the examination involves looking for a possible cause, including the site of infection or of a primary malignancy. Special attention should be paid to the presence or absence of enlargement of the liver and spleen and the haemopoietic system, including features such as bruising, purpura or petechiae.

In clinical practice the lymph nodes are examined piecemeal and regionally. At this stage they are considered together.

Table 3.13 Some causes of pathological lymphadenopathy

Generalised	
Viral	Epstein–Barr virus, cytomegalovirus and HIV
Bacterial	Brucellosis, syphilis
Protozoal	Toxoplasmosis
Neoplastic	Lymphoma, acute or chronic lymphocytic leukaemia
Others	Rheumatoid arthritis, systemic lupus erythematosus, sarcoidosis
Localised	
Infective	Acute or chronic, including viral, bacterial and other agents
Neoplastic	Secondary metastatic
	Primary haematological, including Hodgkin's and non-Hodgkin's lymphoma

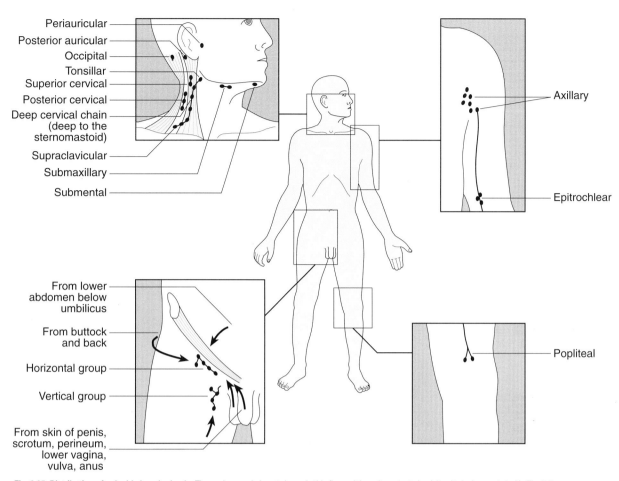

Fig. 3.35 Distribution of palpable lymph glands. The scalene node is not shown in this figure. It is an important gland. Its site is demonstrated in Fig. 5.3.

Consistency. The consistency of the glands may provide important information. For example, in Hodgkin's disease the glands are characteristically 'rubbery'. In tuberculosis they may be 'matted' and in metastatic carcinoma they feel 'craggy'. Calcified glands feel stony hard.

Tenderness. Tenderness is usually a feature of acute bacterial infection. With tender cervical lymphadenopathy the possibilities include dental sepsis, tonsillitis and mastoiditis.

Fixation. Glands which are fixed to deep structures or skin are usually malignant.

Examination

☐ Inspect for any obvious lymphadenopathy.
☐ Palpate one side at a time using the fingers of one hand.

☐ In turn compare the findings in a group of glands on one side with the contralateral side.
☐ Assess the site, size and consistency of any palpable gland. Note tenderness and determine if the gland is fixed to surrounding structures.
☐ Examine the cervical and axillary glands with the patient sitting.
☐ Lie the patient down to examine for the abdomen, inguinal and popliteal glands.
☐ Cervical glands. From behind, examine the submental, submandibular, preauricular, tonsillar (Fig. 3.36A and B), supraclavicular and deep cervical glands in the anterior triangle of the neck. Palpate deeply for the scalene nodes (Fig. 5.4 p. 143). From in front of the patient, examine the posterior triangles, up the back of the neck and for the posterior auricular and occipital nodes (Fig. 3.36C).
☐ Axillary glands. Sit in front of the patient, supporting the arm on the side under examination.

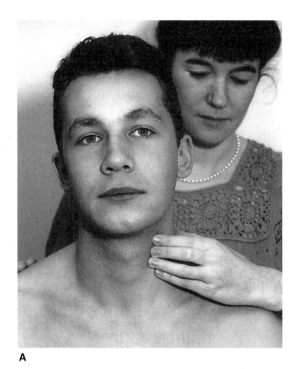

A

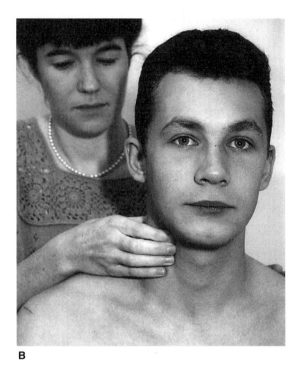

B

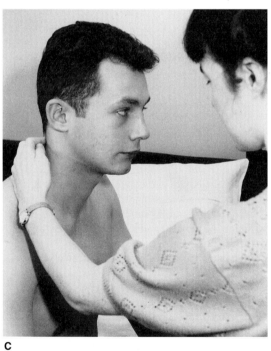

C

Fig. 3.36 Palpation of the cervical glands. Examine the glands of the anterior triangle from behind (**A** and **B**) using one hand at a time. Examine the posterior glands from the front (**C**).

Palpate the right axilla with the left hand and vice versa. Insert the fingertips into the vault of the axilla and then draw them downwards while palpating the medial, anterior and posterior axillary wall in turn

(Fig. 3.37A and B).

❑ Epitrochlear glands. While supporting the patient's right wrist with the left hand, grasp the partially flexed elbow with the right hand and use the

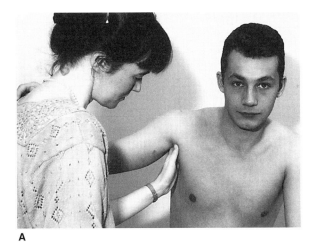

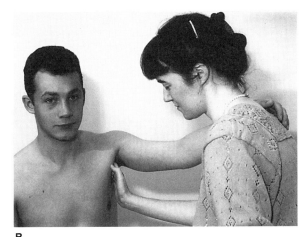

A

B

Fig. 3.37 Palpation of the axillary glands. **A.** Right side. **B.** Left side.

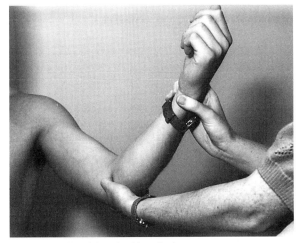

Fig. 3.38 Palpation of the epitrochlear gland.

thumb to feel for the epitrochlear gland. Examine the left epitrochlear gland with the left thumb (Fig. 3.38).

☐ Inguinal glands. Palpate in turn over the horizontal chain, which lies just below the inguinal ligament, and then over the vertical chain along the saphenous veins.

☐ Popliteal glands. Use both hands to examine the popliteal fossa with the knee flexed to about 45°.

THE NECK

Physical abnormalities in the neck are common. In addition to the general inspection of the neck for any skin lesions or visible tumours, various other structures should be examined. These are:

- thyroid gland
- lymph glands (p. 75)
- salivary glands
- neck movements (p. 284)
- carotid and subclavian arteries (p. 207)
- jugular veins (p. 99).

The thyroid gland

The thyroid consists of two symmetrical lateral lobes joined together by a central isthmus that normally covers the second and third tracheal rings. Occasionally, the gland may extend into the superior mediastinum, or may be entirely retrosternal. Rarely, the gland may be located along the line occupied by the thyroglossal duct. When situated near the origin on the dorsum of the tongue, it is referred to as a lingual goitre.

The gland is normally ensheathed by the pretracheal fascia and moves on swallowing. The normal thyroid is palpable in about 50% females and 25% of males.

Disorders of the thyroid gland may present in three different ways.

1. Symptoms of thyrotoxicosis

The features include weight loss with increased appetite, heat intolerance, emotional lability, excessive sweating and palpitations. There may be a change in the menstrual cycle and in bowel habit as a consequence of intestinal hurry. In elderly patients many of these features may be missing and the presenting features may relate to the development of atrial fibrillation.

2. Symptoms of hypothyroidism

These comprise weight gain and constipation, apathy

and forgetfulness, gruffness of voice and cold intolerance. In the elderly, symptoms tend to develop insidiously and may be unrecognised or wrongly attributed to ageing processes.

3. Goitre

Significant enlargement of the thyroid gland (goitre) is common. By definition, the lateral lobes of the thyroid have a volume in excess of the terminal phalanges of the thumbs of the subject. Goitre may be noted by the patient or by relatives and friends, but many subjects are unaware of its presence. The vast majority are asymptomatic. Tenderness may be associated with various forms of thyroiditis and acute pain may occur following bleeding into a thyroid cyst. Dysphagia is rare except when there is marked swelling of the gland. Its presence suggests a malignant process.

The size of any goitre should be assessed clinically and the gland examined for the following features:

Shape. Simple goitres may be relatively symmetrical in their earlier stages but usually become irregular with time. The gland is usually symmetrical in primary hyperthyroidism (Graves' disease), whereas it is irregular in secondary or nodular toxic goitre.

Mobility. Most goitres move with swallowing, however an invasive thyroid carcinoma may lead to fixation of the gland to other surrounding structures and very large goitres may be immobilised because they expand to occupy all the available space in the root of the neck.

Consistency. The consistency, texture and the smoothness of the surface of the gland may vary from one part to another. Nodules in the substance of the gland may be large or small, single or multiple. If the consistency is 'stony hard', carcinomatous change is likely. The presence of large, firm or hard lymph nodes near a goitre also suggests the possibility of a thyroid malignancy.

Tenderness. Diffuse tenderness usually implies thyroiditis; localised tenderness may occur following bleeding into a cyst.

Colour changes. These are most unusual unless the goitre is very big, when distended veins may be responsible for a dusky, blue appearance.

Auscultation. A bruit indicates an abnormally large blood flow and is sometimes associated with a palpable thrill. Increased blood flow occurs in hyperthyroidism, but the use of anti-thyroid drugs may also increase the vascularity of the gland sufficient to produce a murmur. A thyroid bruit should be distinguished from a murmur arising in the carotid artery or transmitted from the aorta and from a venous hum originating in the internal jugular vein.

Table 3.14 Some signs of thyroid disease

Thyrotoxicosis	Lid lag (p. 259) Tachycardia and high pulse pressure Hands hot and sweaty Increase in physiological tremor Hyperactive movements Proximal myopathy
Hypothyroidism	Bradycardia Skin coarse and dry Gruff voice Delay in tendon relaxation time (p. 235)
Autoimmune thyroid disease	Proptosis, exophthalmos and ophthalmoplegia Pretibial myxoedema

Other features. The presence or absence of a goitre is a poor index of thyroid function, but the facial appearance may be an excellent guide to the diagnosis (Fig. 3.39). Some of the systemic features of thyroid disease are summarised in Table 3.14.

Examination

❑ Inspect the neck from the front.
❑ Identify a thyroid swelling while asking the patient to swallow a sip of water with the neck slightly extended.

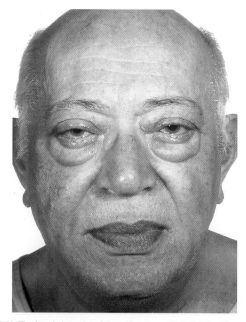

Fig. 3.39 The face in hypothyroidism. (Courtesy of Dr D.H.A. Boyd.)

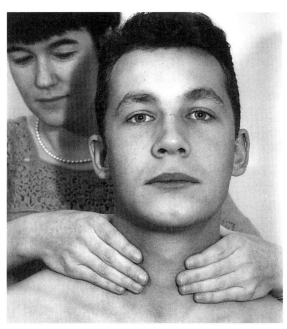

Fig. 3.40 Palpating the thyroid gland from behind.

❏ With the patient sitting or standing, palpate for the thyroid gland from behind (Fig. 3.40). If necessary, confirm its presence by asking the patient to swallow again while palpating over the gland.
❏ Note shape, size and other characteristics of any goitre and the presence or absence of a thrill.
❏ Auscultate for a thyroid bruit.
❏ During the general examination look specifically for systemic features of thyroid disease (see Table 3.14.).

Thyroid function

Where there is a clinical suspicion of abnormal thyroid function, this should be assessed biochemically. In thyrotoxicosis the level of thyroid-stimulating hormone (TSH) will be reduced. Total thyroxine and free thyroxine values are usually raised but may be normal in patients with T3 thyrotoxicosis.

Primary failure of the thyroid gland is associated with elevated TSH. Circulating thyroid hormones will be reduced. In secondary hypothyroidism, TSH will be low.

Other investigations of the thyroid gland may be of value in assessing structure.

• *Plain X-ray.* Identifies calcification within the gland and narrowing or displacement of the trachea.

• *Ultrasonography.* To distinguish between cystic and solid 'nodules'.
• *Radionuclide scanning.* Determines the size and site of the gland and whether nodules are 'hot', taking up radioiodine, or 'cold'.
• *Aspiration cytology.* May help in assessing the pathology of cold nodules.

THE BREASTS

The stages in the development of the female breast are illustrated in Figure 3.41. The adult breast may be divided into the nipple, the areola and four quadrants, upper and lower, inner and outer, with the axillary tail projecting from the upper and outer quadrant (Fig. 3.42). The nipple consists of erectile tissue covered with pigmented skin, which also covers the areola. The openings of the lactiferous ducts may be seen near the apex of the nipple. The size and shape of the breasts in healthy women vary widely, and are influenced by hereditary factors, sexual maturity, the phase of the menstrual cycle, parity, pregnancy and lactation and the general state of nutrition. The amount of fat and stroma surrounding the glandular tissue largely determines the size of the breast, except during lactation, when the enlargement is almost entirely glandular.

The breast is a hormonally responsive gland, and in premenopausal women its consistency may vary considerably in response to fluctuations in oestrogen and progesterone levels during the menstrual cycle and in pregnancy. Swelling and tenderness due to fluid retention and prominence of the glandular elements of the breast are more common in the premenstrual phase. With age there is a reduction in the amount of glandular tissue with a corresponding increase in the amount of relative fat. The breasts are therefore softer in consistency and are more pendulous. The breasts of lactating women are swollen and engorged with milk and are best examined after breastfeeding or milk expression.

The history

The common symptoms of breast disease are lumps, skin changes, nipple inversion, nipple discharge and pain. Men may present with gynaecomastia. Breast tumours may present with signs and symptoms of acute inflammation. The UK Breast Screening Programme invites women between the ages of 50 and 64 to attend for single oblique mammography at 3-year intervals. An increasing number of asymptomatic women present with mammographic abnormalities.

1 Pre-pubertal

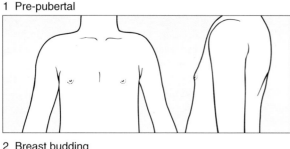

2 Breast budding

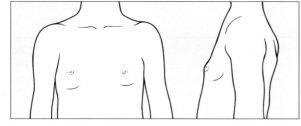

3 Enlargement

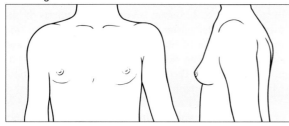

4 Secondary mound formed by areola

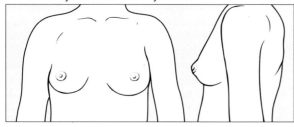

5 Single contour of breast and areola

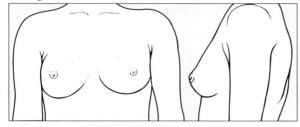

Fig. 3.41 Stages of breast development.

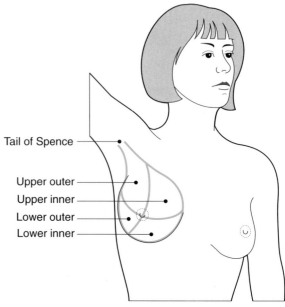

Fig. 3.42 The adult right breast.

Breast lump

The commonest cause of a breast lump varies with age (Fig. 3.43).

Carcinoma of the breast. This affects 1 in 12 women. Its incidence increases with age, but any mass must be regarded as potentially malignant until proven otherwise. Cancer of the male breast is uncommon and is likely to be genetic in origin.

Characteristically carcinomas are solid masses with an irregular outline, often painless but firm or hard, contrasting in consistency with the surrounding breast tissue. The tumour may be confined within the breast tissue or extend into overlying tissues such as skin, pectoral fascia, pectoral muscle or metastasise to intramammary lymphatics, regional lymph nodes or the systemic · circulation. The current TNM (Tumour, Nodes, Metastases) classification of breast tumours is given in Table 3.15.

Fibrocystic changes. Fibrocystic change or irregular nodularity of the breast is common, especially in the upper outer quadrant in young women. Usually the tissue is rubbery in texture and varies in size with the hormonal cycle, being at its largest before menstruation. The changes are usually bilateral.

Fibroadenomas. These are abnormalities of normal development and involution due to overgrowth of elements derived from terminal duct lobules. Characteristically they present as smooth mobile discrete

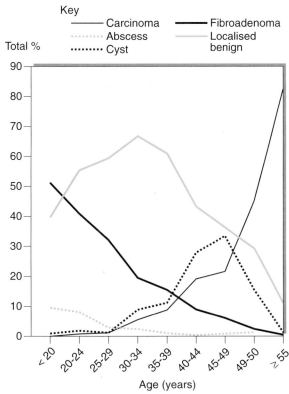

Key
— Carcinoma   — Fibroadenoma
...... Abscess   — Localised benign
.... Cyst

Total %

Fig. 3.43 Percentage of patients in 5-year age groups with a discrete breast lump who have common benign conditions and breast cancer. Localised benign refers to localised nodular areas of breast tissue.

Table 3.15 TNM malignant classification of breast cancers

Tumour

Tx	Cannot be assessed
T0	No evidence of primary tumour
Tis	Carcinoma in situ, intraductal carcinoma, lobular carcinoma in situ, Paget's disease of nipple with no tumour
T_1	Tumour ≤ 2 cm in greatest dimension
	a ≤ 0.5 cm
	b $> 0.5 \leq 1$ cm
	c > 1 cm ≤ 2 cm
T_2	Tumour > 2 cm ≤ 5 cm greatest dimension
T_3	Tumour > 5 cm greatest dimension
T_4	Tumour any size with direct extension to chest wall or skin
	a extension to chest wall
	b oedema including *peau d'orange* or ulceration of skin of breast or satellite skin nodules on same breast
	c 4a + 4b
	d inflammatory carcinoma

Nodes

Nx	Regional lymph nodes cannot be assessed
N0	No regional lymph node metastasis
N_1	Metastasis with moveable ipsilateral axillary nodes
N_2	Metastases with ipsilateral axillary nodes fixed to one another or to other structures
N_3	Metastases to ipsilateral internal mammary nodes

Metastases

Mx	Presence of distant metastases cannot be assessed
M0	No distant metastases
M_1	Distant metastases including supraclavicular nodes

This classification with appropriate modification forms the basis for classification of other primary malignancies.

rubbery lumps in young women. They are second only to localised benign breast disease as the commonest cause of a breast mass in a woman under the age of 35. The distinction between a juvenile fibroadenoma and phyllodes tumour (giant fibroadenoma) is made on pathological grounds and the two are best regarded as distinct pathological entities.

Breast cysts. The aetiology of breast cysts remains obscure, but they are a feature of the involuting breast which is still subject to hormonal stimulation. They are the commonest cause of a breast lump in women between the ages of 35 and 50. Their clinical picture depends on the intracystic pressure. They present as smooth lumps, which may be soft and fluctuant or even impalpable when the intracystic pressure is low, or hard and painful when the intracystic pressure is high. Cysts may occur in multiple clusters. Occasionally a cyst may be associated with malignant disease. For this reason any cyst in which the aspirate is blood-stained, in which there is a residual mass following aspiration or which recurs after several aspirations should be excised to exclude malignancy.

Breast abscesses. There are two distinct types of breast abscesses. Lactational abscesses occur in women who are breastfeeding and are usually peripheral in nature. Non-lactational abscesses occur as an extension of periductal mastitis and have a classical distribution at the edge of the nipple, often associated with nipple inversion. They usually occur in young female smokers. Occasionally a non-lactating abscess may discharge spontaneously, giving an abnormal communication between the inflamed duct and the skin. The classical position of this fistulae is at the areolocutaneous border.

Skin changes

It is important to differentiate between simple skin dimpling due to retraction of the skin and indrawing of the skin due to infiltration of the dermis by tumour. In the former the skin remains mobile over the tumour; in the latter the tumour is fixed to the skin. Likewise in tethering to the chest wall the tumour is solid with the chest wall when the pectoral muscle is contracted, but when it is relaxed it is possible to move the lesion separately. Tumours which infiltrate the chest wall are fixed when the pectoral muscle is both relaxed and contracted.

Obstruction of the intramammary lymphatics with tumour results in lymphoedema of the breast. The skin is attached at the hair follicles but swollen in between, giving the appearance of the skin of an orange ('peau d'orange').

Eczematous changes of the nipple may be part of a generalised skin disorder, however when confined to a nipple they should raise the possibility of Paget's disease of the nipple. In this condition there is invasion of the epidermis by cells from an underlying intra-ductal carcinoma. A skin biopsy should be performed.

Nipple inversion

Retraction of the nipple due to shortening of the nipple ducts from periductal inflammation and fibrosis is a common finding. The characteristics of benign nipple inversion are a symmetrical slit-like inversion. Nipple retraction due to malignant disease is asymmetrical and distorting, pulling the nipple away from its central position (Fig. 3.44).

Nipple discharge

A small amount of clear fluid expressed from multiple ducts of the breast on massage is normal. Persistent single duct discharge or blood-stained (macroscopic or microscopic) discharge should always be investigated. The differential diagnosis includes duct ectasia, intraduct papilloma or rarely intraduct carcinoma.

Galactorrhoea. Galactorrhoea is characterised by a milky discharge from multiple ducts in both breasts and is a feature of hyperprolactinaemia. There is usually associated Montgomery tubercle hyperplasia. Spontaneous milk production is uncommon and often galactorrhoea is found only by trying to express milk. The causes of hyperprolactinaemia include physiological processes (pregnancy, post partum), drugs (dopamine antagonists, dopamine-depleting agents), pituitary tumours, hypothalamic and stalk lesions, primary hypothyroidism and renal failure.

Gynaecomastia

Gynaecomastia (enlargement of the male breast) occurs in about 50% of pubertal boys probably because of the relatively high oestradiol levels. Many drugs can cause enlargement (e.g. spironolactone, cimetidine and oestrogens used in the treatment of prostatic cancer) (Fig. 3.45). Gynaecomastia is also found in cirrhosis of the liver and in conditions associated with increased oestrogen production (interstitial cell tumours of the testis, some adrenal tumours, thyrotoxicosis) or decreased androgen production (hypergonadotrophic hypogonadism, Klinefelter's syndrome, orchitis).

Examination

❑ Take care to avoid upsetting any patient, particularly the more modest, by explaining the purpose of the examination. Male clinicians should be chaperoned.
❑ Ask the patient to sit upright on a well-illuminated chair, undressed to the waist and with the hands resting on the thighs so that the pectoral muscles are relaxed (Fig. 3.46A).

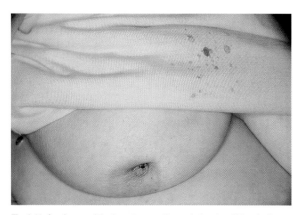

Fig. 3.44 Carcinoma of the breast presenting as indrawing of the nipple.
Note the bloody discharge on the underclothing.

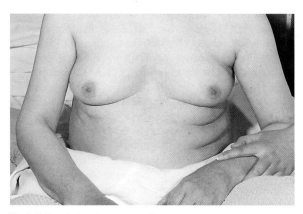

Fig. 3.45 Drug-induced gynaecomastia.

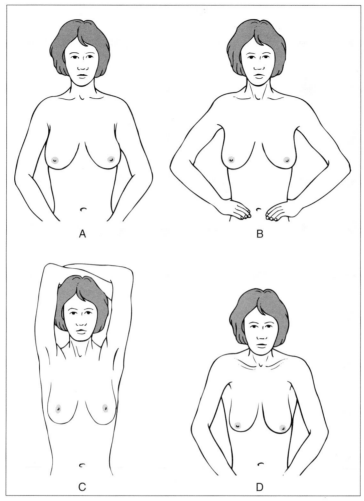

Fig. 3.46 Positions for inspecting the breasts.   **A.** Hand resting on thighs. **B.** Hand pressed onto hips. **C.** Arms above head. **D.** Leaning forward with breasts pendulous.

❏ Sit facing the patient and carefully inspect the breasts for asymmetry, local swelling or changes in the skin or nipples.

❏ Repeat the inspection with the patient's hands pressed firmly on their hips (Fig. 3.46B), thereby contracting the pectoral muscles, then with arms raised above the head (Fig. 3.46C) to stretch the pectoral muscles and the skin over the breasts, and finally leaning forward so that the breasts become pendulous (Fig. 3.46D). Such actions expose the whole breast and exacerbate skin dimpling.

❏ Ask the patient to lie with the head supported on one pillow and with the hand on the side to be examined under the head (Fig. 3.47).

❏ With the hand held flat to the skin, palpate the breast tissue using the palmar surface of the middle three fingers, compressing breast tissue gently against the chest wall.

❏ Consider the breast as the face of a clock and carefully examine each hour of the clock from outside towards the nipple, not forgetting the tissue directly under the nipple. Compare the texture of one breast with that of the other.

❏ Define the characteristic of any mass, including fixation to underlying tissues or tethering to skin, which may become apparent as a dimpling overlying the tumour when the breast is gently elevated by a hand.

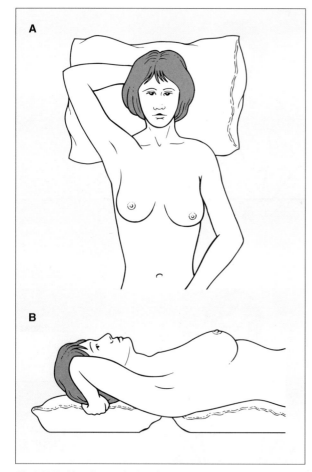

Fig. 3.47 Positions for examination of the right breast.

❑ Examine the axillary tail between finger and thumb as it extends towards the axilla.
❑ To palpate the nipple, hold it gently between index finger and thumb and attempt to express any discharge.
❑ Complete the examination by palpating the regional lymph nodes, including the supraclavicular group. Examine the axillae with the arms relaxed in order to expose the apex of the axilla and then with the hands on the hips to tense the pectoral fascia and contract the pectoral muscles.

Investigation

Diagnosis of most breast lesions relies on a combination of clinical examination, fine-needle aspiration (FNA) and either mammography and/or breast ultra-sound. In some lesions the ultimate diagnosis requires excision biopsy.

Fine-needle aspiration. This involves the passage of a green needle (21G) on suction through a breast lesion. It allows immediate diagnosis of breast cysts and in experienced hands will yield sufficient cells for the diagnosis of 95% of malignancies and 85% of benign lesions.

Mammography. The classical characteristics of a breast cancer are an irregular opacity with spiculated edges, often in association with irregular micro-calcification. Owing to the high fat content mammography is more sensitive in the breasts of older women, in whom it can detect a lesion before it becomes clinically palpable. The mammograms of younger women are more opaque and more difficult to read.

Ultrasound. This is particularly helpful in women under the age of 35. It is possible to differentiate solid from cystic lesions by ultrasound, and also to discriminate between benign and malignant lesions sometimes.

KEY POINTS

- A swelling which is suddenly found may not have recently developed.
- The shape and size of any swelling should be defined and measured.
- In healthy subjects small lymph glands can usually be detected in the axilla and groin.
- Localised lymphadenopathy is common and usually infective.
- The lymph glands are best examined one side at a time in turn, comparing the findings on one side with the contralateral side.
- The normal thyroid gland is palpable in up to 50% of women, fewer men. The presence or absence of a goitre is a poor guide to thyroid function.
- A thyroid bruit is an indication of increased vascularity of the gland.
- Carcinoma of the breast is the commonest malignancy in women. Any breast lump must be regarded as potentially malignant until this has been excluded.
- Examination of the breasts involves careful inspection in various positions as well as a thorough and systematic palpation of the gland and of the regional lymph nodes.

D. P. de Bono • D. S. Macpherson

4

The cardiovascular system

THE HISTORY

The principal symptoms of heart disease are dyspnoea, pain, oedema and palpitation (Table 4.1). Some heart disease is asymptomatic, and only detected during routine examination, or when a complication develops. Heart disease may be one of many causes of a non-specific symptom such as tiredness.

Dyspnoea

Dyspnoea literally means 'unhappy breathing' – better translated as shortness of breath. When a patient complains of shortness of breath the clinician has to find out exactly what is meant, what the circumstances are which cause the symptoms to occur and how severe is the resulting disability. Useful questions include the following:

- Do you feel short of breath?
- What makes you short of breath?
- Do you get short of breath climbing stairs or hills?
- What do you do when you get short of breath?
- Do you feel short of breath when you lie down?
- Do you ever wake up gasping for breath?
- What do you do then?

Some of the mechanisms involved in the development of cardiac dyspnoea are shown in Figure 4.1.

Dyspnoea on effort is breathlessness brought on by physical exertion. It is a symptom of disease if it occurs at exercise levels below those expected for the patient's age and previous degree of fitness.

Paroxysmal nocturnal dyspnoea is sudden, severe breathlessness which wakes the patient from sleep.

Characteristically, the patient sits up gasping for breath, has a cough producing frothy sputum and may have other features of *acute pulmonary oedema*. Paroxysmal nocturnal dyspnoea is a feature of acute left heart failure; the mechanism is explained in Figure 4.2. Paroxysmal nocturnal dyspnoea has to be distinguished from nocturnal asthma and from the kind of sleep disturbance seen in sleep apnoea syndrome (p. 138).

Dyspnoea at rest, or on minimal exertion, is a feature of severe heart failure, though it may also be due to respiratory disease. Patients with heart failure are usually more comfortable sitting upright, and may become breathless on lying flat. This is called *orthopnoea*; the mechanism is similar to that already described for paroxysmal nocturnal dyspnoea. The most severe form of dyspnoea at rest is seen in *acute pulmonary oedema* (Fig. 4.3). There is severe, persistent breathlessness at rest, the patient is unable to lie flat, there is a cough and frothy white sputum which may later become blood tinged and the patient is, understandably, very anxious. Physical findings in acute pulmonary oedema are discussed on page 88.

Acute pulmonary oedema is usually due to acute left heart failure; very occasionally it can be due to other causes such as toxic gas inhalation. It is *not* a feature of chronic left heart failure, because these patients develop chronic pulmonary vasoconstriction, which protects them from a sudden rise in left atrial pressure. Sometimes it can be hard to distinguish acute pulmonary oedema from a severe asthma attack: some of the distinguishing features are listed in Table 4.2.

Sudden severe breathlessness developing at rest may be a feature of *acute pulmonary embolism*. Unlike patients with acute pulmonary oedema, these patients are more

Table 4.1 Principal symptoms of heart disease

Symptom	Cardiac causes	Other causes
Dyspnoea	Heart failure Ischaemic heart disease Pulmonary embolism Pulmonary hypertension	Respiratory disease Anaemia
Chest pain	Ischaemic heart disease Pericarditis Dissecting aneurysm	Oesophageal pain Pneumothorax Musculoskeletal pain
Oedema	Heart failure Venous stasis Constrictive pericarditis	Nephrotic syndrome Liver disease Malnutrition Drugs
Palpitation	Arrhythmias Vasodilatation	Thyroid disease Drugs Perimenopausal Anxiety

Table 4.2 Differential diagnosis: pulmonary oedema *vs* asthma

Pulmonary oedema	Asthma
Severely breathless Dry cough White frothy sputum Sputum may be pink or blood flecked	Severely breathless Cough variable Sputum variable Sputum seldom pink or blood flecked
Patient wants to sit up	Patient restless, may want to sit up
Cyanosis, if severe	Cyanosis, if severe
Pale, cold, sweaty	May sweat if severe
Shallow, rapid breathing inspiration = expiration	Expiration phase > inspiration
Widespread crackles (creps) may be wheezing	Wheezing (not invariable)
Past history of heart disease	History of asthma

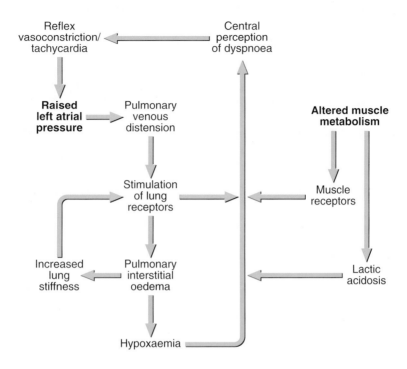

Fig. 4.1 Mechanisms of cardiac dyspnoea.

comfortable lying flat, and indeed may become un-conscious through hypotension if made to sit up.

Anxiety may manifest itself as breathlessness; acti-vation of the sympathetic nervous system alters aware-ness of breathing and, in an extreme form, anxiety may lead to *hyperventilation* (p. 27). A feeling of sudden breathlessness, particularly in crowded environments, may also occur as a menopausal symptom.

Pain

Types of cardiac pain are listed in Table 4.3.

Angina. Angina pectoris is a characteristic chest pain occurring on exertion and relieved by rest. It is the main symptom of *myocardial ischaemia*. By extension, angina is also used to describe any other pain caused by myocardial ischaemia, for example during coronary spasm. Angina, without qualification, implies angina of effort. Useful questions in eliciting a history of angina are:

- Do you ever feel tightness or discomfort in the chest?
- What brings on the discomfort?
- Do you get discomfort climbing stairs or hills?
- How much can you do before you have to stop?

- What do you do when you get the discomfort?
- What happens when you stop? How soon?
- Is there anything which makes you more likely to get the discomfort?
- Is it influenced by exercise after a meal?
- Is it influenced by cold weather?
- Do you ever get discomfort at rest? When?
- Is there anything which makes it better?

Table 4.3 Types of cardiac pain

Type	Cause	Characteristics
Angina	Coronary stenosis (rarely aortic stenosis, hypertrophic cardiomyopathy)	Precipitated by exertion, eased by rest Characteristic distribution (Fig. 4.4, p. 90)
Myocardial infarct	Coronary occlusion	Similar sites to angina, more severe, persists at rest
Pericarditic pain	Pericarditis	Sharp, raw or stabbing Varies with movement or breathing
Dissecting aneurysm	Dissecting aneurysm	Severe, sudden onset, felt first in back, persists at rest

Mechanism

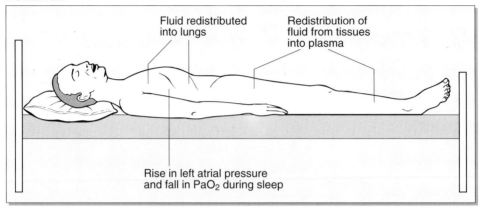

Features

Causes

- Ischaemic heart disease
- Aortic valve disease
- Hypertension
- Cardiomyopathy
- Atrial fibrillation
- Rarely in mitral disease or atrial tumours

Fig. 4.2 Paroxysmal nocturnal dyspnoea.

Site. The pain is characteristically retrosternal. In describing it the patient often places both hands on the chest with fingers meeting on the lower sternum, or presses a palm or a clenched fist there (Fig. 4.4).

Radiation. The pain of angina may radiate to either arm, hand or wrist, to the jaw (in which case it may be described as 'like toothache'), to the ear, to the back or to the epigastrium.

Character. The pain may be described as 'like a tight band round the chest', or a feeling of constriction or heaviness. Or it may be described as discomfort or 'wind'.

Severity and duration. Usually begins about the same place during a regular walk. Severity is usually enough to make the patient stop, or slow down. With rest, the pain disappears in 2–3 minutes. Sometimes patients get a 'second wind' and are able to increase exertion after 'warming up'.

Unstable or crescendo angina is the term used to describe angina of rapidly increasing severity. The pain may occur on minimal exertion or at rest. Without treatment it often culminates in myocardial infarction.

Aggravating factors. The single most characteristic feature of angina is that it is brought on by exertion and relieved by rest. Other factors which may exacerbate angina are listed in Table 4.4.

Relieving factors. Angina is characteristically relieved by rest; pain persisting for longer than a few minutes after stopping exertion is unlikely to be angina. It is also relieved by medication such as glyceryl trinitrate, but this is not specific: nitrates can also relieve oesophageal pain.

Causes	Mechanism	Manifestations

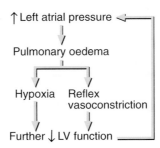

Causes

1. Acute left heart failure
   Myocardial infarct
   Mitral valve disease
   Aortic stenosis
   Arrhythmia
   Cardiomyopathy
   Overtransfusion

Mechanism

↑ Left atrial pressure

Pulmonary oedema

Hypoxia   Reflex vasoconstriction

Further ↓ LV function

Manifestations

Severe dyspnoea
Cough
Frothy white sputum (may be blood-flecked)
Shallow inspiration
Widespread lung crepitation
Usually reflex tachycardia and vasoconstriction

2. Rarely:
   Acid aspiration (Mendelsohn's syndrome)
   Toxic gases (e.g. phosgene)
   Adult Respiratory Distress syndrome

Failure of lung capillary permeability

As above; can be distinguished by normal left atrial pressure (Swann-Ganz catheter)

Fig. 4.3 Acute pulmonary oedema.

Table 4.4 Factors worsening or relieving angina

Worsening	Relieving
Physical exertion	Rest
Emotional exertion/excitement	Peace
Cold	Warm weather
Exercise after meal	'Warming up' before exercise

Associated phenomena. Angina is often accompanied by breathlessness and a feeling of 'wind' or belching.

The distinction between angina and other *cardiac* causes of pain is discussed below. The two commonest *non-cardiac* chest pains which can be mistaken for angina are musculoskeletal chest pain and oesophageal pain (Table 4.5).

Myocardial infarction. Myocardial infarction causes pain which is *similar* to angina in site, radiation and character, but *differs* in that it is not necessarily precipitated by exertion, it persists at rest, and it is usually much more severe (Table 4.6). However, painless, even asymptomatic, myocardial infarction is not uncommon, particularly in elderly patients and diabetics.

Pericarditic pain. Pericarditis causes pain which is retrosternal and may radiate to the shoulders or upper arm. It is accentuated by, or may only be present in, inspiration and also varies with posture (Table 4.7). It may be made worse by exertion but is not reliably relieved by rest. It is often described as a stabbing pain or a soreness.

Table 4.5 Differential diagnosis: angina *vs* oesophageal pain

Angina	Oesophageal pain
Usually precipitated by exertion	Can be worsened by exertion, but often present at other times
Rapidly relieved by rest	Not rapidly relieved by rest
Retrosternal and radiates to arm and jaw	Retrosternal and epigastric, sometimes radiates to arm
Seldom wakes patient from sleep	Often wakes patient from sleep
No relation to heartburn (but patients often have 'wind')	Sometimes related to heartburn
Relieved by nitrates	Often relieved by nitrates

Table 4.6 Differential diagnosis: angina *vs* myocardial infarction

Angina	Myocardial infarction
Site: retrosternal, radiates to arm, epigastrium, neck	As for angina
Precipitated by exercise or emotion	Often no obvious precipitant
Relieved by rest, nitrates	Not relieved by rest, nitrates
Mild/moderate severity	Usually severe (may be 'silent')
Anxiety absent or mild	Severe
No increased sympathetic activation	Increased sympathetic activity

Pericardial effusion may cause retrosternal chest pain at rest very similar to that of myocardial infarction.

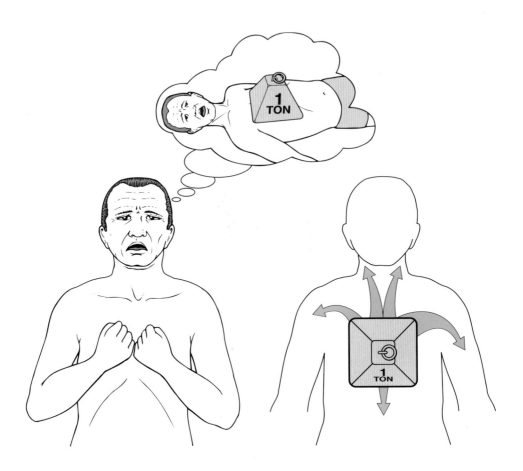

Fig. 4.4. Symptoms of angina.

Table 4.7 Characteristics of pericarditic pain

Site	Retrosternal, may radiate to left shoulder or back
Onset	No obvious initial precipitating factor; tends to fluctuate in intensity
Nature	May be stabbing or 'raw' – 'like sandpaper'. Often described as sharp, rarely as tight or heavy*
Made worse by	Changes in posture, respiration
Helped by	Analgesics
Accompanied by	Pericardial rub

* A feeling of retrosternal oppression may be a feature of a *pericardial effusion*.

Dissecting aneurysm. Dissecting aneurysm of the aorta causes pain that is usually of sudden onset. It is severe, often described as 'tearing' in nature, and is often felt initially in the back between the shoulder blades (Table 4.8).

Precordial catch. This is a characteristic sudden jab of pain at the cardiac apex; it is a common experience in normal subjects and is not a feature of organic heart disease.

Table 4.8 Characteristics of pain caused by dissecting aortic aneurysm

Site	Often first felt between shoulder blades, may be felt retrosternally, in neck or in abdomen
Onset	Usually sudden. May follow sudden twist or exertion
Nature	Severe pain, often described as 'tearing' in nature
Relieved by	Tends to persist. Patients often restless with pain
Accompanied by	Asymmetric pulses, unexpected bradycardia, early diastolic murmur, weakness in legs

Oedema

Oedema is tissue swelling as a consequence of excess extracellular fluid. *Pulmonary* oedema is a characteristic feature of acute left heart failure and presents with breathlessness (p. 88). Oedema is fully described on page 47. Oedema in the absence of other symptoms such as breathlessness is an *uncommon* presentation of heart failure.

Palpitation

Palpitation is an abnormal awareness of the heartbeat. It may be due to:

- a cardiac arrhythmia
- sudden vasodilatation, either as a consequence of perimenopausal vasomotor instability or following exposure to medications or solvent
- abnormal awareness of a normal heartbeat, for example in anxiety.

It is important to determine the exact nature of the palpitation by asking a series of questions:

- What do you mean by palpitation?
- Can you tap out on the table how your heart is beating when you have an attack? Please do so.
- Is it regular or irregular?
- How fast does it go?
- Have you noticed anything which sets off an attack?
- How long does an attack last?
- Do you get other symptoms with an attack?
- Do you ever get chest pain with an attack?
- Do you ever feel dizzy or black-out with an attack?

Asking the patient to 'tap out' the arrhythmia on the table is often helpful. Some characteristic descriptions of arrhythmias are given in Table 4.9.

Other symptoms

Symptoms which involve other systems may be rele-

Table 4.9 Descriptions of arrhythmias

Arrhythmia	Patient's description
Ventricular or atrial extrasystoles	'Heart misses a beat' Heart 'jumps' or 'flutters'
Atrial fibrillation	Heart 'jumping about' or 'racing' May be unnoticed
Supraventricular tachycardia	Heart racing or fluttering

Asystole, complete heart block and ventricular tachycardia often present as syncope rather than as palpitation

Table 4.10 Cardiac disease presenting with 'non-cardiac' symptoms

System	Symptom	Cause
Central nervous system	Syncope	Arrhythmia Hypotension Aortic stenosis
	Stroke	Embolism from heart Endocarditis Hypertension
Gastrointestinal	Abdominal pain Jaundice	Liver congestion secondary to heart failure
Renal	Oliguria	Heart failure

vant to cardiac disease. Some of these are listed in Table 4.10.

Undue tiredness may be a feature of ischaemic heart disease, (see p. 25) and the symptoms of infective endocarditis are often non-specific. They include weight loss, tiredness and night sweats.

Family history

Always ask whether there is any family history of heart disease. Apart from conditions which are thought to result from a single gene with dominant or recessive expression (Table 4.11), there is a familial element in many common cardiac conditions which is probably due to the interaction of several genes of weak effect (Table 4.12). Sometimes, it may be relevant that a parent died suddenly at a young age, even if the cause (e.g. hypertension, cardiomyopathy) was not recognised at the time. Remember that asking about family history may increase the patient's anxiety about their own health and that of their children. Once a diagnosis has been reached its genetic implications may need to be carefully explained.

Table 4.11 'Single-gene' cardiovascular diseases

- Marfan's syndrome
- Hypertrophic cardiomyopathy
- Polycystic kidney disease
- Holt–Oram syndrome
- Myotonic dystrophy
- Familial hypercholesterolaemia
- Ehlers–Danlos syndrome

Table 4.12 Cardiovascular diseases in which several genes may interact

- Ischaemic heart disease
- Hypertension
- Rheumatic heart disease
- Abdominal aortic aneurysm

Occupational history

Occupational illness affecting the heart is relatively uncommon, but it is important to take a full occupational history as this may influence management as well as diagnosis (Table 4.13).

Medication

A complete list of all medication, both prescribed and obtained 'over the counter' is essential (p. 16). Some important associations between medication and symptoms consistent with cardiac disease are listed in Table 4.14.

KEY POINTS

- Acute pulmonary oedema is not a feature of chronic left heart failure. It is usually due to acute left heart failure and very occasionally to another cause such as toxic gas inhalation.

- The diagnosis of angina is made from the history.

- The single most characteristic feature of angina is that it is brought on by exertion and relieved by rest.

- Crescendo, or unstable, angina may culminate in myocardial infarction and is an indication for urgent assessment.

- Ischaemic heart disease may present as unexplained tiredness; various cardiac conditions may present as neurological problems.

- The severity of symptoms often depends upon normal daily activity; hence the occupational history may exert a major influence on management.

- Left heart failure problems (e.g. aortic stenosis) may present as right heart failure because of reflex pulmonary vasoconstriction.

- It is important to ask patients to explain what they mean by palpitations; it is often helpful for the patient to 'tap out' the sensation on the table.

THE PHYSICAL EXAMINATION

The approach to physical examination will depend on the condition of the patient. Cardiovascular *triage* divides patients into

Table 4.13 Occupational aspects of heart disease

Occupational exposure associated with cardiovascular disease	
Organic solvents	Arrhythmias, Cardiomyopathy
Vibrating machine tools	Raynaud's phenomenon
Publicans	Alcoholic cardiomyopathy
Occupational exposure exacerbating pre-existing cardiac condition	
Cold exposure	Angina, Raynaud's disease
Deep-sea diving	Embolism through foramen ovale
Occupational requirements for high standards of cardiovascular fitness	
Pilots	
Public transport/heavy goods drivers	
Armed forces	
Police	

Table 4.14 Symptoms related to medication

Dyspnoea	Beta-blockers in patients with asthma
Exacerbation of heart failure by beta-blockers, calcium antagonists, non-steroidal anti-inflammatory agents
Pain	Oesophageal pain from medication (e.g. tetracyclines)
Oesophageal reflux exacerbated by nitrates, calcium antagonists
Oedema	Fluid retention from corticosteroids, non-steroidal anti-inflammatory agents
Oedema from calcium antagonists (e.g. nifedipine)
Palpitation	Tachycardia and/or arrhythmia from sympathomimetics (ephedrine), salbutamol, methylxanthines (aminophylline), digoxin toxicity, hypokalaemia from diuretics

- those with cardiac or respiratory arrest requiring resuscitation
- those who are severely ill and require immediate treatment
- those who are haemodynamically stable.

Characteristics of patients who are *severely ill and require immediate treatment* are summarised in Table 4.15. Assessment of such patients involves the following steps:

- Does the patient complain of pain? Where?
- Is a pulse palpable? (Use a large artery such as femoral or carotid to assess the pulse)
- Is the pulse inappropriately slow or excessively fast?
- Is there peripheral vasoconstriction?
- What is the blood pressure?

Table 4.15 Characteristics of patients with severe circulatory failure

Hypotension	Systolic blood pressure < 100 mmHg
Tachycardia	Pulse usually > 100/min
Peripheral vasoconstriction	Cold, pale or cyanosed peripheries
Reduced urine output	< 30 ml/h

- If the blood pressure is low, is there a possibility, considering the history, of major haemorrhage?
- Is the patient cyanosed?
- Does the patient have pulmonary oedema?
- Are there any heart murmurs?

Using this basic approach it is possible to narrow down the diagnostic options (Fig. 4.5) and enable investigations to be used efficiently.

For patients who are haemodynamically stable at the time of examination, it is important to have a scheme or routine of physical examination. An example is shown in Table 4.16. The emphasis given to different aspects of the examination will depend on the history.

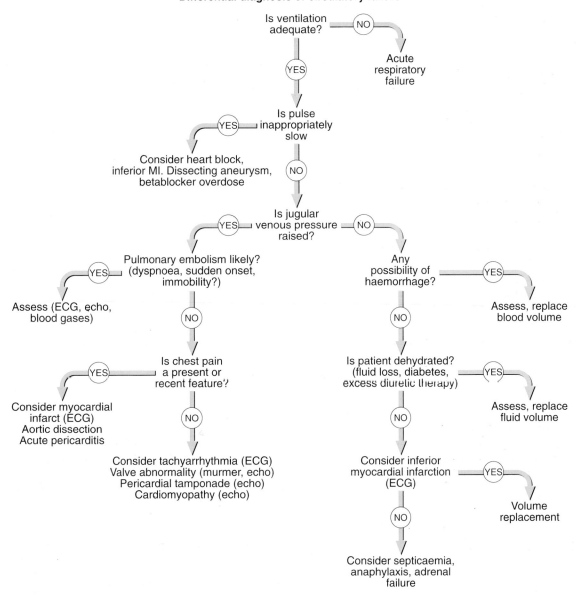

Differential diagnosis of circulatory failure

Fig. 4.5 **Flow chart for diagnosis in severe circulatory failure.**

Table 4.16 Scheme of cardiovascular examination

1. Get a general impression of the patient: look for cyanosis, signs of anxiety, excessive breathlessness
2. Shake hands: assess peripheral circulation (warmth), sweating, look for clubbing, splinter haemorrhages
3. Palpate radial pulse: measure rate, assess rhythm
4. Palpate brachial pulse: assess quality. Measure blood pressure
5. Palpate carotid pulse. Listen for bruits
6. Assess jugular venous pulse
7. Examine face: look for features of hypercholesterolaemia, examine tongue for cyanosis
8. Examine chest: assess cardiac impulse, locate apex beat
9. Auscultate the heart
10. Examine back of chest: listen for crepitations. Look for sacral oedema
11. Examine abdomen: palpate liver, look for renal enlargement or aortic aneurysm. Listen for renal bruits
12. Assess femoral pulses: look for radiofemoral delay
13. Examine legs: palpate pulses, assess oedema
14. Examine the optic fundi

Table 4.17 Facial abnormalities in cardiac disease

Features of hypercholesterolaemia
   Corneal arcus
   Xanthelasma

Transverse ear crease (associated with ischaemic heart disease)

Genetic syndromes
   Down's syndrome
   Marfan's syndrome
   Myotonic dystrophy
   Paget's disease
   Velo-facio-cardiac syndrome
   Leopard syndrome

Endocrine disease
   Acromegaly
   Hyperthyroidism
   Hypothyroidism
   Cushing's syndrome

The *general inspection* of patients has been discussed on page 41. Some of the features apparent on general inspection which are relevant to cardiac diagnosis include evidence of cyanosis (p. 141) or of tobacco or alcohol abuse (p. 16) and whether or not the patient appears comfortable, distressed or anxious.

THE HANDS

The hands may provide important signs to suggest cardiac disease. Nonspecific changes include vasodilation and sweating. Specific clues include finger clubbing (Table 5.6, p. 141), splinter haemorrhages (Fig. 3.9A p. 54), which may occur in infective endocarditis and xanthoma (palmar or tendon) which are a feature of hyperlipidaemia (p. 15).

Examination

❑ Shake hands with the patient.
❑ Note whether the hand is warm (vasodilation) or cold (vasoconstriction), and whether the palm is dry or moist (clammy hands may indicate anxiety or sympathetic activation).
❑ Look for tobacco staining.
❑ Examine the fingernails for clubbing and, if infective endocarditis is a possibility, for splinter haemorrhages.
❑ Look for swellings (xanthomas) in the extensor tendons of the fingers.

THE FACE

Many of the facial features of syndromes associated with cardiac disease are listed in Table 4.17.

Cyanosis is best appreciated by looking at the tongue and mucous membranes. *Central* cyanosis results when the oxygen saturation of arterial blood falls below 80–85%. It may be due to respiratory disease (p. 141). The commonest cardiac cause is pulmonary oedema, when it is invariably accompanied by dyspnoea. A less common cause is a 'right-to-left shunt', in which venous blood bypasses the lungs and is 'shunted' into the arterial circulation. Examples are listed in Table 4.18. Cyanosis due to an extrapulmonary right-to-left shunt is not corrected even by giving 100% oxygen to breathe. Very rarely, cyanosis is due to abnormal pigments, methaemoglobin or sulphaemoglobin in the blood. Features of the different kinds of cyanosis are summarised in Table 4.19.

There are three important clues to the possible existence of *ischaemic heart disease* which may be seen on examining the face (Fig. 4.6):

Table 4.18 Types of right-to-left shunt

At atrial level	Fetal shunt through foramen ovale
	Patent foramen ovale plus raised right-sided pressures (e.g. pulmonary embolism)
	Atrial septal defect plus pulmonary hypertension (more common with AV canal defects)
At ventricular level	Ventricular septal defect plus pulmonary stenosis (Fallot's tetralogy)
	Ventricular septal defect plus pulmonary hypertension (Eisenmenger's syndrome)
At pulmonary artery level	Fetal shunt through arterial duct
	Persistent arterial duct plus pulmonary hypertension
	Pulmonary arteriovenous fistula

Table 4.19 Types of cyanosis

1.	Peripheral	Hands and feet cyanosed, cold, poor circulation, pulses weak or impalpable, arterial PaO_2 normal
	Causes	Low cardiac output Peripheral vasoconstriction (Raynaud's phenomenon, ergot poisoning)
2.	Central cyanosis	Central mucous membranes cyanosed, arterial PaO_2 reduced

	Causes	a. Impaired pulmonary gas exchange (respiratory disease, pulmonary oedema)
		Giving oxygen improves saturation
		b. Right-to-left shunting
		  i. Intracardiac
		  ii. Intrapulmonary
		Giving oxygen has little effect

3.	Methaemoglobinaemia/ sulphaemoglobinaemia	From nitrites, sulphites, etc. Greyish pigmentation, PaO_2 normal, oxygen saturation reduced

- *Corneal arcus* is due to precipitation of cholesterol crystals at the periphery of the cornea. In young people it is strongly associated with hyper-cholesterolaemia, but the association gets weaker with increasing age.
- *Xanthelasma* is a yellowish eruption at the inner side of the eyelids, again strongly associated with hyper-cholesterolaemia in people under the age of 50.
- *Transverse ear crease.*

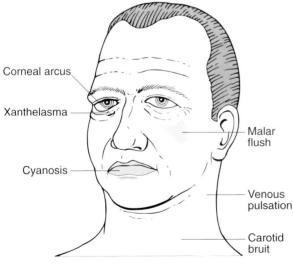

Corneal arcus

Xanthelasma

Cyanosis

Malar flush

Venous pulsation

Carotid bruit

Fig. 4.6 Facial clues to heart disease.

Dental or gum disease (or its treatment) may be responsible for infective endocarditis (p. 61). The optic fundi should be examined (p. 266) in patients with hypertension or in patients suspected of endocarditis.

THE PULSE

The radial pulse

The radial pulse is readily felt just lateral to the tendon of the flexor carpi radialis muscle (Fig. 4.7). It is useful for assessing the *rate* and *rhythm* of the pulse – pulse character is better assessed from larger arteries such as the brachial and carotid. The pulse rate in a normal healthy adult may vary from as low as 40 per minute while at rest, particularly in fit subjects, to 160 or even greater during exercise, or 80 to 200 per minute in a child. Causes of slow and fast pulse rates are shown in Table 4.20.

The normal rhythm of the heart is called sinus rhythm, because it is controlled from the sino-atrial node. Sinus rhythm is seldom completely regular, because the heart speeds up during inspiration and slows at the beginning of expiration. This *sinus arrhythmia* is most obvious in children, fit young people and athletes. Whenever an irregular or slow pulse is felt at the wrist, it is important to try to confirm the cause. Some common causes of an irregular pulse are listed in Table 4.21. One of the

Table 4.20 Causes of a slow and fast pulse

Fast heart rate (tachycardia, > 100/min)
Sinus tachycardia
  Exercise
  Emotional excitement/anxiety
  Fever
  Hyperthyroidism
  Medication
    Atropine
    Sympathomimetics
    Vasodilators
  Heart failure (compensation for impaired ventricular function)
Arrhythmias
  Atrial tachycardia
  Supraventricular tachycardia
  Atrial fibrillation
  Ventricular tachycardia

Slow heart rate (bradycardia, < 60/min)
  Sleep
  High vagal tone (athletes)
  Fainting reflex
  Carotid sinus overactivity
  Sick sinus syndrome
  Complete heart block
  Second degree heart block
  Medication (beta-blockers, calcium antagonists)

Note: *Apparent* bradycardia can be due to frequent extrasystoles.

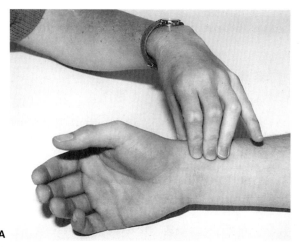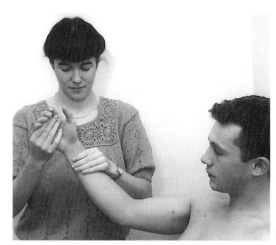

A   **B**

Fig. 4.7 The radial pulse.   **A.** Locating and palpating the radial pulse; **B.** Feeling for a collapsing radial pulse.

commonest is extrasystoles, or ectopic beats (Fig. 4.8A). The extra beat 'resets' the cardiac cycle; frequently the pulse wave produced by the ectopic beat is too weak to be felt at the wrist, and the impression is of a missed beat followed by an unusually powerful beat. Sometimes ectopic beats occur regularly after every normal beat (Fig. 4.8B) – this is called 'bigeminy' (from the Latin word for twins) and may give the impression of a very slow pulse.

A further common cause of an irregular pulse is *atrial fibrillation* (Fig. 4.8C). This is often described as an 'irregularly irregular' rhythm. Common causes are shown in Table 4.22. It is usually easy to distinguish from sinus rhythm plus ectopics when the pulse rate is fast, but harder when the pulse rate is relatively slow. When in doubt, record an electrocardiogram.

The brachial pulse (Fig. 4.9)

Because the brachial artery is larger than the radial artery, it is better for assessing pulse character: a large-volume pulse occurs in patients with vasodilatation or aortic reflux (p. 110), a small-volume pulse when the peripheral arteries are constricted, or the cardiac output is low. A pulse with two 'humps', called a bisferiens

Table 4.21 Causes of an irregular pulse

- Sinus arrhythmia
- Atrial extrasystoles
- Ventricular extrasystoles
- Atrial fibrillation
- Atrial tachycardia with variable response
- Second degree (Wenckebach) heart block

Table 4.22 Common causes of atrial fibrillation

- Ischaemic heart disease
- Alcohol-related heart disease
- Mitral valve disease
- Thyrotoxicosis
- Impaired ventricular function
- Anaesthetic agents
- Atrial septal defect
- Idiopathic

pulse, is sometimes felt at the elbow in patients with aortic stenosis and incompetence: its mechanism is controversial. Another reason for locating the brachial pulse at the elbow is to use it in measuring the blood pressure.

Examination

Radial pulse

- ❑ Apply three fingers over the radial pulse at the wrist (Fig. 4.7A).
- ❑ Use the pulp of the middle finger to assess the rate and rhythm.
- ❑ To feel for a collapsing pulse, raise the arm while feeling across the pulse with the fingers of the other hand (Fig. 4.7B).

Brachial pulse

- ❑ Use the thumb (right thumb for right arm and vice versa) with the fingers cupped round the back of the elbow (Fig. 4.9).
- ❑ Feel just medial to the tendon of the biceps muscle to detect the artery.

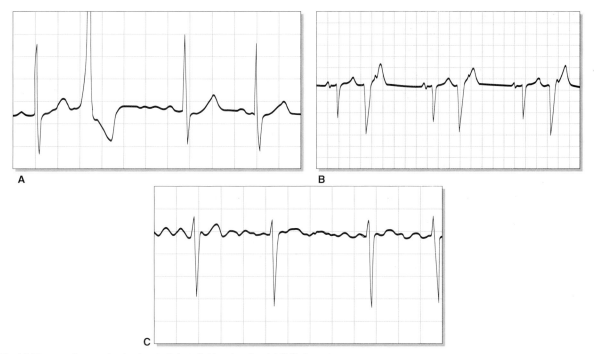

Fig. 4.8 Electrocardiogram showing A. ectopic beat, B. bigeminy, C. atrial fibrillation.

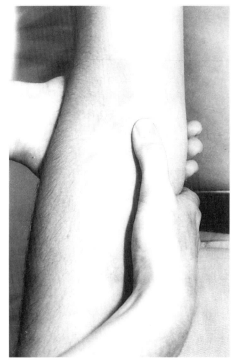

Fig. 4.9 Assessing the brachial pulse.

Measuring the blood pressure

Blood pressure is usually measured using a sphygmo-manometer cuff wrapped around the upper arm. This is shown in Figure 4.10. It is important to use the right size of cuff (Table 4.23).

Examination

- ❏ Support the arm comfortably at about heart level.
- ❏ Feel the brachial pulse or the pulse at the wrist with the fingers of one hand.
- ❏ Inflate the cuff till the pulse is impalpable. Note the pressure on the manometer. This is a rough estimate of systolic pressure.
- ❏ Now inflate the cuff another 10 mmHg, and apply the stethoscope over the brachial artery.

Table 4.23 Cuff sizes for blood pressure measurement

Neonate	5 cm
Child	5–7 cm
Normal adult	14–15 cm
Obese adult	20 cm
Thigh	20–25 cm

Note: The air bag within the cuff should extend for at least two-thirds of the circumference of the arm

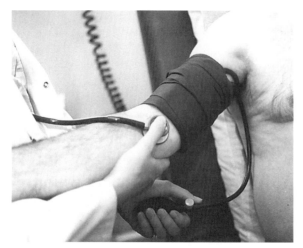

Fig. 4.10 Measuring the blood pressure.

❑ Deflate the cuff slowly until regular sounds (called the Korotkoff sounds, after their discoverer) can just be heard through the stethoscope. (If these were available on first listening, inflate the cuff till they disappear, then deflate it gradually.)

❑ Note the systolic pressure as accurately as possible.

❑ Continue to deflate the cuff slowly (about 1 mmHg per second). The sounds get louder, then suddenly become muffled, then disappear.

❑ Record the point at which the sounds just disappear as diastolic pressure (Fig. 4.11).

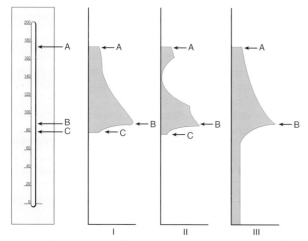

Fig. 4.11 Different patterns of the Korotkov sounds.   At A. sounds are first heard, B. sounds become muffled (phase 4) and C. sounds disappear (phase 5). I. is normal, II. show 'silent gap' phenomenon between systole and diastole, and in III. muffled sounds persist with no phase 5.

Blood pressure is usually recorded as systolic pressure/diastolic pressure: 145/92 means the systolic pressure was 145, the diastolic 92 mmHg.

Attention to detail is needed for accurate blood pressure measurement: a checklist is given in Table 4.24. Blood pressure varies with excitement, stress, and environment – repeated measurements are required before a patient should be identified as hypertensive. The population distributions of systolic and diastolic blood pressure are smooth and unimodal, and any 'definition' of high blood pressure is arbitrary. Table 4.25 shows the proportion of an adult population with diastolic blood pressures above a given value. If the blood pressure appears to be high, look specifically for possible causes and for evidence of 'end-organ' damage (Table 4.26).

The carotid pulse

The carotid pulse is the closest point to the heart at

Table 4.24 Checklist for blood pressure measurement

Patient	Relaxed
	Arm supported at heart level
	Clothing removed from arm
Cuff	Neatly applied
	Correct size for arm
	No leaks
Manometer	Well supported
	Upright
	If aneroid manometer, regularly calibrated
Operator	Check systolic pressure by palpation
	Release pressure slowly
	Avoid parallax error (eye same level as manometer)
	Avoid end-digit preference
	Use phase 5 as diastolic

Table 4.25 Proportions of an adult population with diastolic blood pressure greater than a given value

> 90 mmHg	25.3%
> 95 mmHg	14.5%
> 100 mmHg	8.4%
> 105 mmHg	4.7%
> 110 mmHg	2.9%
> 115 mmHg	1.4%

Data from HDFP Cooperative (*Circulation Research* 1977; 40: 1–106)
Notes:
1. Any 'cut-off point' between normal and hypertensive populations is arbitrary.
2. Life expectancy is progressively reduced with increasing blood pressure.
3. Risks of systolic and diastolic pressure increases are additive.
4. The older the patient, the more important the systolic pressure in predicting risk of cardiovascular disease (30% increase in risk per 10 mmHg rise in systolic pressure).

Table 4.26 End-organ damage in hypertension

Heart	Left ventricular hypertrophy
	Heart failure
	Increased risk of coronary atheroma, myocardial
	infarction
Eye	Hypertensive retinopathy (p. 267)
Kidney	Hypertensive nephropathy
Brain	Increased incidence of transient ischaemic attacks
	(TIAs) and stroke
	Hypertensive encephalopathy
	Subarachnoid haemorrhage
Great vessels	Aortic dilatation and aortic valve reflux
	Abdominal aortic aneurysm
	Dissecting aneurysm of the aorta

which the arterial pulse can easily be felt (Fig. 4.12). It gives more information about *pulse character* than other pulses. Abnormalities which can be detected in the carotid pulse are summarised in Figure 4.13. Although it has been common practice to feel for a collapsing pulse at the radial artery, this can give spurious results, especially in the elderly with a rigid arterial system. A more reliable method of detecting a collapsing pulse is by palpation of the carotid artery. Auscultation of the carotid arteries is described on page 207.

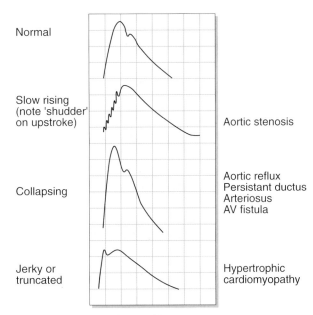

Fig. 4.13 Abnormalities of the carotid pulse.

Examination

- Always feel the carotid pulse with the patient lying on a bed or couch, as pressure on the carotid sinus can sometimes cause marked bradycardia and hypotension (carotid sinus syncope).
- Never compress both carotids simultaneously.
- Use the left thumb for right carotid, and vice versa.
- Place the tip of the thumb against the larynx.
- Press the thumb gently *backwards* to feel the pulse against the front of the cervical vertebrae (Fig. 4.12).

The jugular venous pulse

Just as the carotid pulse is the nearest to the 'output' side of the heart, the jugular venous pulse provides much information about the input side of the heart. There are no valves between the right atrium and the internal jugular vein. This lies deep to the sternal and clavicular heads of the sternomastoid. This muscle needs to be relaxed to examine the internal jugular pulsation clearly.

The internal jugular vein is more reliable than the external, because the latter is sometimes kinked or partially obstructed where it traverses the deep fascia in the neck. It is impossible to see jugular pulsation with a patient lying flat, because the vein is then completely distended. (Note that veins are pliable but inelastic, whereas arteries are elastic – the difference is

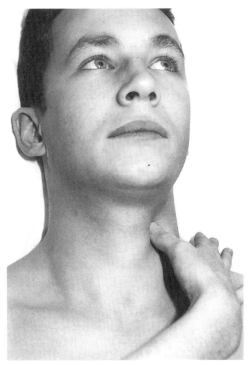

Fig. 4.12 Locating the carotid pulse.

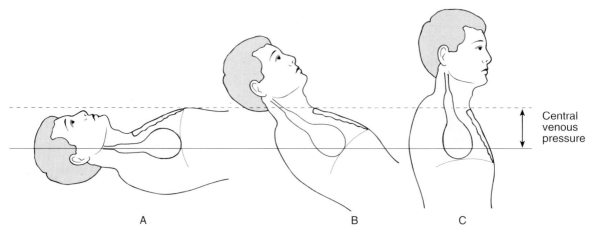

Fig. 4.14 Jugular venous pressure in a normal subject. A. Supine: jugular vein distended, pulsation not visible. **B.** Reclining at 45 degrees: point of transition between distended and collapsed vein can usually be seen to pulsate just above the clavicle. **C.** Upright: upper part of vein collapsed and transition points obscured by sternum.

like that between a paper bag and a balloon.) Conversely, when a normal subject sits or stands upright the pulsatile part of the internal jugular is hidden behind the clavicle and sternum. Indeed, if jugular venous pulsation can be seen with the patient sitting upright, then jugular venous pressure is raised. This is illustrated in Figure 4.14. If jugular venous pressure is very high, then the point of pulsation may be invisible (because it is within the skull!). Causes of a raised jugular venous pressure are given in Table 4.27. The

Table 4.27 Causes of a raised jugular venous pressure

Causes	Comment
Fluid overload	Overtransfusion
Primary or secondary right heart failure	Often with peripheral oedema
Pulmonary embolism	May be very high and missed in the supine patient
Pericardial tamponade	With prominent y descent
Constrictive pericarditis	Often very high, prominent y descent
Superior vena caval obstruction	Distended non-pulsatile

Table 4.28 Differences between carotid and jugular pulse

Carotid	Jugular
Usually felt rather than seen	Usually seen rather than felt
Most obvious movement outward	Most obvious movement inward
One peak per heartbeat	In sinus rhythm, two peaks per heartbeat
Independent of position	Varies with posture, breathing and abdominal pressure

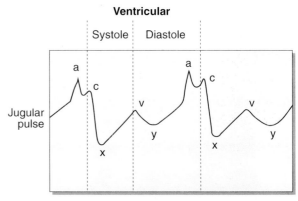

Fig. 4.15 Form of the venous pulse wave tracing from internal jugular vein: a = atrial systole; c = transmitted pulsation of carotid artery at onset of ventricular systole; v = peak pressure in right atrium immediately prior to opening of tricuspid valve: a – x = x descent, due to atrial relaxation; v – y = y descent at commencement of ventricular filling.

main points of difference between jugular venous and carotid arterial pulsation are shown in Table 4.28.

When the patient is in sinus rhythm, there are characteristically two peaks and troughs in the jugular waveform for every heartbeat (Fig. 4.15). Some abnormalities of the jugular waveform are shown in Table 4.29.

Examination

❏ Position the patient reclining supine at 45° (the usual examination position). Inspect from the side (Fig. 4.16).

Table 4.29 Common abnormalities in jugular venous pulsations

Condition	Features
Atrial fibrillation	Absent 'a' waves
Atrial flutter	'Flutter' waves replacing 'a' waves
Complete heart block	'Cannon waves'
Pulmonary stenosis	Often prominent 'a' waves
Chronic pulmonary hypertension	Often prominent 'a' waves
Tricuspid incompetence	Giant 'v' wave
Tricuspid stenosis	Slow *y* descent, and giant 'a' waves
Chronic constrictive pericarditis	Exaggerated *y* descent

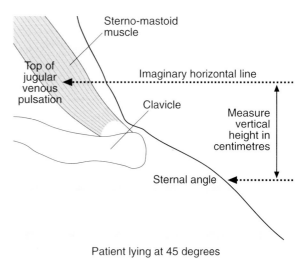

Patient lying at 45 degrees

Fig. 4.17 Measuring the height of the JVP.

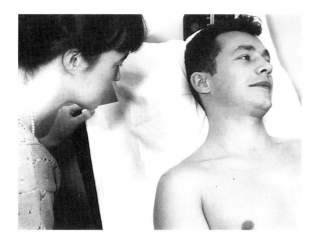

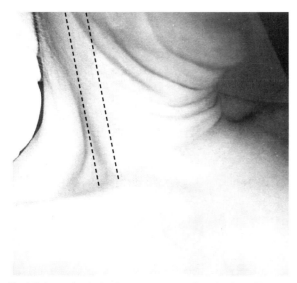

Fig. 4.16 Inspecting the jugular venous pressure from the side. (The dotted lines outline the course of the internal jugular vein lying deep to the sternomastoid muscle.)

❑ Identify the internal jugular pulsation.
❑ Measure the vertical height in centimetres between the mid-point of the venous pulsation and the sternal angle to give the venous pressure (Fig. 4.17).
❑ Now identify the waveforms of the pulsation and note any abnormality.

THE CHEST

Inspection

Much can be learnt by inspecting the praecordium. An 'active' heart may indicate ventricular dilatation from aortic or mitral regurgitation, or a shunt such as atrial septal defect. Features such as a double apex beat in hypertrophic cardiomyopathy or a diffuse apical impulse associated with anterior myocardial infarction are often easier seen than felt. Epigastric pulsation transmitted from the abdominal aorta is a normal finding, particularly in slim people.

Palpation

Palpation is important. The cardiac impulse, which can usually be felt over the left side of the chest, is the result of the heart rotating, moving forward and striking against the chest wall during systole. The *character* of the cardiac impulse is often more important than its precise position. Different types of cardiac impulse are listed in Table 4.30. The *apex beat* is defined as the further point outwards and downwards from the manubrium sterni at which the cardiac

Table 4.30 Abnormalities of the apex beat

Diffuse or dyskinetic	Post infarction; left ventricular aneurysm
Sustained or 'heaving'	Left ventricular hypertrophy
Double impulse	Hypertrophic cardiomyopathy
Hyperkinetic	Mitral reflux; shunts

Table 4.31 Lesions which cause thrills

Systolic thrills	*Diastolic thrills*
Aortic stenosis	Mitral stenosis
Ventricular septal defect	Tricuspid stenosis
Pulmonary stenosis	

impulse can be palpated. The normal apex beat lies in the fifth left intercostal space, within the mid-clavicular line.

Palpation of the chest may also reveal *thrills*, which are palpable vibrations in time with the cardiac cycle. Thrills are the palpable counterpart to murmurs. Any murmur may be associated with a thrill; the common lesions are listed in Table 4.31. The diastolic thrill of mitral stenosis is best felt at the apex with the patient rolled onto the left side. The thrill itself feels rather like placing one's hand on a purring cat; like murmurs, thrills can be timed against the carotid pulse. Thrills may also be present with aortic or pulmonary stenosis or a ventricular septal defect: these are often best felt by asking the patient to sit up, lean forward and exhale.

Auscultation of the heart

Use a good stethoscope and take care of it. The ear-pieces must fit comfortably; the tubing should be about 25 cm in length and thick enough to reduce external sound. The diaphragm of the stethoscope filters out low-pitched sounds and helps to identify high-pitched ones, such as the second heart sound. The bell is essential for listening to low-pitched sounds such as the murmur of mitral stenosis. It is helpful to *time* what is heard against the carotid pulse. Work out a routine for auscultation but be prepared to modify it to suit the particular patient. A knowledge of the surface anatomy of the heart is important (Fig. 4.18). However, the auscultating areas do not correspond with the surface markings of the heart valves. Some clinicians first auscultate at the base where the second heart sound is usually recognisably louder. Many others start at the apex.

It is usually easy to hear two sounds when auscultating a normal heart. They sound rather like 'lub-dup'. The 'lub' is the first heart sound. It coincides with the upstroke of the carotid pulse and it is caused by the closure of the mitral and tricuspid valves (Fig. 4.19). The 'dup' is a higher pitched sound, it comes after the peak of the pulse wave and is caused by closure of the aortic and pulmonary valves. Careful listening to the second heart sound, especially in older children or fit young adults, will reveal that it changes slightly in time with respiration: when the subject

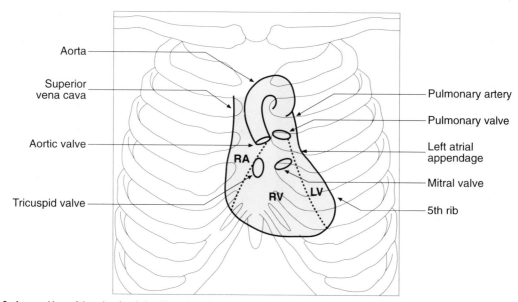

Fig. 4.18 Surface markings of the valves in relationship to the radiological outline of the heart. The directions in which murmurs are preferentially conducted from the valves are described in Table 4.41 on page 112.

breathes in, it becomes 'lub da-dup' and reverts to 'lub-dup'. when the subject exhales. This is called 'physiological splitting of the second heart sound'. This occurs because the intrathoracic pressure falls during inspiration and blood tends to pool in the pulmonary veins, thus reducing left ventricular filling. As a result the aortic valve closes earlier. During expiration ventricular filling equalises and the aortic and pulmonary valves close simultaneously (Fig. 4.19).

Examination

Inspection

❏ Ask the patient to lie semirecumbent with the shoulders horizontal.

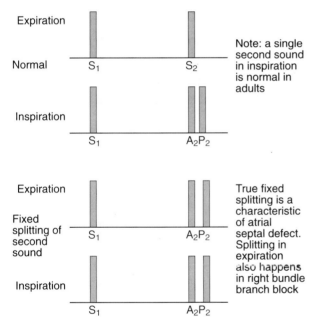

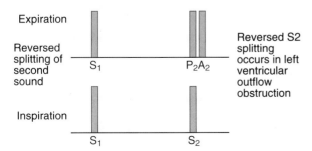

Fig. 4.19 The first and second heart sounds.

❏ Inspect the chest for skeletal abnormalities such as pectus excavatum or kyphoscoliosis.
❏ Look for and identify any pulsation.

Palpation

❏ Lay the whole hand flat on the chest to get a general impression of cardiac activity (Fig. 4.20A).
❏ Now localise the apex beat (Fig. 4.20B) and assess its character.
❏ If necessary, ask the patient to roll onto the left side (Fig. 4.20C).
❏ Identify any other pulsation particularly in the parasternal area (Fig. 4.20D).

Auscultation

❏ Auscultate all over the praecordium, listening in turn to the apex, upper and lower left sternal edge, the upper right sternal edge. If appropriate, also auscultate over the carotids and into the axilla.
❏ At each site identify the first and second heart sounds and assess the character with regard to intensity and splitting.
❏ Now listen to the interval between heart sounds for added sounds and murmurs.
❏ Roll the patient onto the left side and listen at the apex using the bell pressed lightly onto the skin to detect the murmur of mitral stenosis (Fig. 4.21A).
❏ Sit the patient up, leaning forward and listen with the diaphragm for the murmur of aortic incompetence and for pericardial friction (Fig. 4.21B).
❏ Note the features of any murmur heard.
❏ If a murmur is present, palpate again for an accompanying thrill with the patient leaning forward (Fig. 4.21C) and rolled onto the left side.

The heart sounds

The first heart sound. Abnormalities of the intensity of the first heart sound are listed in Table 4.32. A *loud* first heart sound is often heard when cardiac output is

Table 4.32 Abnormalities of intensity of the first heart sound

Quiet	Low cardiac output
	Poor left ventricular function
	Low filling pressure
Loud	Increased cardiac output
	Large stroke volume
	Mitral stenosis
	Atrial myxoma (rare)
Variable	Atrial fibrillation
	Extrasystoles
	Complete heart block

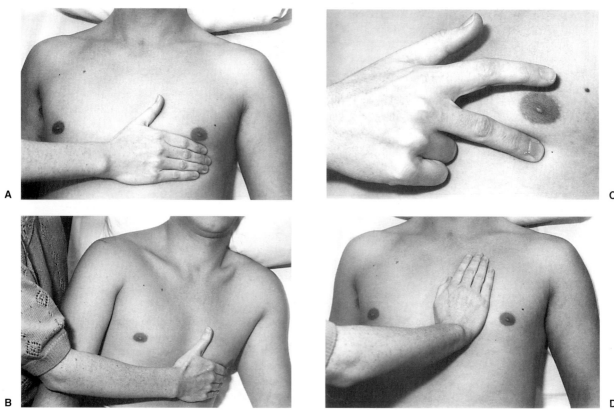

Fig. 4.20 Palpating the heart. **A.** Use the hand flat to palpate the cardiac impulse. **B.** If necessary, roll the patient into the left lateral position. **C.** Localise the apex beat with a finger. **D.** Palpate from apex to sternum for parasternal pulsations.

increased. The other important cause of an unusually loud first heart sound is *mitral stenosis*; the thickened mitral valve cusps form a diaphragm which is forced back towards the atrium when the ventricle contracts.

The second heart sound. Abnormalities of the second heart sound are listed in Table 4.33. They are best heard using the diaphragm of the stethoscope applied just to the left of the sternum in the third or fourth intercostal space. Splitting of the second heart sound which persists throughout the respiratory cycle is commonly due to right bundle branch block, which delays activation of the right ventricle and so delays the pulmonary component of the second sound. The splitting still gets wider in inspiration, though this can be hard to detect with a stethoscope. Wide *fixed* splitting of the second sound is a feature of atrial septal defect (Fig. 4.22) – splitting is wide because the right ventricle is dealing with a larger blood volume than the left, and it is fixed because the defect equalises pressure between the atria throughout the heart cycle.

Third heart sound. This is not heard in all subjects. It is a low-pitched sound (lub-dup-*dum*, lub-dup-*dum*) which comes after the second sound, (Fig. 4.23), and is

Table 4.33 Abnormalities of the second heart sound

Quiet	Low cardiac output
	Calcific aortic stenosis
	Extreme vasodilation
Loud	Systemic hypertension
	Pulmonary hypertension
	Corrected transposition of the great vessels
Split	1. Widens in inspiration (enhanced physiological splitting)
	Right bundle branch block
	Pulmonary stenosis
	Pulmonary hypertension
	Ventricular septal defects
	2. Fixed splitting (unaffected by respiration)
	Atrial septal defect
	3. Widens in expiration (reverse splitting)
	Left ventricular outflow obstruction
	Hypertrophic cardiomyopathy
	Left bundle branch block

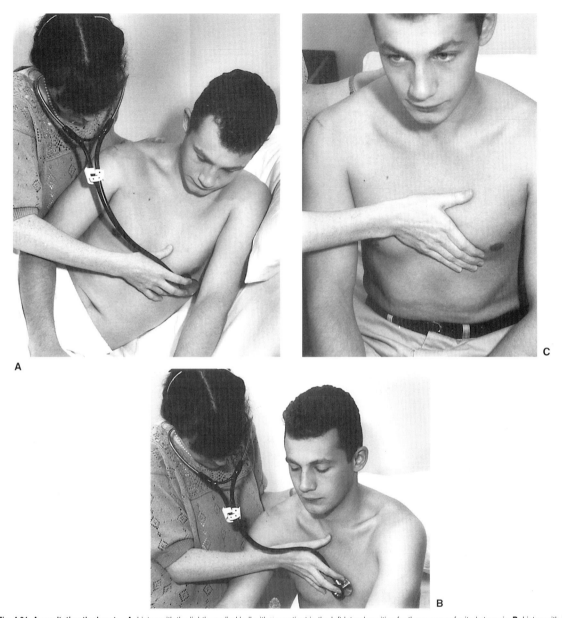

Fig. 4.21 Auscultating the heart.   A. Listen with the lightly applied bell with the patient in the left lateral position for the murmur of mitral stenosis. **B.** Listen with the diaphram with the patient tearing forward for the murmur of aortic incompetence. **C.** If there is a murmur at the base of the heart, feel for a thrill with the patient leaning forward.

best heard with the bell. It coincides with the initial passive filling of the ventricles. It is heard *physiologically* in children, healthy young adults, athletes and during pregnancy, when it is associated with a large stroke volume. It is heard *pathologically* in patients with a large, poorly contracting ventricle (for example dilated cardiomyopathy) or when ventricular stoke volume is increased as a result of a leaking heart valve (Table

4.34). A pathological third heart sound is often associated with a fast heartbeat and quiet first and second sounds; the resulting 'triple rhythm' is sometimes called a gallop rhythm because it is said to resemble the sound of a galloping horse.

Fourth heart sound.   The fourth heart sound is a soft, low-pitched sound which occurs just before the first sound (da-lub dup, da-lub dup). It is produced by a trial

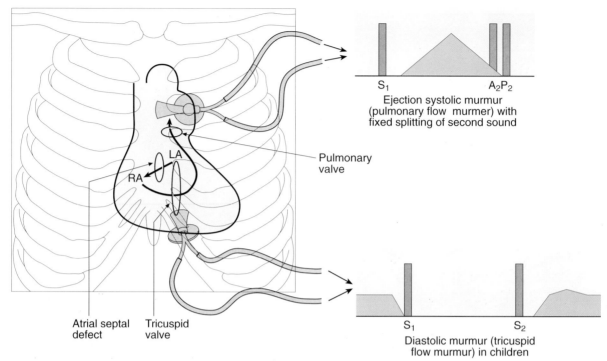

Fig. 4.22 Auscultatory features of atrial septal defect.

Table 4.34 Causes of a third heart sound

Physiological	Healthy young adults
	Athletes
	Pregnancy
	Fever
Pathological	Large, poorly contracting heart (cardiomyopathy)
	Mitral reflux, aortic reflux (large stroke volume)

contraction and does not occur in atrial fibrillation. It is the sound of rapid emptying of a hypertrophied atrium and really 'belongs' to the next beat (Fig. 4.23). It is associated with conditions such as hypertension and hypertrophic cardiomyopathy (Table 4.35). It is not heard in mitral stenosis because, although hypertrophied, the left atrium cannot eject blood rapidly through the narrowed mitral valve.

Auscultatory notation

A standard 'shorthand' notation for recording heart

Table 4.35 Causes of a fourth heart sound

- Systemic hypertension
- Hypertrophic cardiomyopathy
- Aortic stenosis
- Ischaemic heart disease

sounds, added sounds and murmurs has evolved from phonocardiography (a technique for recording the heart sounds graphically). Figure 4.24 shows a phonocardiogram recorded from a normal heart. The first and second heart sounds appear as vertical 'blips' on

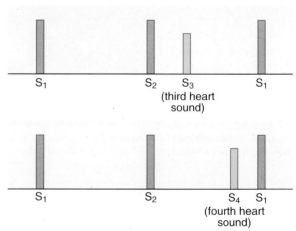

Fig. 4.23 Third and fourth heart sounds. The third sound coincides with the onset of ventricular filling, and the fourth sound with the ventricular filling which results from atrial contraction. The third and fourth sounds are heard at the cardiac apex when they arise in the left ventricle, and to the left of the lower sternum when their origin is in the right ventricle. (Diagrammatic representations of phonocardiograms.)

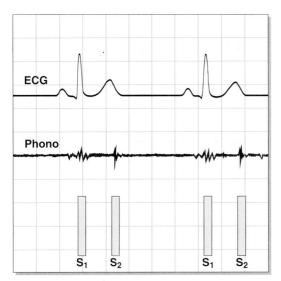

Fig. 4.24 Auscultatory notation. The relationship between a phonocardiogram (the graphic recording of the heart sounds) and the conventional 'shorthand' auscultatory notation.

either side of a baseline. The height of a 'blip' depends on the loudness of a sound, and the width on its duration. The conventional notation is simply a sketch of what might be seen on the phonocardiogram, using vertical lines or oblongs to represent sounds and shading to represent murmurs.

Murmurs

A heart *murmur* (Table 4.36) is a more or less musical sound made by turbulent blood flow in the heart. Murmurs are produced either by a normal volume of blood passing through an abnormal valve or by an increased volume of blood passing through a normal valve.

Timing. The first thing to decide about a murmur is whether it is *systolic* (occurs during ventricular systole) or *diastolic* (occurs during diastole). The safest way to do this is to *time* the murmur against the carotid. Murmurs which *accompany* the pulse are systolic, murmurs which *follow* the pulse are diastolic. With experience, common murmurs will be recognised with-

Table 4.36 Features of a murmur

- Timing
- Character
- Intensity
- Site
- Radiation
- Pitch

Table 4.37 Causes of systolic murmurs

Ejection systolic murmurs
Increased flow through normal valves:
  'Innocent systolic murmur'
    Fever
    Athletes (bradycardia → large stroke volume)
    Pregnancy (cardiac output maximum at 15 weeks)
  Atrial septal defect (pulmonary flow murmur)
  Aortic reflux (aortic flow murmur)

Normal or reduced flow through stenotic valve
  Aortic stenosis
  Pulmonary stenosis
  Hypertrophic obstructive cardiomyopathy
    (obstruction at subvalvar level)

Pansystolic murmurs
All caused by a systolic leak from a high to a lower pressure chamber
  Mitral reflux
  Tricuspid reflux
  Ventricular septal defect
  Leaking mitral or tricuspid prosthesis
  Mitral valve prolapse

out needing to time them, but experienced clinicians have been known to make mistakes!

Systolic murmurs. If a murmur is *systolic*, it is usually *either* an ejection murmur *or* a pansystolic murmur (Table 4.37).

Ejection systolic murmurs. These commence *after* the first heart sound. They increase in amplitude to a peak about mid-systole, and then become quiet towards the end of systole, stopping *before* the second heart sound. The crescendo–decrescendo cadence is a bit like the sound of a handsaw cutting wood. On a phonocardiogram trace the murmur is 'diamond shaped', and this is used as shorthand for recording the murmur.

Ejection systolic murmurs are due *either* to the ejection of a *normal* quantity of blood through a narrowed (stenosed) aortic or pulmonary valve *or* to the ejection of an *increased* volume of blood through a normal valve. For example, 'flow murmurs' occur during pregnancy, in fit athletes (in whom stroke volume may be further increased by resting brady-cardia) and in patients with an atrial septal defect, in whom increased flow at the pulmonary valve causes a murmur (Fig. 4.22). Ejection systolic murmurs (Fig. 4.25) which result from stenosed valves are usually harsher and higher pitched, and there are often other diagnostic clues (Fig. 4.26).

Pansystolic murmurs. These extend throughout systole, right up to, or indeed beyond, the second heart sound. The result is a 'blowing' or 'tearing' sound. The phonocardiogram shows a relatively constant amplitude throughout systole (there is usually a slight accentuation in mid systole) (Fig. 4.27).

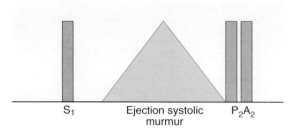

Fig. 4.25 Ejection systolic murmur (aortic stenosis). The aortic element of the second heart sound is delayed and a reversed splitting of the second heart sound may result.

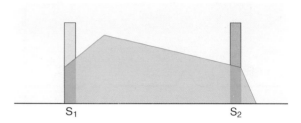

Fig. 4.27 Pansystolic murmur.

Pansystolic murmurs are caused

- by leakage (regurgitation) through the mitral (Fig. 4.28) or tricuspid valves
- by a congenital or acquired ventricular septal defect.

Late systolic murmurs are variants of pansystolic murmurs in which the murmur does not start immediately after the first heart sound, but starts later in systole. This is common in *mitral valve prolapse*, in which the valve is competent in early systole, but pro-

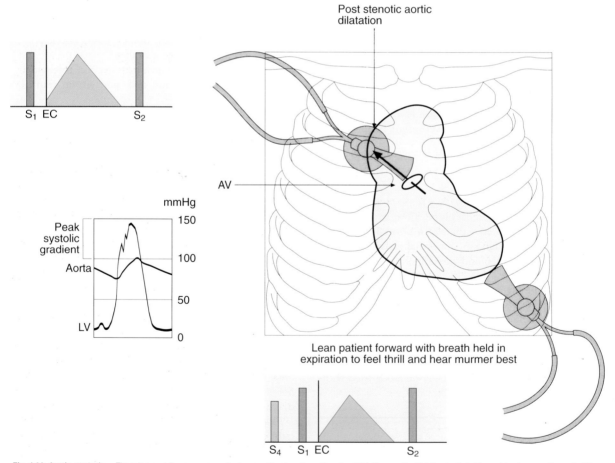

Fig. 4.26 Aortic stenosis. There is a systolic pressure gradient across the stenotic aortic valve (AV). The resultant high velocity jet (arrow) impinges on the wall of the aorta and the diaphragm placed near to this on the chest detects the murmur best. Alternatively the bell may be placed in the suprasternal notch. The diagrammatic representation of phonocardiogram show the ejection systolic murmur preceded by an ejection sound (EC). A fourth heart sound may be heard at the apex.

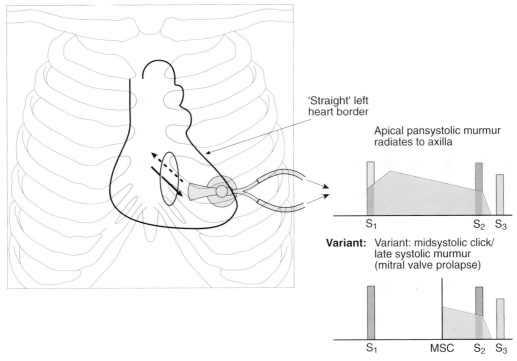

'Straight' left
heart border

Apical pansystolic murmur
radiates to axilla

S_1 S_2 S_3

Variant: Variant: midsystolic click/
late systolic murmur
(mitral valve prolapse)

S_1 MSC S_2 S_3

Fig. 4.28 Features of mitral regurgitation.

lapses into the atrium and becomes incompetent as systole continues (Fig. 4.28).

Innocent systolic murmurs. Soft systolic murmurs can be heard in many people who have no cardiac abnormality detectable by echocardiography, and who have no cardiac symptoms. It is important not to label such people as having a cardiac problem. The characteristics of innocent systolic murmurs are summarised in Table 4.38.

Diastolic murmurs. Diastolic murmurs can be divided into early diastolic murmurs, mid-diastolic murmurs and presystolic murmurs.

Early diastolic murmurs. These are usually due to aortic or pulmonary valve regurgitation. The murmur starts immediately after the second heart sound, and becomes quieter as diastole proceeds ('decrescendo murmur'). It often sounds like a whispered letter 'r'.

Aortic regurgitation is the most important cause of an early diastolic murmur, which is usually best heard

Table 4.38 Features of innocent systolic murmurs

- Systolic
- Soft (≤ 2/6)
- Upper sternal edge
- Normal splitting of second sound
- Normal pulses

along the left sternal border. As the murmur is high pitched, it is best heard with the diaphragm while the patient sits up, leans forward (Fig. 4.21B) and breathes out fully. The murmur radiates in the direction of the regurgitant blood flow. The commonest reason for failing to hear it is to apply the stethoscope too high (Fig. 4.29).

Pulmonary regurgitation is relatively uncommon. An early diastolic murmur originating from the *pulmonary* valve is sometimes heard in patients with pulmonary hypertension (and may be called a 'Graham Steell' murmur), or after a pulmonary valvotomy.

Mid-diastolic murmurs. These are best exemplified by the murmur of mitral stenosis (Fig. 4.30).

Mitral stenosis. The murmur starts just after the second heart sound; it is often preceded by an 'opening snap', which is a sound made by the rigid mitral valve as it moves forwards towards the apex of the left ventricle. The opening snap is high pitched; it sounds rather like the second component of a widely split second heart sound. An opening snap will not be audible if the valve is heavily calcified. The murmur of mitral stenosis is low pitched and rumbling, and best heard with the bell of the stethoscope (Fig. 4.31) and with the patient rolled onto the left-hand side

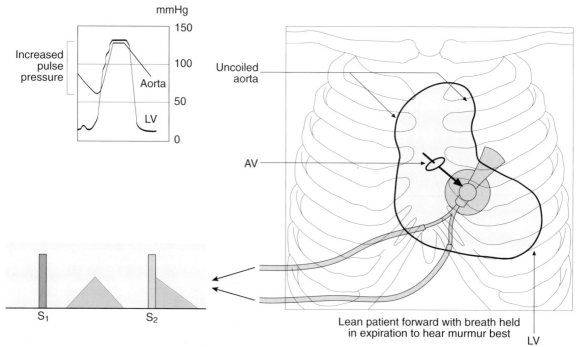

Fig. 4.29 Features of aortic regurgitation.   The pulse pressure is usually increased; the jet from the aortic valve (AV) impinges on the interventricular septum (arrow) during diastole, producing a high pitched murmur which is best heard with the diaphragm. The diagrammatic representation of phonocardiogram also shows the systolic murmur which is common because of the increased flow through the aortic valve in systole.

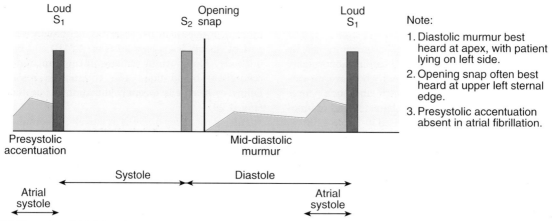

Fig. 4.30 The murmur of mitral stenosis.

(Fig. 4.21A). The area over which it can be heard is often restricted to the cardiac apex. The whole cadence sounds like 'lup-ta-ta-rou', where 'lup' is the loud first sound, 'ta-ta' the second sound and opening snap and 'rou' the rumbling mid-diastolic murmur. Presystolic accentuation occurs if the patient is in sinus rhythm because of the increase in blood flow produced by atrial contraction. It follows that there is no presystolic accentuation if the patient has atrial fibrillation. Sometimes the murmur only becomes audible if the patient's cardiac output is increased by exercise.

An Austin Flint murmur is a mid-diastolic murmur. It is not associated with an opening snap, presystolic accentuation or a loud first heart sound. It occurs in patients with aortic reflux, and it is due to vibration of

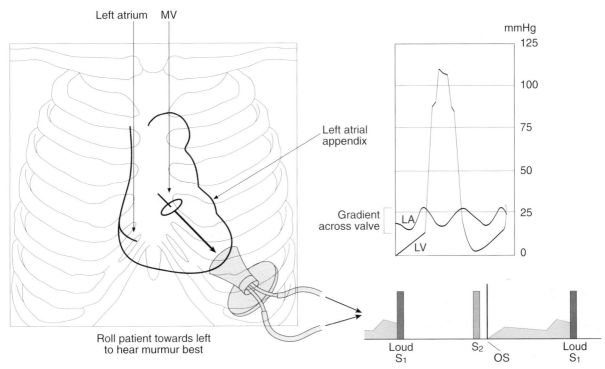

Left atrium   MV

Left atrial appendix

mmHg
125
100
75
50
25
0

Gradient across valve

LA

LV

Roll patient towards left to hear murmur best

Loud S₁   S₂   Loud S₁
                 OS

Fig. 4.31 Features of mitral stenosis. There is a pressure gradient across the mitral valve; in this example it continues throughout diastole. This causes a sharp movement of the tethered anterior cusp of the mitral valve at the time when flow commences and the opening snap (OS) results. The jet through the stenotic valve (arrow) strikes the endocardium at the cardiac apex. The murmur which results is best heard with the bell lightly applied there.

the anterior mitral valve cusp in the turbulence of the regurgitant bloodstream.

Tricuspid stenosis is rare: it produces a murmur similar in timing to mitral stenosis but higher pitched, and best heard to the left of the lower sternum. There is also a characteristic abnormality of the jugular venous pulse (Table 4.29).

Continuous murmurs. A continuous murmur is one which bridges systole and diastole. The most important cause is a *persistent arterial duct* (persistent ductus arteriosus). This connects aorta and pulmonary artery, and normally closes just after birth. A persistent arterial duct causes a continuous murmur usually loudest in the second left intercostal space (Fig. 4.32). In infants it may be accompanied by other features of a systemic arteriovenous fistula (Table 4.39), but in older children or adults these are usually absent.

A venous hum may be heard, usually in children, as a continuous roaring noise above either clavicle. It is loudest when the child is sitting up, and usually disappears when the child is laid head-down. It is of no pathological significance.

Intensity of murmurs. This is often described in terms of 'grades' (Table 4.40). It is common to use six grades

to describe systolic murmurs, but diastolic murmurs are only exceptionally louder than grade 4.

Changes in intensity are often of prognostic significance. For example, an increase in the intensity of an aortic early diastolic murmur implies increasing valvular

Table 4.39 Features of an arteriovenous fistula

- Hyperdynamic circulation
- Large-volume pulses (including dorsalis pedis in infants)
- Third heart sound and possible 'flow' ejection murmur
- Continuous murmur over fistula
- May cause heart failure

Table 4.40 Grades of intensity of murmurs

1. Heard by an expert in optimum conditions
2. Heard by a non-expert in optimum conditions
3. Easily heard; no thrill
4. A loud murmur, with a thrill
5. Very loud, often heard over wide area, with thrill
6. Extremely loud, heard without stethoscope

Optimum conditions require the room to be quiet, the patient to be properly positioned and the clinician to listen with the correct part of the stethoscope over the correct site

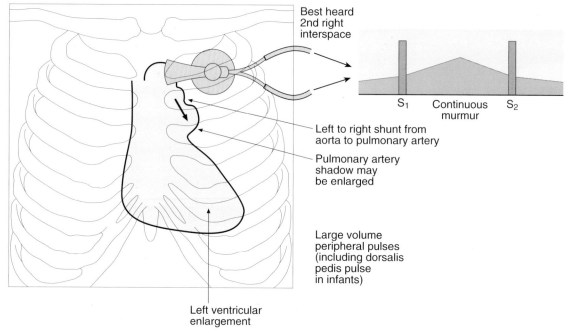

Best heard
2nd right
interspace

S_1 Continuous
murmur S_2

Left to right shunt from
aorta to pulmonary artery

Pulmonary artery
shadow may
be enlarged

Large volume
peripheral pulses
(including dorsalis
pedis pulse
in infants)

Left ventricular
enlargement

Fig. 4.32 Features of a persistent arterial duct.

incompetence. However, a reduction in intensity may also indicate deterioration, the fall in intensity being associated with reversal of flow in a right-to-left shunt or a fall in cardiac output, as in critical aortic stenosis.

The site and radiation of murmurs. As a general rule, murmurs are heard over the lesion causing them, and radiate in the direction of the turbulent blood flow. Surface markings of the heart valves are shown in Figure 4.18, and the radiation of murmurs is described in Table 4.41.

Pitch of murmur. As a principle, the higher the pitch the greater the pressure gradient. Thus the murmur of aortic incompetence is high pitched and best heard with the diaphragm, whereas that of mitral stenosis is low pitched and best identified using the bell.

Table 4.41 Radiation of murmurs

General rule: Murmurs radiate in the direction of the blood flow causing the murmur

Aortic stenosis	To upper right sternal edge and neck
Aortic reflux	Down left sternal border and towards apex
Mitral stenosis	To apex (very localised)
Pulmonary stenosis	To upper left sternal border, beneath left clavicle and to back
Pulmonary reflux	Down left sternal border
Tricuspid stenosis	Lower left sternal border (localised)
Tricuspid reflux	Lower left and right sternal border and epigastrium
Ventricular septal defect	Lower sternal edge

Added sounds

Added sounds is a term used to describe a variety of sounds distinct from murmurs and the four heart sounds. These are summarised in Figure 4.33. They include valve opening sounds, mid-systolic clicks as in mitral valve prolapse (Fig. 4.28), the sounds of artificial heart valves and pericardial rubs.

Normal heart valves open silently, but the thickened valve in mitral stenosis produces an opening snap as described above. Thickened aortic and pulmonary valves also produce an opening sound, which occurs immediately after the first sound, before any ejection murmur, and is called an *ejection click*. Ejection clicks are sometimes heard when the valve is normal but the ascending aorta or pulmonary artery is abnormally dilated.

Prosthetic heart valves usually have a quiet opening sound and a louder closing sound. A *mitral* prosthesis has an opening sound which corresponds to the opening snap and a closing sound which corresponds to the first heart sound. An *aortic* prosthesis opens with a sound corresponding to an ejection click, and closes with a sound which coincides with the second heart sound.

A *pericardial rub* is the characteristic physical sign of acute pericarditis (Table 4.42). It is generally best heard to the left of the lower sternum with the patient

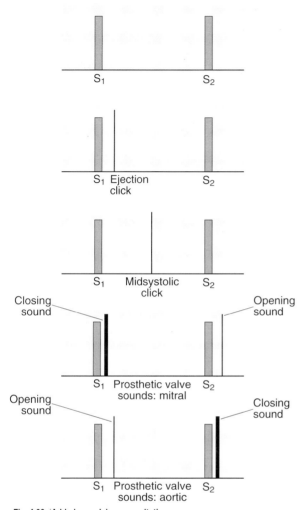

Fig. 4.33 'Added sounds' on auscultation.

Table 4.42 Features of pericardial disease

Acute pericarditis	Pericardial pain
	Pericardial friction rub
Pericardial effusion	Retrosternal 'oppressive' feeling
	Raised JVP
	Rub variable or absent
Pericardial tamponade (pericardial effusion under pressure)	Raised JVP
	Hypotension
	Paradoxical pulse (pulse volume smaller on inspiration)
	Postural hypotension
	Oliguria
Chronic constrictive pericarditis	Exertional dyspnoea
	Peripheral oedema
	Raised JVP with exaggerated *x* descent
	JVP rises on inspiration (Kussmaul's sign)

breathing out, using the diaphragm of the stethoscope. It sounds like friction between rough surfaces, often has two or three components ('chi-cha-cha, chi-cha-cha'), and seems near to the stethoscope. Like the pain of pericarditis, it may vary from hour to hour in intensity and its intensity may alter with the position of the patient.

KEY POINTS

- The approach to physical examination will depend upon the condition of the patient.

- When measuring the blood pressure, it is important to use the correct size of cuff.

- Never palpate both carotids simultaneously.

- Pulsatile elevation of the internal jugular venous pressure is a reliable sign of right heart failure or fluid overload.

- Roll the patient onto the left lateral position and use the bell while auscultating for the murmur of mitral stenosis.

- Sit the patient upright and use the diaphragm while listening for the murmur of aortic incompetence.

- Murmurs are produced either by a normal volume of blood passing through an abnormal valve or by an increased volume of blood passing through a normal valve.

- Systolic murmurs extending up to or beyond the second heart sound must be regurgitant in nature.

- Murmurs radiate in the direction of the blood flow.

- Change in the intensity of a murmur may be of considerable prognostic significance.

- The fourth heart sound is pathological. It is the sound of rapid emptying of a hypertrophied atrium.

Respiratory and abdominal signs

The detailed examination of chest and abdomen are described on pages 141–157 and 170–183.

The *pattern of breathing* is frequently altered in patients with cardiac problems (see p. 26). Pulmonary congestion leads to increased lung stiffness and hence to rapid shallow breathing with a short inspiratory phase and rapid expiration. Patients with severe heart failure may have periodic (Cheyne–Stokes) breathing. Patients

Table 4.43 Cor pulmonale

Definition	Heart failure secondary to chronic lung disease
Causes	Chronic respiratory failure Emphysema Cystic fibrosis
Mechanisms	Increased pulmonary vascular resistance Pulmonary vasoconstriction Right and left ventricular failure from hypoxaemia
Features	Fluid retention (often massive) Effort dyspnoea Raised JVP Right ventricular hypertrophy (right parasternal heave) Central cyanosis common

Table 4.44 Congenital valve lesions

Aortic stenosis	Common, may present with heart failure. May be associated with coarctation
Bicuspid aortic valve	May present as aortic reflux or aortic systolic murmur in late childhood or early adult life. Aortic valve replacement may eventually be needed. Common (1:120)
Aortic reflux	Rare as isolated lesion
Mitral reflux	Rare as isolated lesion. May be part of atrioventricular canal defect
Mitral stenosis	Relatively rare
Pulmonary stenosis	Fairly common, either as isolated defect or with ventricular septal defect and overriding aorta (tetralogy of Fallot)

with pulmonary disease may have secondary cardiac problems. These are largely the result of pulmonary hypertension and the condition is called 'cor pulmonale' (Table 4.43).

Crepitations at the lung bases which persist after the patient has been asked to take a deep breath or to cough may occur in early pulmonary oedema. As pulmonary oedema becomes more severe the crepitations become more extensive, and eventually can be heard all over the chest. Lung crepitations are seldom the only evidence of left heart failure. In the absence of other features of heart failure, they are usually caused by pulmonary disease such as interstitial fibrosis (see p. 155).

Pleural effusions are a feature of severe heart failure, usually accompanied by lung crepitations and ankle oedema. They may be unilateral or bilateral, and their position may vary with the posture in which the patient has been lying.

In the abdomen, hepatic enlargement may be due to venous congestion resulting from cardiac failure: if so, the jugular venous pressure will also be elevated. Expansile pulsation of the liver is a feature of tricuspid regurgitation. Abdominal palpation may also reveal an aortic aneurysm. In patients with hypertension, there is a need to palpate for *polycystic kidneys* and adrenal masses, and to auscultate for *renal bruits*.

Congenital heart disease

The examination of the cardiovascular system in neonates, infants and children is described in Chapter 10 (p. 336). It is increasingly common to encounter adults with congenital heart disease, either in its original form, or modified by surgery. Such patients can be divided into those with valve lesions, aortic abnormalities, shunts or complex abnormalities.

Valve lesions. Congenital valve lesions are listed in Table 4.44. Their clinical features are usually similar to those of acquired valve lesions already discussed. If possible, valve replacement surgery is avoided until the patient is large enough for an adult-sized valve. Until then the valvotomy or balloon valvuloplasty is preferred either as a definitive or palliative procedure.

Aortic abnormalities. The commonest aortic abnormality is coarctation of the aorta (Fig. 4.34). The

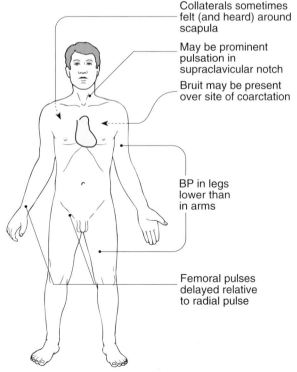

Collaterals sometimes felt (and heard) around scapula

May be prominent pulsation in supraclavicular notch

Bruit may be present over site of coarctation

BP in legs lower than in arms

Femoral pulses delayed relative to radial pulse

Fig. 4.34 Coarctation of the aorta.

characteristic features are the femoral pulses, which are weak and delayed in timing when compared with the radial pulses, and a lower blood pressure in the legs than the arms. There may be exaggerated carotid pulsation, and sometimes dilated collateral vessels can be felt and heard over the chest wall and around the scapulae. The commonest site for coarctation is just distal to the left subclavian artery, and a systolic or continuous bruit is often audible just medial to the left scapula. There is an association between aortic coarctation and a bicuspid aortic valve or congenital aortic stenosis.

Shunts. A 'shunt' is an abnormal communication between the left side and the right side of the heart, or between the aorta and pulmonary artery. Shunts can be classified into left to right and right to left, and further classified according to the level of the communication.

The commonest *left-to-right shunts* are atrial septal defect, ventricular septal defect and persistent ductus arteriosus (Table 4.45). Patients with left-to-right shunts are not cyanosed, tend to have a hyperdynamic cardiac impulse and may develop heart failure. There are two principal varieties of atrial septal defect. The more common is called a 'secundum-type' defect and

Table 4.45 Left-to-right intracardiac shunts

Atrial level	
Atrial septal defect	Secundum type
	Primum type (atrioventricular canal defect)
Ventricular level	
Ventricular septal defect	Inflow septum
	Outflow septum
	Muscular
Great vessel level	Persistent arterial duct

involves only the atrial septum. The less common variety is called a 'septum primum type', or more correctly an atrioventricular canal defect. It is more common in patients with Down's syndrome. The defect involves not only the atrial septum but also the mitral valve, which is malpositioned and sometimes incompetent. Unlike secundum-type atrial septum defects, atrioventricular canal defects and other large left-to-right shunts in children often lead to the development of Eisenmenger's syndrome.

Pressures on the left side of the heart are normally higher than on the right side, so for right-to-left shunting to occur there must either be obstruction of

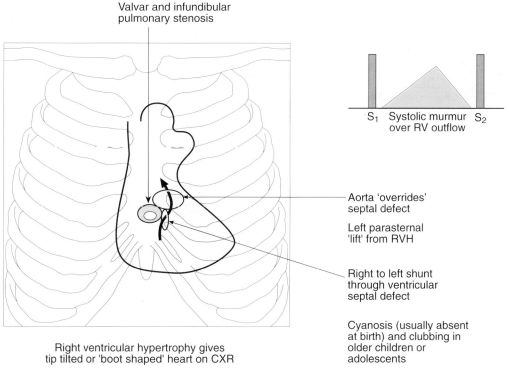

Fig. 4.35 Features of the Tetralogy of Fallot.

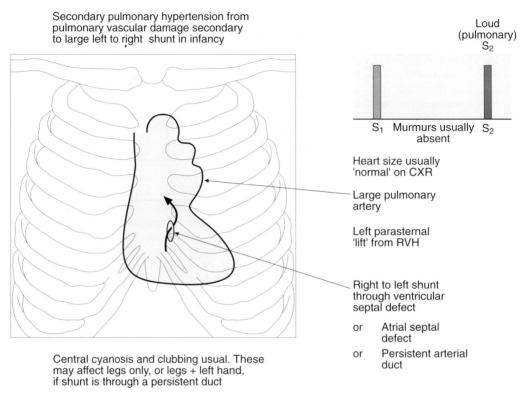

Secondary pulmonary hypertension from pulmonary vascular damage secondary to large left to right shunt in infancy

Loud (pulmonary) S₂

S₁   Murmurs usually absent   S₂

Heart size usually 'normal' on CXR

Large pulmonary artery

Left parasternal 'lift' from RVH

Right to left shunt through ventricular septal defect

or   Atrial septal defect

or   Persistent arterial duct

Central cyanosis and clubbing usual. These may affect legs only, or legs + left hand, if shunt is through a persistent duct

Fig. 4.36 Features of Eisenmenger's syndrome.

right ventricular outflow, as in the *tetralogy of Fallot* (Fig. 4.35) or severe pulmonary hypertension.

Large left-to-right shunts in infancy will produce severe pulmonary hypertension. This may subsequently result in 'reversal' of the shunt, with right-to-left shunting, so-called Eisenmenger's syndrome (Fig. 4.36).

Patients with right-to-left shunts are centrally cyanosed, and the cyanosis is not fully corrected with oxygen. Finger clubbing is common.

Complex abnormalities. Complex congenital heart lesions are made up of different combinations of shunts and valve lesions. They are often incompatible with long-term survival unless corrected surgically, but increasing numbers of patients with corrected congenital heart defects are now reaching adulthood.

Patients who have had cardiac surgery

Approximately 300 people per million of the population undergo cardiac surgery per year in the United Kingdom, and the proportion is higher in some other countries. About 75% of the operations are for coronary artery disease and 20% for valve replacement. The majority of heart operations are performed through a

median sternotomy incision. Patients who have had saphenous vein used for coronary bypass grafts will also have scars on their legs. Replacement heart valves are usually *prosthetic valves* made of metal, plastic or

KEY POINTS

- 'Cor pulmonale' is a phrase used to describe patients with primary pulmonary disease who develop a secondary cardiac problem.

- Lung crepitations are seldom the only evidence of left heart failure.

- Expansile pulsation of the liver is a feature of tricuspid regurgitation.

- The commonest left-to-right shunts are atrial septal defect, ventricular septal defect and a persistent arterial duct.

- It is increasingly common to find adults with congenital heart disease which has been modified by surgery.

- Murmurs are usually absent in patients with Eisenmenger's syndrome.

carbon fibre, and have a distinctive clicking sound (Fig. 4.33). Sometimes 'tissue valves' – usually preserved animal valves – are used, and these give normal heart sounds. If a patient with a replacement heart valve suddenly develops heart failure and the usual 'clicks' are inaudible, it must be assumed that the valve has become stuck or detached and the patient must be sent to a cardiac surgical unit with the utmost urgency.

FURTHER INVESTIGATIONS

The standard aids to clinical diagnosis are electrocardiography, radiography and ultrasound. These can be supplemented with radionuclide studies and cardiac catheterisation. This section briefly describes how best to integrate these techniques with the clinical examination.

Electrocardiography

The standard resting electrocardiogram is recorded

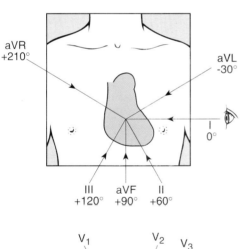

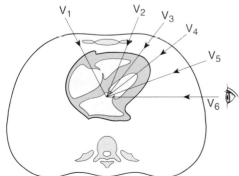

Fig. 4.37 Electrocardiography.   Diagram to show the directions from which the 12 standard leads 'look at' the heart. The transverse section is viewed from below like a CT scan.

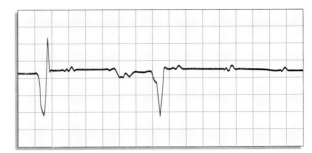

Fig. 4.38 ECG showing complete heart block.   There are regular 'p' waves and only occasional ventricular complexes.

using 12 'leads'. Each lead is a set of electrode positions which 'looks' at the heart from a particular direction (Fig. 4.37).

Arrhythmias. If the patient has an abnormal heart rhythm at the time of examination, the diagnosis can usually be made from a 12-lead ECG (Fig. 4.38). In patients at risk of dangerous arrhythmia (for example after myocardial infarction) the ECG can be continuously monitored at the bedside. In patients with intermittent symptoms the ECG can be monitored over 24 or 48 hours using a small tape recorder (Holter monitoring).

Intracardiac electrophysiology is a technique in which the heart is stimulated to produce extra beats using a pacemaker electrode passed through a vein, and the resulting arrhythmias analysed. It is helpful in the diagnosis and subsequent management of patients with recurrent and life-threatening arrhythmias.

Hypertrophy. The ECG may show characteristic changes in hypertrophy of each of the cardiac chambers (Fig. 4.39). Usually echocardiography is a better method of detecting chamber hypertrophy or dilation.

Ischaemia. The ECG gives information about heart muscle, *not* about the coronary arteries! Many patients with angina and severe coronary disease have a *normal* resting electrocardiogram and *exercise electrocardiography* is often a more reliable way of detecting, and assessing the severity of angina of effort. In myocardial infarction, the ECG changes are usually the most useful confirmation of the diagnosis (Fig. 4.40).

Radiography

The plain chest radiograph is an important cardiac investigation. One method of assessment involves asking the following questions:

- Is the film technically satisfactory?
- Is it a posteroanterior film?

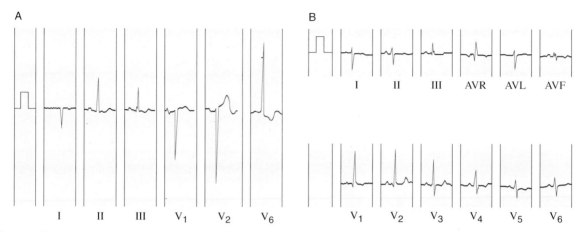

Fig. 4.39 ECG showing ventricular hypertrophy. **A.** Left ventricular hypertrophy from a woman with aortic stenosis. Leads I, II and III show only T wave inversion. Note the enormous voltages, broadened QRS complex and T wave inversion and V_2 and V_5. **B.** Right ventricular hypertrophy from a woman with pulmonary hypertension. Note the dominant R wave in lead V_1 and V_2 and predominant S wave in lead I and V_6.

- Has the patient taken an adequate inspiration?
- Is the heart size normal (cardiothoracic ratio < 0.5)?
- Is the upper mediastinum normal?
- Is the aortic knuckle normal?
- Is the pulmonary artery normal?
- Is the cardiac contour normal?
- Is there any abnormal cardiac calcification?
- Are the lung fields normal?
- Is there upper lobe venous diversion?
- Is there pulmonary oedema?
- Are there pleural effusions?

Technical quality. Film should be properly exposed and the patient should have taken a good breath in and should not be rotated.

Heart size. The cardiothoracic ratio (widest part of heart/widest part of lung fields) should be < 0.5. Spurious appearances of cardiac enlargement may be visible on radiographs during expiration or on antero-posterior (portable) radiographs.

Heart contour (Fig. 4.41). Check size and position of upper mediastinum and aortic knuckle (e.g. dissecting aneurysm), pulmonary artery, left atrial appendage and left ventricular border.

Lung fields. Normally vascular markings are more apparent at the lung bases. Prominence of upper lobe vascular markings is an early sign of left heart failure. More advanced left heart failure causes pulmonary interstitial oedema, with prominent septal markings (Kerley B lines) and finally frank alveolar oedema

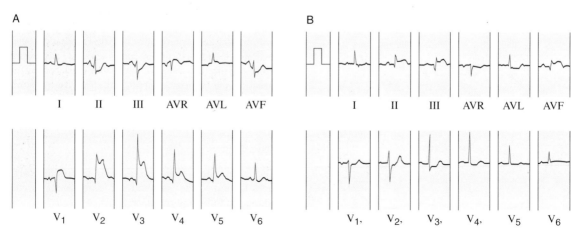

Fig. 4.40 ECG showing acute myocardial infarction. **A.** Acute anterior. Note the ST elevation in leads V 1–5.
B. Acute inferior. Note ST elevation in leads II, III and AVF.

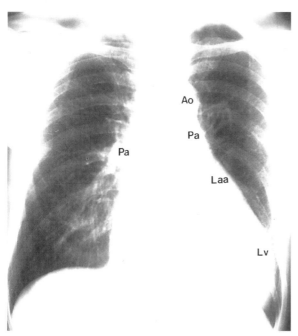

Fig. 4.41 **Chest radiograph from a patient with mitral valve reflux showing the 'landmarks' of the cardiac contour.** Ao = aortic knuckle; Pa = pulmonary artery; Laa = left atrial appendix; Lv = left ventricle. Both the left atrial appendage and the left ventricle are enlarged.

(Fig. 4.42). Fluid retention may also cause pleural effusions.

Other features. These include artificial heart valves, pacemaker electrodes and clips used in cardiac surgery.

Cardiac ultrasound investigations

Cardiac ultrasound encompasses

- *echocardiography*, which uses reflection of ultrasound to produce a two-dimensional image of the heart and
- *Doppler ultrasound*, which uses the frequency shift of sound reflected from moving blood cells to detect and measure blood flow velocity.

Ultrasound waves are emitted from and picked up by a transducer, which is usually applied to the chest wall (transthoracic ultrasound); special transducers may also be passed down the oesophagus (transoesophageal echocardiography) to provide excellent images of posterior cardiac structures.

Echocardiography. Echocardiography is useful in detecting abnormalities of cardiac structure. It is the definitive technique for assessing abnormalities of heart valves, cardiac hypertrophy, the size and arrangement of the cardiac chambers, the presence of pericardial effusions and intracardiac masses such as endocarditic vegetations or thrombi (Fig. 4.43).

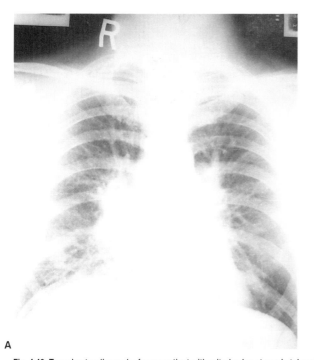

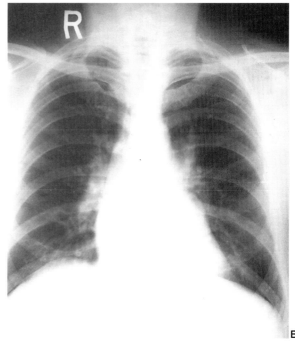

A   B

Fig. 4.42 **Two chest radiographs from a patient with mitral valve stenosis taken 48 hours apart.** **A.** shows pulmonary oedema. **B.** shows clearing of the oedema following treatment.

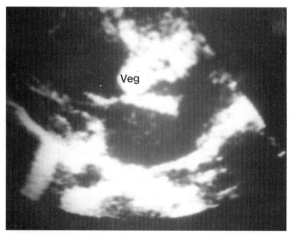

Fig. 4.43 Echocardiogram showing a large endocarditic vegetation (veg) attached to the aortic valve.

Doppler ultrasound. This is a method of detecting valve abnormalities and of measuring blood flow. It can detect forward and reverse flow through the valves and chambers of the heart. Doppler ultrasound is very sensitive and will often pick up valve regurgitation which is clinically and prognostically trivial.

Radionuclide studies

Radionuclide studies use short-lived radioactive isotopes and detection apparatus which produces and analyses an image of the radiation within the body (Table 4.46).

Blood pool scanning. Blood pool scanning uses a gamma-emitting radionuclide (technetium-99m), which mixes with, and 'labels' the circulating blood. Blood pool scanning gives a numerical measure of left ventricular function, and is also useful for detecting abnormalities of left ventricular wall movement as a result of ischaemia.

Lung perfusion scanning. This uses similar blood-labelling techniques, but scanning images the distribution of blood flow to the lungs. Its main use is

Table 4.46 Cardiac radionuclide studies

Type	Isotope	Use
Blood pool scan	Technetium, tantalum	LV function RV function
Lung scan	Technetium, xenon (gas)	Suspected pulmonary embolism
Myocardial scan	Thallium technetium/MIBI	Suspected ischaemia
Positron emission tomography (PET)	Various	Myocardial metabolism

in detection of suspected pulmonary embolism. Reliability is enhanced, particularly in patients who have an abnormal chest radiograph, by simultaneously using another isotope, in the form of radioactive gas (xenon) to measure gas distribution (ventilation–perfusion or 'V/Q' scanning).

Myocardial scanning. Myocardial scanning uses isotopes which are taken up by myocardial cells and give an indication of their viability or metabolism.

- Using *Thallium* in an exercising subject, ischaemic parts of the heart show up as 'holes' on the scan.
- *Technetium-labelled pyrophosphate* (or iodine-labelled *anti-myosin antibodies*) detects dead or damaged myocytes after infarction.
- Direct measurement of myocardial metabolism is possible using short-lived isotopes of oxygen or nitrogen, but these need special (and expensive) detection systems (positron emission tomography).

Computed tomography and magnetic resonance imaging

In cardiology, the main uses of CT scanning are in detecting dissecting aneurysm of the aorta and in analysing complex vascular malformations. Magnetic resonance imaging is also an excellent technique for studying vascular anatomy; it provides accurate images of all the cardiac chambers and information about flow in the great vessels.

Cardiac catheterisation

Cardiac catheterisation is an 'invasive' procedure. Although the complication rate is very low, wherever possible non-invasive techniques are preferred.

Catheters can be used to measure the pressures in the various chambers of the heart (Fig. 4.44), and thus to assess the severity of obstruction from valve disease. Oxygen saturation can be measured and used to calculate left-to-right or right-to-left shunts. Radio-opaque contrast can be injected to study the function of the different chambers.

Coronary angiography. Coronary angiography uses specially shaped arterial catheters to inject radio-opaque dye into the mouths of the right and left coronary arteries (Fig. 4.45). It provides information about the site, nature and severity of coronary stenoses and is an essential prelude to coronary bypass grafting or coronary angioplasty.

Bedside right heart catheterisation. This can be performed using the Swann–Ganz catheter, which has a small balloon on the end to allow blood flow to guide it into the pulmonary artery. With the balloon deflated, it measures pulmonary artery pressure; when the

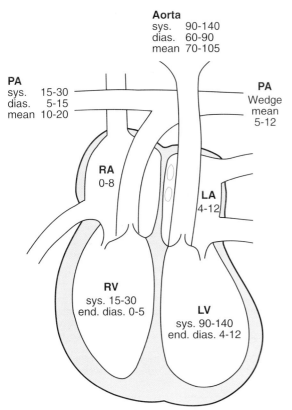

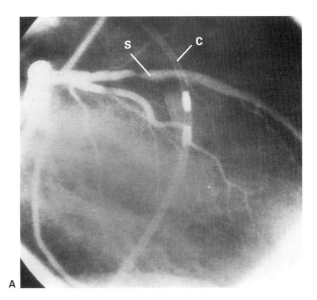

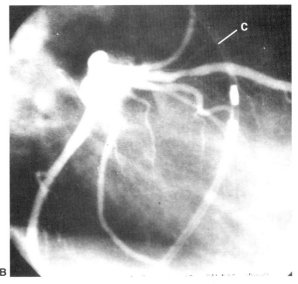

Fig. 4.44 Normal resting pressures in mm mercury in the chambers of the heart.

balloon is inflated, the pressure measured is the 'wedged pulmonary artery pressure', which reflects left atrial pressure.

KEY POINTS

- Patients with severe coronary artery disease may have a normal resting electrocardiogram.

- Echocardiography is a valuable technique for assessing abnormalities of heart valves, cardiac hypertrophy, the size and arrangement of the cardiac chambers and the presence of pericardial effusions.

- Doppler cardiography is a sensitive method of detecting and measuring abnormal blood flow.

THE METHODS IN PRACTICE

This section discusses three common cardiac problems: angina, cardiac failure and hypertension.

Fig. 4.45 Coronary artery angiography.   A. Showing a stenotic lesion in the left anterior descending artery B. Note the improvement following angioplasty. C = catheter; S = stenosis in LAD.

Angina

The diagnosis of angina is made on the basis of a careful history (p. 87). The object of examination and investigation is to evaluate its severity, possible causes and most appropriate treatment. During the examination of the patient with angina, emphasis should be placed on looking for the presence or absence of various features (see Fig. 4.46). Previous varicose vein surgery may be relevant if coronary bypass grafting is to be contemplated.

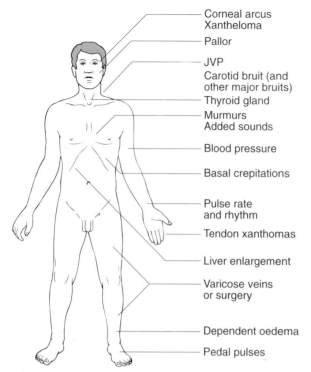

Corneal arcus
Xantheloma

Pallor

JVP

Carotid bruit (and other major bruits)

Thyroid gland

Murmurs
Added sounds

Blood pressure

Basal crepitations

Pulse rate and rhythm

Tendon xanthomas

Liver enlargement

Varicose veins or surgery

Dependent oedema

Pedal pulses

Fig. 4.46 Features to look for in angina.

Baseline investigations are shown in Table 4.47. The resting electrocardiogram is often normal but, if abnormal, indicates a worse prognosis.

If symptoms are severe or unstable, or if the resting electrocardiogram is markedly abnormal, it may be appropriate to proceed straight to treatment or to further investigation by angiography, but in other cases the severity is assessed by means of a treadmill exercise test. The most commonly used 'protocol' is that devised by Bruce (Table 4.48). The important questions to ask about an exercise test include the following:

Table 4.47 Investigations in suspected angina

- Resting 12-lead ECG (often normal)
- Blood glucose and urinalysis
- Haemoglobin
- Cholesterol (total and HDL cholesterol)
- Triglycerides
- Exercise electrocardiogram
- Fibrinogen*
- Thallium scan*
- Gated blood pool scan*
- Coronary arteriography*

*Selected patients only.

Table 4.48 Exercise tolerance test procedure using the Bruce protocol

1. Patient is fasted for minimum of 2 hours prior to test
2. The procedure is explained by the technician and the patient is encouraged to ask any questions
3. Resting 12-lead ECG and blood pressure are taken and checked by the attending physician, who also discusses any queries the patient may have regarding the test
4. The patient is shown how to use the treadmill and is asked to inform the technical/medical staff if any of the following occur:
    - chest pain or discomfort
    - breathlessness
    - dizziness
    - fatigue

The patient is told to terminate the test immediately if unable to continue for any reason.

Bruce protocol

Stage 1	3 min	1.7 m.p.h.	10% gradient
Stage 2	3 min	2.5 m.p.h.	12% gradient
Stage 3	3 min	3.4 m.p.h.	14% gradient
Stage 4	3 min	4.2 m.p.h.	16% gradient
Stage 5	3 min	5.0 m.p.h.	18% gradient

The physician and technician observe the ECG, blood pressure and the patient's reactions to the exercise very closely during the test to ensure maximum exercise and workload achieved without undue discomfort to the patient.

The *target heart rate* for all patients is *220 minus age. 80% of this is acceptable.*

The ECG is recorded at 1-minute intervals throughout the test, during peak exercise and 1-minute intervals post exercise up to a minimum of 6 minutes post test.

Blood pressure is measured at the end of each stage of the Bruce protocol and at the end of the test.

- What exercise protocol was used?
- What medication was the patient taking?
- How much exercise did the patient achieve?
- Why did the patient stop?
- Were symptoms reproduced?
- What happened to the pulse, blood pressure?
- Were there any ECG changes?

Patients in whom the exercise test is negative can be reassured that their prognosis is very good; patients who develop characteristic symptoms and ischaemic ECG changes at low workloads may have severe coronary disease and may need coronary arteriography with a view to bypass grafting or angioplasty. The final decision will also depend upon other factors, including age and occupation, severity of symptoms and the presence or absence of widespread vascular disease and other unrelated pathology. Exercise radionuclide studies, e.g. exercise thallium scanning, may have an important role in patients with pre-existing ECG abnormalities which may be due to a different cause such as hypertension. The 'flow chart' of investigation is shown in Figure 4.47.

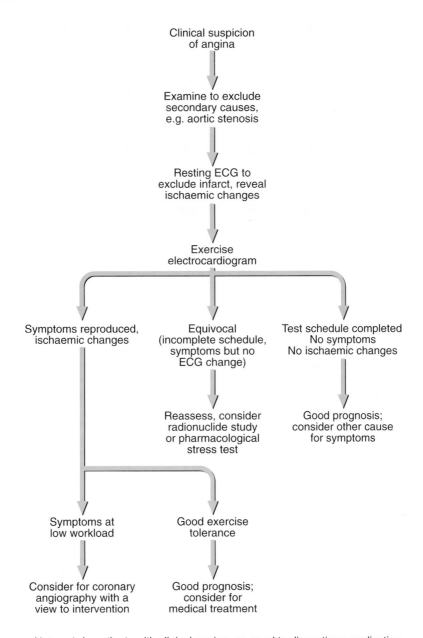

Fig. 4.47 Flowchart of investigation in suspected angina.

Cardiac failure

The initial assessment of patients in cardiogenic shock has been described on page 92. Once the patient has been resuscitated, or in patients who present with less severe symptoms, it is important to make an accurate physiological and pathological diagnosis. The possible physiological causes of heart failure are:

- volume overload
- myocardial failure
- inflow obstruction
- outflow obstruction

Each process can affect the right heart (right atrium and ventricle), left heart (left atrium and ventricle) or both sides of the heart.

Volume overload

This occurs when a patient with a healthy heart is overtransfused with blood or blood substitutes, or when renal failure prevents excretion of excess fluid. There is a raised jugular venous pressure, tachycardia, large-volume pulses and an active apical impulse. Basal crepitations develop, and the patient may suddenly develop frank pulmonary oedema.

More insidious examples of volume overload may occur as a result of an excessively low peripheral resistance over a prolonged period, as a result of persistent arterial duct (p. 111), Paget's disease of bone or generalised skin disease. The kidneys respond to the chronically low perfusion pressure as evidence of volume depletion, and retain fluid. Heart failure under these conditions is sometimes called 'high-output failure'. Congenital atrial septal defect (Fig. 4.22, p. 106) causes 'high-output failure' that is confined to the right side of the heart. Echocardiography in high-output failure shows dilated, vigorously contracting ventricles. The chest radiograph shows an enlarged heart, and pulmonary oedema or pleural effusions may be present.

Myocardial failure

Myocardial disease is one of the commonest causes of heart failure. It may be secondary to coronary artery disease, to a specific viral infection (for example Coxsackie viral myocarditis), to toxic drugs or to an uncertain aetiology, in which case the term 'cardiomyopathy' is used. It may also follow long-standing volume overload or outflow obstruction.

Physical signs are often unimpressive.

- There is a tachycardia (because stroke volume is limited the heart rate must increase to maintain output).
- Jugular venous pressure may be raised.
- In long-standing myocardial failure the heart enlarges, and the cardiac apex is displaced and may be hard to localise ('dyskinetic apex').

- The first and second heart sounds tend to be quiet, and there may be a third sound or gallop rhythm (p. 104).

Useful investigations include:

- The electrocardiogram is often abnormal and may indicate previous myocardial infarction.
- The chest radiograph often shows generalised cardiac enlargement.
- Echocardiography shows dilated, poorly contracting ventricles.

Inflow obstruction

The inflow of blood to the ventricles may be obstructed at the level of the tricuspid or mitral valves – the latter is much more common. Characteristic features of mitral stenosis are shown in Figure 4.31, (p. 111). Dilatation of the left atrium 'upstream' of the obstruction may lead to ECG features of left atrial hypertrophy and to atrial fibrillation. Initially, a rise in left atrial pressure tends to cause pulmonary congestion or pulmonary oedema. If it develops gradually, there is reflex pulmonary vasoconstriction, and pulmonary oedema is prevented at the cost of developing right-sided cardiac failure.

A different form of inflow obstruction occurs if ventricular filling is limited by excessive stiffness of the ventricle, as a result of cardiomyopathy or of ventricular damage from ischaemic heart disease or hypertension. The atria hypertrophy to compensate for the stiffness, and this may produce a fourth heart sound (p. 105).

The final form of inflow obstruction is when the ventricles are compressed from outside, as in the case of a pericardial effusion under pressure: *pericardial tamponade*. Pericardial tamponade usually compresses the thinner walled right ventricle more than the left, and produces symptoms of predominantly right-sided heart failure with a high jugular venous pressure. Echocardiography is invaluable in detecting the causes of inflow obstruction. Because the ventricles are underfilled, they are usually small and contract vigorously. The chest radiograph may show dilatation of the chambers 'upstream' of the obstruction, for example left atrial enlargement in mitral stenosis (Fig. 4.42).

Outflow obstruction

The load against which the ventricles have to contract ('afterload') may be increased either because ventricular outflow is 'throttled' by stenosed aortic or pulmonary valves or because the resistance in the

Table 4.49 Features of pulmonary hypertension

- Dyspnoea
- Loud S2
- Prominent 'a' wave in JVP
- Right parasternal heave
- Right ventricular hypertrophy on ECG

pulmonary or systemic circulation is high, as in pulmonary or systemic hypertension. Initially, the ventricle responds by becoming hypertrophied – later myocardial failure and increasing inflow obstruction from ventricular stiffness will develop.

- Left ventricular outflow obstruction may be indicated by a slow-rising pulse.
- Ventricular hypertrophy is often palpable as an alteration in the character of the cardiac impulse: a 'heaving' apex for left ventricular hypertrophy, a right parasternal heave for right ventricular hypertrophy.
- An ejection systolic murmur in the absence of increased cardiac output may indicate right or left ventricular outflow obstruction (p. 107). If cardiac output is reduced, an ejection murmur may become soft or inaudible.
- Whereas systemic hypertension can be readily diagnosed, pulmonary hypertension is less easy to detect. Some of its features are listed in Table 4.49.

Useful investigations include:

- The electrocardiogram frequently shows evidence of left or right ventricular hypertrophy.
- The chest radiograph may show cardiac enlargement. Post-stenotic dilatation of the pulmonary artery or aorta may be seen in pulmonary or aortic stenosis.
- Echocardiography will detect valve abnormalities and ventricular wall hypertrophy.
- Doppler ultrasound (p. 119) will provide a measure of the severity of any obstruction.

Hypertension

Systemic hypertension is common, has no specific symptoms but, if untreated, can lead to death or morbidity from stroke or heart disease. The clinical examination of the hypertensive patient has two aims:

- to seek a specific cause
- to evaluate the extent of damage already done.

In particular, the presence of cardiac failure will influence the choice of hypotensive agents.

A specific cause for hypertension is more likely in younger subjects (Table 4.50). In the history import-

Table 4.50 Causes of secondary hypertension

Cause	Clues	Test
Aortic coarctation	Radiofemoral delay Bruits	Ultrasound Angiography
Cushing's syndrome	Facial and bodily appearance, striae Fluid retention	Plasma and urinary cortisol Dexamethasone suppression, CT scan
Conn's syndrome	Polyuria, muscle weakness	Electrolytes, renin, Aldosterone Abdominal scan
Phaeochromocytoma	History, disproportionately severe ocular changes	Urine metanephrins Abdominal CT scan
Polycystic kidneys	Abdominal masses	Ultrasound
Renal disease	History, proteinuria	Creatinine clearance, urography, angiography
Congenital adrenal hyperplasia	Primary amenorrhoea with or without virilisation	Hormone assays

ant questions to ask include a history of paroxysmal headaches, vomiting, sweating and weight loss which may indicate phaeochromocytoma. Recurrent urinary tract infections, nocturia or enuresis or other urinary symptoms may indicate renal disease. Excessive analgesic abuse may cause analgesic nephropathy, and enquiry should also be made concerning alcohol intake (see p. 16).

Examination

❑ Record the blood pressure (p. 97).
❑ Look for radiofemoral delay in the pulses, which indicates aortic coarctation (p. 114).
❑ Examine the optic fundi for hypertensive retinopathy (p. 267). Its presence may indicate intermittent hypertension even if the blood pressure is normal at the time of examination.
❑ Look for features of Cushing's syndrome (Fig. 3.4, p. 47) or virilisation.
❑ Palpate the abdomen for adrenal masses and for enlarged kidneys (p. 179).
❑ Examine the heart for features of left ventricular hypertrophy; a heaving apex beat and sometimes a fourth heart sound.
❑ Look for evidence of cardiac failure.

Investigations will vary from patient to patient but might include:

- urinalysis for protein, and microscopy for blood cells and casts.

- measurement of plasma urea and creatinine concentration. Plasma potassium concentration may be reduced in primary or secondary hyperaldosteronism.
- Plasma glucose and lipid measurements to assess the risk of ischaemic heart disease.
- The ECG and chest radiograph as useful 'baseline' investigations in determining prognosis.
- Echocardiography is a more reliable method for investigating left ventricular mass than the electrocardiogram.
- Ambulatory blood pressure monitoring is helpful in distinguishing patients with labile blood pressure or 'white coat' hypertension from those with sustained hypertension.
- Renography and other renal investigations may be indicated when history, examination or other investigations point to the possibility of renal disease.
- Renal arteriography may be indicated in selected patients to investigate possible renal artery stenosis.
- A 24-hour urine collection for catecholamine metabolites as a screening test for phaeochromocytoma in patients with severe or paroxysmal hypertension.

PERIPHERAL VASCULAR SYSTEM

ARTERIAL DISEASE

The history

Arterial disease is common. Sometimes symptoms are caused by arterial emboli; more frequently they are the consequence of arterial luminal narrowing. Atheroma may be extensive without causing symptoms and is a 'systemic' problem which can cause diffuse narrowing in many vessels. Atheromatous deposits in arteries may also cause symptoms without major obstruction of the lumen, such as an ulcerating lesion in the internal carotid giving rise to microembolic stroke or transient ischaemic attacks or the small distal emboli associated with aneurysms, particularly those of the popliteal artery.

Peripheral arterial disease is frequently associated with coronary heart disease, cardiovascular disease, hypertension, diabetes and smoking. For this reason the general history should focus on these factors, the family history of vascular disease and hyperlipidaemia, the current drug treatment and any history of possible contra-indications to specific therapy, e.g. asthma or peptic ulcer disease.

The main symptom of peripheral arterial disease is pain, especially in the leg. Pain is due to an inadequate supply of nutrients to muscle and/or skin, secondary to atheromatous obstruction to blood flow in the arteries supplying the area. Pain may occur with exercise (claudication) or be present at rest (severe ischaemia).

Limb pain

Claudication.   This pain typically occurs in the calf, but may also be felt in the buttock or thigh if the main obstruction to flow is sufficiently proximal. It is often described as a tightness or 'cramp like'. The patient usually has a normal gait before the onset of pain. Characteristically the pain develops after a relatively constant distance, and this will be shorter if walking uphill. It goes completely with rest within 5–10 minutes. The actual claudication distance described by the patient is often inaccurate, but a useful guide to severity may be obtained by asking specific questions, such as 'did it come on while walking to the clinic from the car park or bus stop or while walking from waiting area to consulting room?' It is important to try to obtain an accurate assessment of this distance and to put this in context with the patient's occupation. For example, claudication after 200 metres may be a real problem for a postman, but not for an elderly man who can get down the road to the local pub for his daily pint before it develops. Other important aspects of the history are:

- nature of onset: acute or insidious
- severity of disability in context of lifestyle
- site of pain
- smoking habit, past and present
- drug treatment – especially beta-blockade
- other symptoms – especially angina
- associated symptoms including male impotence.

Severe limb ischaemia.   Typically these patients are older than those with claudication. There is a greater incidence of diabetes in this population and it is less skewed towards the male sex. Often there is no previous history of claudication. Patients present with pain at rest, with or without ischaemic ulceration or gangrene.

Frequently the onset is insidious, gradually worsening over a period of weeks or months, and the patient may delay seeking advice. The pain is often worse in bed at night, and patients find relief from hanging the leg dependently or even walking a few steps. The pain becomes constant, severe, and is usually only relieved by opiate drugs. If untreated there is a real risk of infection, extending gangrene and eventual limb loss. There is a high incidence of associated medical conditions, especially heart and lung disease, diabetes and hypertension.

Acute limb pain.   The onset of pain is typically sudden and the patient may remember the exact time it started.

Pain may be related to emboli becoming detached from the heart and obstructing a major blood vessel to the limb, or may be due to thrombosis of an already diseased arterial segment. Arterial injury, either due to direct trauma or secondary to a bony fracture, is another cause. In the arm, acute ischaemia is normally embolic. In the lower limb a previous history of claudication makes acute thrombosis the more likely diagnosis.

Neurological symptoms

Vascular disease is responsible for many neurological problems including multi-infarct dementia. A significant proportion of strokes are due to emboli from either the heart or great vessels, especially at the origin of the internal carotid artery. Many patients suffer a minor stroke with full recovery; if recovery is within 24 hours this is known as a transient ischaemic attack (TIA). The importance of recognising these events lies in the possibility of treating the underlying cause, either medically or surgically, and so preventing a more devastating stroke.

TIAs related to the internal carotid territory may present with:

- transient blindness (amaurosis fugax) – often described as a curtain coming down over one visual field
- a mild or partial hemiparesis.

Symptoms such as giddiness, collapse or blackouts are *not* usually related to carotid territory TIAs but may be a feature of vertebro-basilar ischaemia (p. 34).

Visceral symptoms

Mesenteric ischaemia. This underdiagnosed condition may present in a variety of ways. These include:

- post-prandial pain or discomfort
- weight loss – possibly secondary to impaired absorption
- acute abdominal pain, with or without fresh rectal bleeding.

Renal artery ischaemia. Renal infarction is rare and usually causes intense loin pain. Renal artery stenosis is much more common. The symptoms are secondary to the development of hypertension or renal failure.

Secondary to aortic aneurysms. Aortic aneurysms are frequently asymptomatic until they cause an acute complication; when they do present, they often cause atypical symptoms leading to a delay in diagnosis.

Some modes of presentation of abdominal aortic aneurysms are listed in Table 4.51.

Table 4.51 Abdominal aortic aneurysms

- *Acute*
  Collapse ⎫
  Back pain ⎭ (rupture or leak)
  Lower chest pain (?MI)
  Abdominal pain
  Loin pain (? ureteric colic)
  Major or minor emboli to the legs
- *Chronic*
  A pulsatile lump in the abdomen
  Leg swelling (venous obstruction or deep vein thrombosis)
  Back pain
  Symptoms of renal failure

It follows that patients with aortic aneurysms may be seen, either electively or as emergencies, with a wide variety of symptoms, and leaking or expanding aneurysms are now one of the commonest causes of abdominal pain in men over the age of 65; a high index of suspicion must be maintained.

Vasospastic symptoms

Vasospastic disease comprises those conditions in which the common factors are:

- abnormally discoloured or cold hands and feet
- normal peripheral pulses.

Raynaud's disease. This condition of unknown aetiology, most commonly affecting young adult females, is characterised by accentuated vasospasm in a cold environment. The extremities go white and following warming become red and often swollen. In the rewarming phase, the extremity may be described as burning or sometimes actually painful. The hands are affected more often than the feet, and both sides are usually affected symmetrically. Typically all the peripheral pulses are present.

Secondary Raynaud's phenomenon. Here the features of Raynaud's disease are associated with a variety of underlying pathologies:

- connective tissue disorders (especially systemic sclerosis)
- vibration-induced injury
- myeloproliferative disease (including myeloma)
- Arterial disease (especially with microemboli).

The problem is often more severe than with primary Raynaud's disease, sometimes with digital ulceration due to occlusion of small digital arteries. It is important always to look for an underlying cause and to enquire specifically about vibration. If predominantly affecting one hand, a local anatomical abnormality in the neck (such as a cervical rib) should be suspected.

Acrocyanosis. In this 'benign' condition which usually affects females the hands or feet are red or purple in colour most of the time; there is no painful response to cold and rewarming.

Asymptomatic

Much arterial disease is asymptomatic and may be discovered by chance when the patient is being examined for something else, or only after the development of a vascular catastrophe.

KEY POINTS

- Widespread arterial disease may be asymptomatic.

- The significance of intermittent claudication is dependent upon the expected daily activity of the patient.

- Acute limb ischaemia and arterial insufficiency causing rest pain require urgent investigation.

- Leaking or expanding aneurysms are a common cause of abdominal pain in the elderly.

- The possibility of underlying pathology should always be considered in a patient presenting with Raynaud's phenomenon.

The physical examination

Much of the general assessment follows that already described for the heart and includes looking for evidence of anaemia or cyanosis, facial clues to vascular disease (e.g. xanthelasma) and signs of cardiac failure.

Peripheral pulses

This is the key part of peripheral arterial assessment. Pulses are graded according to a simple system:

Normal	+
Reduced	±
Absent	−
Aneurysmal	++

Aneurysms transmit an 'expansile' pulsation, best appreciated by placing both hands over the pulse and feeling them pushed apart. In large patients, however, sizeable aortic aneurysms are easily missed. Femoral or popliteal aneurysms are usually easy to feel. Indeed, if the popliteal pulse is easily felt it is quite likely to be aneurysmal!

The radial, brachial and carotid pulses have already been described (p. 95–98). Examination of the lower limb pulses require knowledge of their anatomy.

Femoral. This artery lies roughly midway between the anterior superior iliac spine and the pubic tubercle, at a site that usually corresponds to the lateral extent of pubic hair.

Popliteal. The pulse is usually felt just lateral to the midline. Most people have difficulty initially, and this is often due to the use of inadequate pressure with the fingers.

Posterior tibial. The position of this artery is variable as it passes behind the medial malleolus.

Dorsalis pedis. This may be absent or abnormally sited in 10% of normal subjects.

Examination

General

- Feel the radial pulse and record rate and rhythm (p. 96).
- Examine the brachial pulse (p. 96).
- Measure the brachial blood pressure in both arms (p. 97) (a difference may indicate associated subclavian disease).
- Look at the legs and feet for changes of ischaemia.
- Examine for peripheral aneurysms.
- Listen for bruits, especially over the carotid and femoral arteries and in the abdomen.
- Feel specifically for the abdominal aorta in anyone with suspected vascular disease.

Femoral

- With the patient supine, press firmly down and cephalad in the groin crease (Fig. 4.48).
- Use the thumb or two or three extended fingers.

Popliteal

- Flex the knee to about 30° and make sure the patient is relaxed.
- Press firmly with the thumbs in front and the four fingers of both hands posteriorly over the popliteal artery below the knee (Fig. 4.49).
- While palpating the artery look specifically for popliteal aneurysm.

Posterior tibial

- Feel for this about 1–2 cm below and behind the medial malleolus (Fig. 4.50A).

Dorsalis pedis

- Feel in the middle of the dorsum of the foot just lateral to the extensor hallucis tendon (Fig. 4.50B).

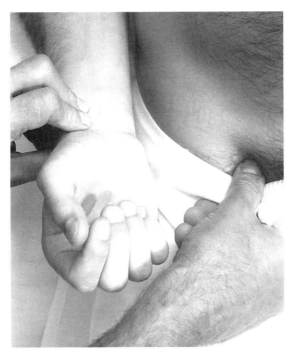

Fig. 4.48 Examination of the femoral artery.   Use the right thumb, while checking for radio-femoral delay with the left hand.

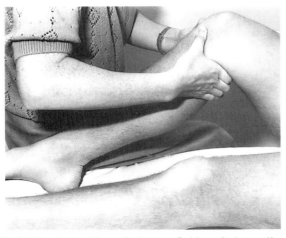

Fig. 4.49 Examination of the popliteal artery.   Feel the popliteal artery with the fingertips, having curled both hands into the popliteal fossa.

Interpretation

It is important to remember that in some normal subjects the dorsalis pedis pulse may be absent and that with age many of the pedal pulses become more difficult to feel. It is useful to record the findings diagrammatically (Fig. 4.51).

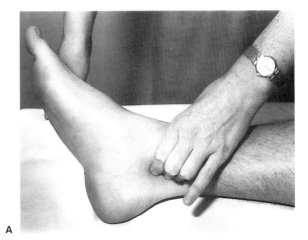

A

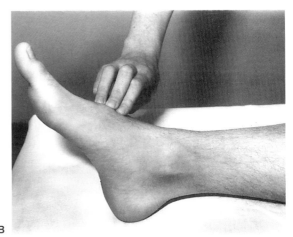

B

Fig. 4.50 Examination of A. the posterior tibial artery and B. the dorsalis pedis artery.

Occasionally foot pulses may feel normal at rest but may disappear on exercise because of the increased flow and consequent decreased distal pulse pressure. If the history is typical of claudication the pedal pulses should be re-examined after the patient has exercised for a few minutes.

The finding of a bruit implies turbulence of blood flow. However, although a carotid bruit is strong evidence of underlying disease, a bruit may occur in its absence; likewise severe disease may be present even without a bruit. An abdominal bruit may suggest some vascular disease, but is very non-specific, and can sometimes be heard in normal subjects.

Intermittent claudication

Arthritis and claudication may coexist in the same

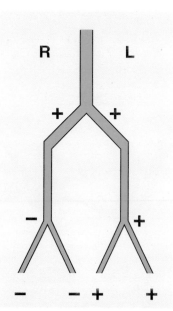

Fig. 4.51 Suggested method of recording peripheral pulses. Clinically this patient has an occluded right superficial femoral artery.

patient, but arthritis pain usually starts as soon as the patient begins to walk, and there is often a limp. Likewise, if the pain is centred over a joint, or down the front of the lower leg, it is probably not due to arterial disease.

The feet and legs often look normal, but there is a spectrum of severity and some patients may have signs of more advanced disease, such as hair loss from the toes and a rather shiny, red skin. There will normally be a pulse deficit on the affected limb.

Severe limb ischaemia

The skin of the foot is red and shiny and there may be arterial ulcers. Initially these are small and occur behind the heel, between the toes, in the bunion area and on the dorsum of the foot. If elevated, the foot quickly becomes pale; if placed dependently, it slowly suffuses as blood pools in the skin capillaries (Buerger's test). There may be evidence of cellulitis or even abscess formation, especially in diabetics. Gangrene of the toes, heel or dorsum of the foot may be present.

- The absence of the femoral pulse, implying major proximal disease, often indicates that reconstructive surgery will be both possible and beneficial.
- The presence of femoral and popliteal pulses, by contrast, suggests predominantly distal disease with poorer prospects for surgical or angioplasty treatment.

- The presence of a popliteal aneurysm is a potentially treatable cause of severe lower limb ischaemia.

Acute limb ischaemia

This is an emergency situation if a functioning limb is to be preserved. The examination comprises:

1. Assess the severity. The characteristic features are:

- pain
- pallor
- pulselessness
- paraesthesia
- paralysis.

Any sensory deficit or motor weakness gives a warning of the severity of the problem and the need for urgent intervention if significant muscle necrosis is to be avoided.

2. Look for a cause. The most frequent associations with peripheral emboli from the heart are arrhythmias, especially atrial fibrillation and recent myocardial infarction: emboli may also arise from a diseased aorta or more peripheral aneurysms.

3. Examine the other leg. A full complement of pulses suggests a relatively normal arterial tree and increases the likelihood of an embolic source.

4. Look at the patient as a whole. Is the patient suitable for surgery and are the medical problems under optimal control?

Investigations

Detailed investigation will depend on many factors, including the patient's age and general condition as well as the specific presenting condition, but most patients with peripheral arterial disease should undergo the basic tests to exclude anaemia, diabetes and ischaemic heart disease.

It is rare to find any underlying abnormality in primary Raynaud's disease or acrocyanosis, but a thorough search should be made in those patients in whom a secondary cause such as a connective tissue disorder may be present.

Specific investigations include the following:

Doppler probe. Ankle pressure measurement, using a simple hand-held Doppler probe and a blood pressure cuff around the calf, will confirm the presence of significant lower limb arterial disease in most patients, and is really an extension of clinical examination which should be used if there is doubt about the foot pulses. Systolic pressure is measured with the patient supine and compared with the arm pressure to give the ankle-brachial pressure index (ABPI). Normal values of this ratio are in the range 1–1.2; most claudicant patients will have ABPI of 0.7–1, while patients with severe ischaemia normally have ratios <0.4 (or absolute values <50 mmHg). As with pulse palpation, a simple exercise test will result in lower ankle pressures. It should be possible to exclude vascular disease in patients with atypical histories without resorting to more invasive tests.

Ultrasound scanning. This often gives accurate diameter measurements in both aortic and peripheral aneurysms.

Duplex scanning. This is indicated in patients who have suffered a carotid territory TIA or minor stroke. It provides non-invasive imaging of the carotid bifurcation, together with Doppler waveform analysis of the disturbed and accelerated flow seen with a stenosis.

Angiography. Indications include:

- acute or severe lower limb ischaemia
- peripheral aneurysms
- aortic aneurysms in which the proximal extent is difficult to determine by ultrasound or CT scanning.

KEY POINTS

- In a large patient sizeable aorta aneurysms are easily missed on examination.
- Bruits are evidence of turbulence of blood flow, but abdominal bruits may be heard in normal subjects.
- Pain which is centred over a joint is probably not arterial.
- The absence of a femoral pulse implies major proximal disease and often indicates that reconstructive surgery would be beneficial in a patient with severe limb ischaemia.

VENOUS DISEASE

The history

The purpose of obtaining a history is twofold.

1. To identify any underlying cause or precipitating factor.
2. To establish the nature and severity of the venous problem.

The cause

The possibilities to consider, and questions to ask, will depend upon the nature of the problem.

Deep venous thrombosis

- recent bed rest or operation (especially to leg or pelvis)
- recent travel (especially air)
- trauma to the leg (especially fractures and immobilisation)
- underlying malignancy
- heart failure
- previous DVT
- pelvic mass
- central venous catheters.

Superficial venous thrombosis

- injury to the vein wall (especially venous infusion)
- sluggish flow (including varicose veins)
- a coagulation problem (including some malignancies).

The severity

The cardinal symptoms of venous disease are pain and discomfort, swelling, discoloration and ulceration. These features frequently coexist. The severity of the symptoms may bear little relationship to the gravity of the underlying condition. Indeed, a life-threatening deep venous thrombosis may be asymptomatic.

Pain

This is a common symptom of venous disease.

- In superficial venous incompetence pain is experienced as an aching or discomfort which is diffuse in nature and aggravated by prolonged standing, becoming more obvious towards the end of the day. It is relieved by rest and elevation.
- In acute superficial thrombosis the pain overlies the affected vein.
- In deep venous thrombosis (DVT), when pain is present it is usually associated with swelling of the limb below the level of the obstruction.

Swelling

Swelling may occur in any venous disorder but is most noted in acute DVT and in chronic deep venous insufficiency – a condition which is usually preceded by an episode of DVT.

Discoloration and ulceration

These are characteristic of chronic deep venous insufficiency. If ulceration is present it is important to consider additional causative factors, because chronic ulceration is frequently multifactorial in the elderly. Factors include:

- major arterial disease
- small vessel disease and vasculitis
- primary skin conditions including malignancy
- neuropathic processes in general and diabetes in particular
- arthritis.

The physical examination

Venous examination is largely dependent on inspection with palpation playing a secondary role.

A simple test (Trendelenburg's test) usually helps to confirm the presence of high saphenofemoral incompetence.

Examination

❑ Expose the patient's limbs and inspect for skin and colour changes, limb swelling and venous dilatation or tortuosity.
❑ Palpate for any difference in temperature.
❑ Elevate the limb to about 15° above the horizontal and look for the rate of venous emptying.
❑ Feel gently and carefully for any localised tenderness.

Trendelenburg's test
❑ Lie the patient flat and elevate the leg.
❑ Place a tourniquet around the upper thigh tight enough to compress the superficial veins.
❑ Ask the patient to stand while observing for any filling of the veins.
❑ Then release the tourniquet and continue to observe.

Interpretation

Varicose veins are usually obvious from inspection. Most cases are confined to either the long (>90%) or short (<10%) saphenous systems. The Trendelenburg test takes experience and practice to perform well. If positive, the veins fill only slowly on standing, but quickly on releasing the tourniquet. A finger over the saphenofemoral junction will also work, although it is less reliable than a tourniquet in the obese.

Acute superficial venous thrombosis (thrombophlebitis) can be readily identified, producing a red, painful area overlying a superficial vein.

Acute deep venous thrombosis occurs most commonly in the leg, but occasionally affects the arm. Life-threatening thrombosis can occur in an apparently

normal limb. In other instances the limb is diffusely swollen and painful beyond the level of the obstruction. The lower leg is warm and red or purplish in colour. If the calf veins are mainly affected, there will be tenderness in the calf muscles; more proximal iliofemoral thrombosis causes swelling and warmth of the whole leg, often with some tenderness over the femoral vein in the upper thigh.

In *chronic deep venous insufficiency* there is swelling and thickening of the skin and subcutaneous tissue of the lower calf. The skin becomes pigmented because of haemosiderin deposits, and ulceration may supervene, especially in the region above the medial malleolus. The foot itself is frequently relatively normal. There may be associated dilated superficial veins, although it is unusual to see severe ankle skin changes in cases of primary varicose veins.

Investigations

Duplex scanning. This may be of value in assessing complex cases of varicose veins by helping to identify the presence and the level of reflux in the femoral, popliteal and superficial veins.

It can also be used to demonstrate the presence of a large proximal deep venous thrombosis.

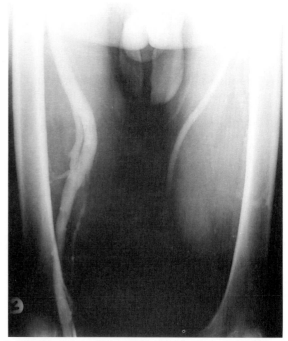

Fig. 4.52 Ascending venogram showing the normal pattern of deep veins on the right and major venous occlusion on the left.
(Courtesy of Dr L. MacDonald).

Ascending venography. This remains the definitive investigation in suspected DVT (Fig. 4.52).

Doppler ankle pressure. The same technique is used to assess the degree of arterial disease in patients with suspected chronic deep venous insufficiency, especially as foot pulses are often difficult to feel. Combined arterial and venous disease is common, and tight bandages must not be applied to the legs in patients with significant arterial disease.

KEY POINTS

- The cardinal symptoms of venous disease are pain and discomfort, swelling of the limb and discoloration with ulceration.

- Life-threatening deep venous thrombosis may be present in the absence of symptoms.

- The Trendelenburg test, properly performed, is an effective method of confirming the presence of high saphenofemoral incompetence.

- Leg ulceration in the elderly is often multifactorial.

G. K. Crompton

5

The respiratory system

Advances in physiology, pathology, immunology, micro-biology, radiology, endoscopy and thoracic surgery have not only permitted the diagnosis of respiratory disease with more precision but also a reappraisal of the value of clinical examination in its various forms. In many instances careful history-taking is more important than the elicitation of elegant, but possibly misleading, physical signs. Indeed, in many disorders the disease process may reach an advanced stage before any abnormal signs can be detected and, unless symptoms are promptly investigated, serious delays in diagnosis and treatment may result.

THE HISTORY

The approach to history-taking in patients thought to have respiratory disease differs according to the nature of the illness, the main distinction being between an acute or subacute illness and a chronic respiratory disorder. The methods used to obtain a coherent account of the patient's symptoms are, however, the same. Firstly, a narrative history is taken, as outlined in Chapter 1. Specific enquiry is then made about any of the principal respiratory symptoms not mentioned in the narrative history. At this stage the clinician should consider all the conditions that might conceivably be responsible for the patient's symptoms. This will seldom be more than perhaps three or four options. A series of supplementary questions designed to provide evidence for and against each possible diagnosis should then be asked. This method of integrating and rationalising the history has an important place in the diagnosis of respiratory disease because it facilitates the recognition of certain characteristic symptom patterns, such as those presented by chronic bronchitis and bronchial asthma, in which physical signs and even specialised investigations may be of limited diagnostic value.

In an *acute respiratory illness* it is important to enquire carefully about the onset of the illness. In pneumococcal pneumonia, for example, systemic disturbance (rigor, pyrexia, malaise) seldom precedes the first respiratory symptom (often pleural pain) by more than a few hours, while in viral pneumonia the patient may be generally unwell for several days before there are any symptoms or signs to suggest pulmonary involvement. Pleural pain may be a manifestation of pneumonia, but when it occurs spontaneously pulmonary thromboembolic disease must always be considered. Acute dyspnoea is a presenting symptom of particular importance since it often demands urgent treatment,

and an error in diagnosis between tension pneumothorax, an acute attack of bronchial asthma and left heart failure may have catastrophic consequences. A carefully taken history, from a relative if the patient is too breathless to give a coherent account of the illness, may enable such a mistake to be avoided. The nature and effect of treatment prescribed before the patient is seen should also be carefully noted.

In *chronic respiratory disorders* history-taking is complex and time-consuming. Care must be taken not only to record major incidents in the illness but also to describe and assess the interval or background symptoms. In the case of acute episodes, such as exacerbations of chronic bronchitis, an enquiry should be made into any preceding events and their apparent effects on the course of the disease. Most chronic respiratory disorders pursue a fairly predictable course and, if a patient exhibits symptoms out of line with the established pattern of the illness, the development of another disease should be suspected. The course of disease may also be adversely influenced by the treatment of coexisting disorders, for example a beta-adrenoreceptor blocking drug for hypertension or angina in a patient with chronic asthma. The influence of occupational and environmental factors should be recorded in detail. Such information, in addition to its diagnostic value, may be relevant to prevention and compensation in the case of occupational lung diseases.

SYMPTOMS OF RESPIRATORY DISEASE

The six principal symptoms of respiratory disease are cough, sputum, haemoptysis, chest pain, breathlessness and wheeze. Most of these may occur in the absence of primary respiratory disease. Certain types of central chest pain, for example, may be cardiac, pericardial or oesophageal in origin: breathlessness may be due to pulmonary oedema secondary to left ventricular failure, and haemoptysis may be the presenting symptom in mitral stenosis or disorders of the blood clotting mechanism. Nevertheless, lateral chest pain and the other five principal symptoms are usually indicative of respiratory disease, and will be discussed in that context.

Cough

This is the most frequent symptom of respiratory disease. It may be caused by stimuli arising in the mucosa of any part of the respiratory tract from the pharynx to the smaller bronchi. Stimuli arising in the parietal pleura may, on rare occasions, also produce cough, for example during the aspiration of a pleural

Table 5.1 Cough

Origin	Common causes	Nature/Characteristics
Pharynx	Post-nasal drip	Usually persistent
Larynx	Laryngitis, tumour Whooping cough, croup	Harsh, barking, painful, persistent, associated with stridor (tumours)
Trachea	Tracheitis	Painful
Bronchi	Bronchitis (acute and chronic)	Dry or productive. Worse in mornings
	Asthma	Dry or productive. Worse at night
	Bronchial carcinoma	Persistent (often with haemoptysis)
	Pneumonia	Dry initially, productive later
	Bronchiectasis	Productive. Changes in posture induce sputum production
	Pulmonary oedema	Often at night (may be productive of pink frothy sputum)
	End-stage interstitial fibrosis	Dry, irritant and distressing

Table 5.2 Sputum

Type	Appearance	Cause
Serous	Clear, watery, frothy, may be pink	Acute pulmonary oedema Bronchioalveolar cell carcinoma (rare)
Mucoid	Clear, grey, white, may be frothy or black (soot)	Chronic bronchitis Chronic asthma
Mucopurulent or purulent	Yellow, green, brown	All types of bronchopulmonary bacterial infection (eosinophils can cause sputum to appear purulent)
Rusty	Rusty, golden yellow	Pneumococcal pneumonia

effusion. The frequency, severity and character of cough are dependent on several factors including (a) the situation and nature of the lesion responsible for the cough, (b) the presence or absence of sputum and (c) coexisting abnormalities such as vocal cord paralysis, impairment of ventilatory function and pleural pain.

Types of cough. Cough can be produced by stimulation of sensory nerves of the mucosa of the pharynx, larynx, trachea and bronchi (see Table 5.1).

Cough in chronic bronchitis, which is frequently accompanied by wheezing, is particularly troublesome when going to bed at night and also when getting up in the morning. Sleep is seldom disturbed. In contrast, cough in asthma causes sleep disturbance in most patients and is usually worse in the early hours of the morning. Prolonged bouts of coughing in chronic bronchitis may give rise to cough syncope (p. 34).

The explosive quality of a normal cough cannot be achieved in patients with very severe airflow obstruction, respiratory muscle paralysis and unilateral vocal cord paralysis. Single vocal cord paralysis, usually the left, gives rise to a prolonged low-pitched inefficient and *bovine cough* – which is accompanied by hoarseness.

Sputum

When a patient has sputum, information should be obtained as to amount, character, viscosity and taste or odour.

Amount. This can seldom be accurately estimated by the patient, although statements that it is very large (e.g. a teacupful per day) or very small (one or two spits per day) are usually reliable. Some patients deny cough while admitting to the presence of sputum, saying that they bring it up merely by clearing the throat. A specific enquiry about sputum should, therefore, be made in every case. Most children and some adults swallow their sputum, even when it is being produced in large amounts. The sound of the cough, if it is loose or moist, will, however, indicate that sputum is present.

Character. This is seldom described accurately and, wherever possible, a specimen should be inspected. Apart from haemoptysis, there are four main types of sputum: serous, mucoid, purulent and mucopurulent (Table 5.2). The term 'dirty spit' used by many patients is misleading as it may refer either to purulent sputum or to mucoid sputum containing soot particles. Mucoid sputum may be copious and frothy in some cases of chronic bronchitis and asthma.

Viscosity. Mucoid sputum is often more viscous than purulent sputum and for that reason is more difficult to cough up. Sputum is particularly viscous in the early stages of pneumococcal pneumonia and in asthma. Serous sputum is watery with a low viscosity.

Taste or odour. When this is described as 'nasty' the patient may merely be referring to the normal taste of purulent sputum. When sputum is foul tasting/smelling this suggests bronchiectasis, lung abscess or infection with anaerobic organisms. The observer's own sense of smell should be used to assess odour.

Haemoptysis

Coughing up blood from the lower respiratory tract

Table 5.3 Causes of haemoptysis

Common	Uncommon	Others
Pulmonary infarction*†	Mitral stenosis	Foreign body inhalation
Bronchial carcinoma*†	Aspergilloma	Chest trauma
Tuberculosis*	Bronchial adenoma	Iatrogenic
Bronchiectasis†	Tracheal tumours	Bronchoscopy
Lung abscess	Metastatic pulmonary	Transbronchial biopsy
Acute bronchitis⁺	malignant disease	Transthoracic lung biopsy
Chronic bronchitis⁺	Laryngeal tumours	
	Connective tissue	
	diseases	
	Idiopathic pulmonary	
	haemosiderosis	
	Goodpasture's syndrome	
	Blood dyscrasias and	
	anticoagulation	
	Hypertension	

* Most important causes.
† Most common causes of frank/massive haemoptysis.
⁺ Diagnosis assumed only after exclusion of other causes.

occurs in many disorders (Table 5.3). When no cause can be found the oropharynx should be examined for a source of bleeding. The blood is bright red at first but may later become dark red. It is often frothy and may be mixed with sputum. Although most patients know whether blood has been coughed up or vomited, haemoptysis is occasionally confused with haematemesis.

Whenever a history of haemoptysis is obtained, questions must be asked about its type, degree, frequency and duration. In some cases the events preceding it may be of importance in diagnosis, e.g. deep venous thrombosis in a lower limb or a respiratory infection.

Frank haemoptysis may be massive and fatal, but usually the blood becomes progressively darker during the 48 hours or even longer after the bleeding ceases. When small amounts of fresh blood are coughed up frequently, for example daily for a week, either as frank haemoptysis or as blood-stained sputum, this strongly suggests a diagnosis of bronchial carcinoma. Regular blood streaking of mucoid sputum, sometimes only in the mornings, should always raise the suspicion of bronchial carcinoma. Recurrent episodes of haemoptysis over many years, usually associated with purulent sputum, are a feature of bronchiectasis.

Chest pain

Chest pain may be central (retrosternal) or lateral (Table 5.4). Retrosternal chest pain is caused by disorders of the mediastinal structures, e.g. trachea, oesophagus, heart and great vessels. The most com-

Table 5.4 Chest pain

Site	Causes
Non-central (lateral)	Pleural pain, rib fractures, direct invasion of chest wall by tumour or rib metastatic lesions, spinal nerve root involvement by vertebral disease (usually vertebral body collapse) and herpes zoster (p. 67), coxsackie B infection (Bornholm disease)
Retrosternal	Tracheitis, mediastinal tumours, acute mediastinitis, mediastinal emphysema, lesions of heart and great vessels (p. 87), oesophageal disorders (p. 162)

mon medical cause of non-central chest pain is pleural disease. Pleural pain is recognised by its sharp, stabbing character and by its relationship to breathing and coughing. It is always made worse by deep breathing and coughing, in contrast to most causes of central chest pain except tracheitis. Disorders of the chest wall, e.g. fractured rib, often produce pain that is similar to pleural pain, but rib fracture produces localised chest wall tenderness, which is uncommon in pleural disease. Spontaneous pneumothorax can give rise to pleural pain and/or central chest discomfort.

Pleural pain is often excruciating and causes shallow breathing and suppression of coughing.

Breathlessness (dyspnoea)

This has been previously discussed on page 26. A clinical assessment of pulmonary function is an essential component of the history of every patient with a respiratory cause of dyspnoea.

Apnoea

Apnoea or cessation of breathing can occur during life in a number of circumstances:

- Breath may be voluntarily held for short periods.
- Periods of apnoea alternate with overventilation in Cheyne–Stokes breathing (p. 147)
- Apnoea during sleep is of two main types:
  1. *Obstructive sleep apnoea* occurs when the upper airway is intermittently obstructed during sleep and is more often seen in obese short-necked adults who snore loudly.
  2. *Central sleep apnoea.* Breathing may occasionally cease for up to 10 seconds in healthy people. Pathological central sleep apnoea is rare but causes prolonged and frequent periods during which there is no activity of the respiratory muscles.

Wheeze

When a patient complains of wheeze it is important to discover what is meant by the term. Some patients use it merely to describe noisy and laboured breathing, while others apply it to the rattling of secretions in the upper air passages. Wheeze should, however, be applied only to the musical sounds produced by the passage of air through narrowed bronchi. It is invariably louder during expiration and is often confined to that phase of the respiratory cycle. It is more conspicuous, and sometimes audible only, during deep breathing. Many patients become so accustomed to wheeze that they cease to be aware of its presence until a relative or friend draws attention to it. Patients with stridor (see below) may describe it as wheeze. Care must be taken to distinguish between these two sounds because stridor is usually caused by partial obstruction of a major airway by a tumour or an inhaled foreign body, and thus demands urgent investigation and treatment.

Upper respiratory tract symptoms

Nose and nasopharynx. The most frequent symptoms of disease in the nose and nasopharynx are obstruction of the nasal airway, and nasal discharge often described by patients as 'catarrh'. Not uncommonly, these two symptoms coexist.

Persistent *nasal obstruction* is usually due to adenoidal enlargement, a deflected septum or to polypi, whereas intermittent obstruction is more often caused by mucosal oedema and excessive secretions. Bilateral nasal obstruction may lead to chronic mouth breathing, which, in children particularly, is often the reason for seeking medical advice.

Factors which precipitate recurrent nasal obstruction and discharge, e.g. the inhalation of dust or grass pollens, should be identified whenever possible. An enquiry should also be made about excessive *sneezing*, a common feature of allergic rhinitis, and *headache*, which may accompany acute infection of the nasal sinuses.

Epistaxis may give rise to apparent haemoptysis if blood in the posterior nares is inhaled and then coughed up.

Larynx. The two chief symptoms of laryngeal disease are hoarseness and stridor, but lesions of the larynx may also produce cough and pain. Stridor, and hoarseness which persist for more than a few days, must be fully investigated.

Hoarseness may vary in degree from a slight harshness of the voice to complete loss (aphonia). The voice may have a gruff quality in hypothyroidism (p. 77). Enquiries should be made about the duration of hoarseness and about events which may have preceded its onset, such as a head cold, abuse of the voice, chronic cough or an operation on the neck or throat. It should be noted whether it is improving, worsening or remaining static.

Cough of a short, dry barking character almost invariably accompanies hoarseness caused by an organic lesion within the larynx. The bovine cough of laryngeal paralysis is described on page (137).

Laryngeal stridor is a high-pitched crowing sound occurring during inspiration. It may be produced by a foreign body lodged between the cords or by laryngeal spasm, exudate or oedema related to acute viral or bacterial infection. The sound is aggravated by coughing.

Laryngeal pain of mild degree occurs transiently in acute laryngitis; constant severe pain is a feature of advanced tuberculous laryngitis and laryngeal carcinoma.

Trachea. Diseases of the trachea may produce pain, cough, stridor and dyspnoea.

Tracheal pain is referred behind the sternal manubrium. In the early stages of acute tracheitis it may be severe and become momentarily intense on coughing but subsides as soon as the cough becomes productive.

Tracheal stridor is usually due to obstruction of the tracheal lumen by a malignant tumour and is always accompanied by breathlessness. It is lower in pitch than laryngeal stridor, is heard best during inspiration and is accentuated by coughing. Stridor may also be present when a tumour partially obstructs one or both main bronchi. If stridor is suspected the patient should be asked to cough and then breathe deeply in and out with the mouth widely open. Listening carefully, close to the patient's mouth during the first few breaths after coughing, can often confirm the presence of stridor at an early stage.

HISTORY OF PREVIOUS ILLNESS

When the present illness appears to involve the respiratory system, information of considerable value in diagnosis, prognosis and treatment may be obtained from the past medical history. Important consequences of some previous medical events are shown in Table 5.5.

Previous radiological examination

If an abnormality is present on the chest radiograph, patients should be asked if they have been X-rayed in the past. Every effort should be made to obtain the earlier films, or at least the reports, since comparison with the current radiograph may be of diagnostic value.

Table 5.5 Previous history

History	Consequences
Tuberculosis	May have relapsed, caused bronchiectasis or a fungus ball (aspergilloma) may have formed in an old TB lung cavity
Pneumonia and pleurisy	May have caused bronchiectasis. Recurrent pneumonia and pleurisy may be caused by bronchiectasis, bronchial tumour, aspiration of oesophageal contents (achalasia of the cardia) or of pharyngeal secretions or vomit (bulbar palsy) and alcoholism. Immunological disorders such as hypogammaglobulinaemia and multiple myeloma should also be considered in patients with recurrent pneumonias
Measles and whooping cough	Can be complicated by pneumonia, particularly in early childhood, and cause subsequent bronchiectasis
Wheezy bronchitis or recurrent bronchitis in childhood	In the past asthma in childhood was often diagnosed as bronchitis. Recurrence of asthma in adults who have a history of childhood asthma is common
Chest injuries	Traumatic haemothorax can give rise to gross pleural thickening which splints the lung ('frozen chest')
Recent general anaesthetic or loss of consciousness	Inhalation (aspiration) of oropharyngeal secretions or foreign body (e.g. tooth) can give rise to aspiration pneumonia or lung abscess
Chest radiograph	Comparison of a recent chest radiograph with one taken in the past may be of great diagnostic value

FAMILY, OCCUPATIONAL AND SOCIAL HISTORY

Family history.

The family history of patients with respiratory disease may be significant in three ways:

- Certain *infections*, notably tuberculosis, may be transmitted from one person to another. Any history of contact with an infected person is, of course, more important than the family relationship.
- In *allergic disorders*, such as bronchial asthma, there is often an inherited predisposition, and a family history of eczema, hay fever and asthma is not uncommon.
- In *chronic bronchitis*, although an inherited predisposition cannot be excluded, the liability of several members of one family to develop the disease is more likely to be related to their living conditions and smoking habits.

Occupational history.

A detailed history of all occupations and hobbies is essential. Numerous chemicals, moulds, organic dusts and animal proteins can cause asthma and allergic alveolitis. Non-organic particles such as silica, coal dust and asbestos are important causes of pneumoconiosis and malignant diseases.

Social history.

A full social history should be taken as described on page 15 and particular care should be taken to enquire about pets (animals and birds) which may be the cause of rhinitis, asthma, allergic alveolitis and pneumonia (psittacosis). Information which should be obtained from all patients with chronic breathlessness also includes the physical effort involved in any employment. With the more severely disabled it is vital to know about hills and steps leading to the home and stairs within it.

Cigarette smoking is the most important cause of bronchial carcinoma and chronic bronchitis. Indeed both are rare in non-smokers though even 'passive smoking' may increase the liability. A smoking history should include details such as the age when regular smoking started, the age when smoking was given up (where applicable) and the average consumption of tobacco (number of cigarettes or cigars per day, amount of tobacco per week). Patients often under-

KEY POINTS

- Cough causing sleep disturbance is common in asthma, rare in chronic bronchitis.
- Small but frequent amounts of frank haemoptysis or blood-stained sputum are very suggestive of bronchial carcinoma.
- Pleuritic pain is stabbing in nature and is aggravated by deep inspiration and coughing.
- Listening carefully close to the patient breathing deeply through an open mouth during the first few breaths after coughing can often confirm the presence of stridor at an early stage.
- The past history often provides valuable information regarding current respiratory symptoms.
- A smoking history should be obtained from all patients.
- A full history of present and previous occupations should be obtained from all patients.

estimate the amount; the number of cigarettes bought each day or week is often a useful guide to the number smoked!

THE PHYSICAL EXAMINATION

THE EXTERNAL FEATURES OF RESPIRATORY DISEASE

Initial impression. A number of features may have become evident during the course of history-taking and should immediately cause the observer to suspect respiratory disease. These are cough, wheeze or stridor and laboured breathing.

The speed with which a patient can dress or undress is often a useful index of respiratory disability. Attention should be paid to any abnormality of the voice and to *fetor* of the breath. The state of nutrition should be roughly assessed and any suggestion of anaemia or polycythaemia should be noted, as these may be relevant findings in certain types of respiratory disease.

Cyanosis. The cardiac causes of cyanosis are described on page 94. Central cyanosis of respiratory origin is most frequently seen in chronic obstructive airways disease. In such cases peripheral vasodilation due to carbon dioxide retention (type II respiratory failure) leads to warm blue hands, but the colour of the tongue is a more reliable indicator of central cyanosis. This may also occur in many other diseases, including pneumonia, bronchial asthma, pulmonary infarction, allergic alveolitis and in any disease causing extensive pulmonary fibrosis.

Peripheral cyanosis affecting the face and neck, and in some cases the upper limbs also, is one of the features of superior vena caval obstruction (see below). Severe chronic hypoxia of either pulmonary or cardiac origin is often associated with polycythaemia and an extreme degree of cyanosis, partly central and partly peripheral, may be seen.

Oedema. The presence of peripheral oedema in patients with chronic obstructive airways disease suggests right ventricular failure. Oedema of a different distribution is seen in *obstruction of the superior vena cava*. This is most commonly a complication of bronchial carcinoma. When the superior vena cava is obstructed the jugular veins become grossly distended but no venous pulsation is visible in the neck. After a few days, dilated superficial veins and venules appear on the anterior and lateral aspects of the chest wall from the clavicles to below the costal margins. These veins convey blood from the territories of the subclavian and axillary veins to the drainage area of the inferior vena cava. The face and neck are swollen and puffy – although the tissues seldom pit on pressure – and conjunctival oedema

Table 5.6 Causes of finger clubbing

Respiratory	*Alimentary*
Bronchial carcinoma	Hepatic cirrhosis
Intrathoracic suppuration	Ulcerative colitis
Bronchiectasis	Crohn's disease
Empyema	Coeliac disease
Lung abscess	
Fibrosing alveolitis	*Congenital*
	Familial clubbing
Cardiovascular	
Cyanotic congenital heart disease	
Bacterial endocarditis	

(chemosis) is often present. There may be pitting oedema of the hands and forearms. The dilated veins on the dorsum of the hand remain full when lifted well above the level of the suprasternal notch.

The hands. Examination of the hands in patients with suspected respiratory disease, apart from the observation of cyanosis, is chiefly concerned with the recognition of *clubbing of the fingers* (see Fig. 3.6A, p. 52). This occurs in a variety of respiratory, cardiovascular and alimentary diseases (Table 5.6). The swelling of the terminal phalanges in clubbing, which usually, but less obviously, affects the toes also, is due to interstitial oedema and dilatation of the arterioles and capillaries. The early features of clubbing comprise loss of the normal angle between the nail and nail bed and fluctuation of the nail bed.

Examination

☐ Inspect the finger laterally for loss of nail bed angle (Fig. 5.1)

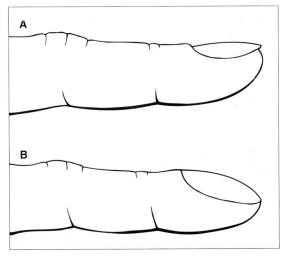

Fig. 5.1 Inspecting the nail bed angle.   Note the difference between **A.** normal and **B.** clubbing, with loss of nail bed angle and increased curvature of the nail.

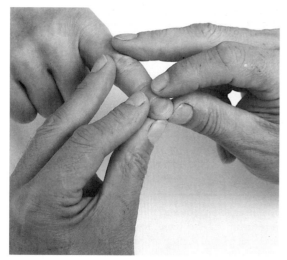

Fig. 5.2 Testing for fluctuation of the nail bed.

To elicit fluctuation place the finger on the pulp of the examiner's two thumbs and hold in this position by gentle pressure with the tips of the middle fingers on the proximal phalangeal joint.

Then palpate the finger over the base of the nail with the tips of the examiner's two index fingers (Fig. 5.2).

The test is positive when the sensation of movement of the nail is greater than the very slight degree of fluctuation which can be detected in normal fingers. When fluctuation is marked, palpation of the nail itself may give the impression that it is floating free on its bed.

With more advanced degrees of clubbing, various visible changes develop progressively.

1. Swelling of the subcutaneous tissues over the base of the nail causes the overlying skin to become tense, shiny and red, with obliteration of the skin creases.
2. Later, as the swelling involves the nail bed, the curvature of the nail, especially in its long axis, increases (Fig. 5.1).
3. Finally, swelling of the pulp of the finger in all its dimensions occurs in fully developed clubbing. In a few cases there may also be *hypertrophic pulmonary osteoarthropathy* causing pain and swelling of the hands, wrists, knees, feet and ankles, with radiographic evidence of subperiosteal new bone formation.

Increased curvature of the fingernails is commonly seen in normal subjects and, as an isolated pheno-menon without other evidence of clubbing, is of no significance.

Flapping tremor. In patients with severe type II respiratory failure a 'flapping' tremor of the hands is often present. To elicit this the patient should be asked to hold the arms outstretched with the wrists cocked. In this position the downward intermittent flap of the hands is exaggerated.

The eyes. It is important to examine the eyes in patients suspected of having respiratory disease (Table 5.10) to look for conditions such as Horner's syndrome (Fig. 3.16B, p. 59).

The neck. A systematic method of examining the neck has been described on page 78. In patients with possible respiratory disease the scalene lymph nodes require careful examination. These nodes are often involved when a pathological process, such as carcinoma, lymphoma, sarcoidosis or tuberculosis, affects the mediastinal nodes, and aspiration or biopsy of an enlarged scalene node may yield diagnostic information. This group of nodes is within a pad of fat on the surface of the scalenus anterior muscle, just in front of its insertion into the scalene tubercle of the first rib (Fig. 5.3).

Examination

Sit the patient on a chair or edge of bed with arms loosely folded and cervical spine partially flexed to relax the anterior cervical muscles.

Examine from behind, one side at a time, the whole supraclavicular and retroclavicular regions from trachea to anterior border of trapezius.

Examine for the scalene node by dipping the palpating finger behind the clavicle, through the clavicular origin of sternomastoid with the patient's neck slightly side-flexed to that side (Fig. 5.4).

When a node is found it should be assessed as indicated on page 74. Nodes which are greater than

Table 5.7 Examples of eye conditions in respiratory disorders

Condition	Disease
Horner's syndrome	Carcinoma of the bronchus
Phlyctenular keratoconjunctivitis	Primary tuberculosis
Iridocyclitis	Tuberculosis Sarcoidosis
Choroidal tubercles	Miliary tuberculosis
Chemosis, conjunctival and retinal vein dilatation (may develop papilloedema)	Hypercapnia Superior vena caval obstruction

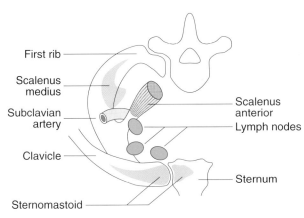

First rib

Scalenus medius

Subclavian artery

Clavicle

Sternomastoid

Scalenus anterior

Lymph nodes

Sternum

Fig. 5.3 Relation of lymph nodes to scalenus anterior.

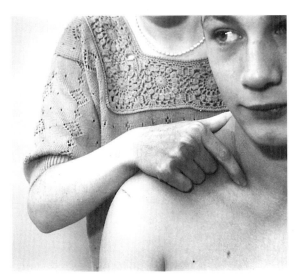

Fig. 5.4 Palpation of the right scalene lymph node. The patient should tilt the head forwards and to the right to relax the sternomastoid during the examination.

Table 5.8 Skin lesions which may yield information of diagnostic importance

Erythema nodosum (Fig 3.25A)	May be the initial clinical manifestation of tuberculosis and sarcoidosis
Metastatic tumour nodules	May be derived from a primary bronchial carcinoma
Cutaneous sarcoids and lupus pernio (Fig 3.21)	May occur in association with intrathoracic sarcoidosis
Rash of lupus erythematosus (Fig 3.16B)	May accompany pulmonary or pleural manifestations of this connective tissue disorder
Herpetic vesicles (Fig 3.27A)	May identify the cause of unilateral chest pain

THE UPPER RESPIRATORY TRACT

The upper respiratory tract extends from the external nares to the junction of the larynx with the trachea. It includes the nasal cavity, the nasopharynx, the nasal sinuses, the oropharynx and the larynx. Infective and allergic disorders of the upper respiratory tract are very common and infection may produce or aggravate disease of the bronchi and lungs. Oral sepsis, particularly suppurative gingivitis, may cause pulmonary disease, such as lung abscess. Clinical examination of the nose, throat and mouth is therefore an essential part of the investigation of all patients with respiratory disease (pp. 60–64).

The larynx

External examination of the larynx seldom yields any useful information, but swelling of the lips, the tongue, around the eyes and on the front of the neck caused by a hypersensitivity reaction (angio-oedema) may be associated with oedema involving the glottis. This may give rise to breathlessness and stridor, which may progress to complete respiratory obstruction.

Examination of the larynx by laryngoscopy is an essential step in the investigation of hoarseness. Fibreoptic laryngoscopes are now used for indirect and direct visualisation of the epiglottis, the arytenoid region and vocal cords. Lesions which can be detected by laryngoscopy include laryngeal tumours, laryngeal tuberculosis and vocal cord paralysis. A paralysed vocal cord adopts a position midway between abduction and adduction and fails to adduct on phonation (Fig. 5.5). Paralysis of abduction may precede complete paralysis of the cord.

The trachea

In normal subjects the upper 4–5 cm of the trachea can be felt in the neck between the cricoid cartilage and the suprasternal notch, but in thick-set or obese

0.5 cm in diameter, firm in consistency and round in shape are usually pathological, many of them containing metastatic deposits from a bronchial carcinoma. Large, fixed masses are present in some of these cases. Hard, craggy nodes may, however, be caused by healed and calcified tuberculosis; in such cases calcification is visible on radiographic examination.

The skin. Examination of the skin may yield information of considerable value in the diagnosis of respiratory disease. Some of the cutaneous and subcutaneous lesions which may be relevant are listed in Table 5.8.

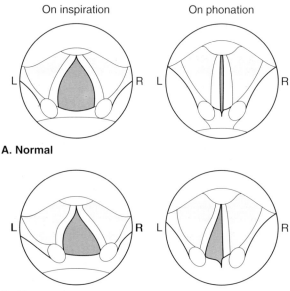

A. Normal

B. Abnormal

Fig. 5.5 The vocal cords. Diagrammatic representation of the laryngoscopic views of vocal cord movements showing **A.** Normal movements. **B.** Movements in the presence of recurrent laryngeal normal paralysis most commonly caused by bronchogenic carcinoma. Note that the paralysed left cord is in the cadaveric position (between inspiration and expiration).

subjects it may be so deeply placed that it is difficult or impossible to feel.

Tracheal displacement by an enlarged thyroid gland should be excluded before attributing any tracheal deviation to intrathoracic disease. Sometimes the trachea is displaced by a superior mediastinal mass including lymphoma and carcinoma, or by a massive effusion. More frequently tracheal deviation is caused by upper lobe collapse or fibrosis pulling the trachea towards the pathological side. Apical fibrosis is most commonly caused by tuberculosis. In patients with chronic airflow obstruction there is a downward movement of the trachea during inspiration. This may greatly reduce the distance between the cricoid cartilage and the suprasternal notch (the cricosternal space) and the cricoid cartilage may be tugged down with sufficient force to squeeze the finger.

Examination

❏ Examine the thyroid gland before localising the trachea (p. 78).
❏ To identify the position of the trachea gently introduce the tip of the index finger into the suprasternal notch exactly in the midline and press downwards (Fig. 5.6).

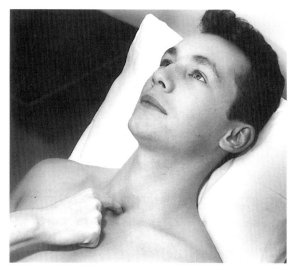

Fig. 5.6 Examining the trachea.

❏ To measure the cricosternal space insert one or two fingers between the cricoid cartilage and the suprasternal notch.

KEY POINTS

- Loss of the nail bed angle and increased fluctuation are early signs of finger clubbing.

- In patients with possible respiratory disease the neck should be examined from the back, one side at a time, for lymphadenopathy with special attention to the scalene regions.

THE CHEST

Physical examination of the chest makes use of the techniques of inspection, palpation, percussion and auscultation.

In health the two sides of the chest move to an equal extent with respiration. The trachea is central and the apex beat is in the normal position. Percussion of the chest wall elicits a resonant note over the lungs. On auscultation the breath sounds are vesicular in type (p. 153). In diseases of the bronchi, lungs and pleura, various changes in these physical signs may be observed.

Examination

❏ Examine the patient with chest and upper abdomen fully exposed and evenly illuminated.

- First examine the front and side of the chest with the patient lying in a semirecumbent position on a bed or couch and with the arm sufficiently abducted to allow access to the axillary regions.
- Then examine the posterior aspect of the chest with the patient sitting upright with arms folded across the chest and remove any pillows to allow unimpeded access to the whole of the back.
- Allow patients too weak to maintain this position to lean forward with arms resting on pillows or hold them forward with assistance.

Inspection and palpation

Abnormalities in the shape of the chest

Those of clinical importance are as follows:

Increase in anteroposterior diameter (barrel chest). The AP diameter may be increased relative to the lateral diameter. In normal subjects the ratio is usually about 5:7, and in flat-chested patients without respiratory disease it may be as low as 1:2. In some patients with emphysema, however, the two measurements may approximate (barrel chest). It should be remembered that an increase in the anteroposterior diameter may be due to thoracic kyphosis unrelated to respiratory disease. Chest deformity in emphysema is not a reliable guide to the severity of the functional defect.

Thoracic kyphoscoliosis. This ranges in degree from the minor changes in spinal curvature seen in many otherwise healthy subjects to grossly disfiguring and disabling deformities (Fig. 5.7). Thoracic scoliosis may alter the position of the mediastinum in relation to the anterior chest wall, with the result that abnormalities in the position of the trachea and the cardiac apex beat may be mistakenly attributed to cardiac or pulmonary disease. Severe kyphoscoliosis may have profound effects on pulmonary function, as the chest deformity reduces the ventilatory capacity of the lungs and increases the work of breathing (p. 26). Many such patients develop hypoxaemia, hypercapnia and heart failure at an early age.

Pectus carinatum (pigeon chest). This is a common sequel to chronic respiratory disease in childhood (Fig. 5.8). It consists of a localised prominence of the sternum and adjacent costal cartilages, often accompanied by indrawing of the ribs to form symmetrical horizontal grooves (*Harrison's sulci*) above the costal margins, which are themselves usually everted. These deformities are thought to result from lung hyper-

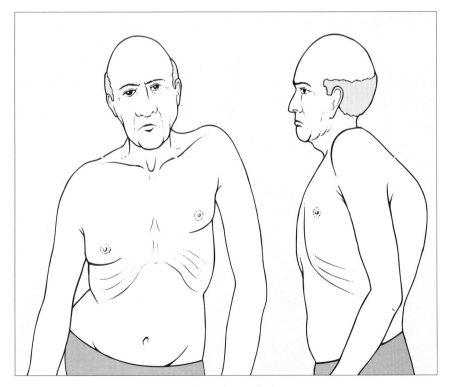

Fig. 5.7 Kyphoscoliosis.

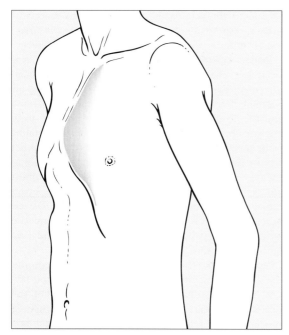

Fig. 5.8 Pigeon chest deformity (Pectus carinatum).

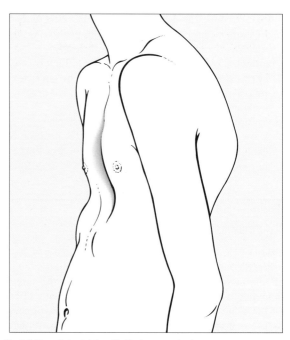

Fig. 5.9 Funnel chest deformity (Pectus excavatum).

inflation with repeated strong contractions of the diaphragm while the bony thorax is still in a pliable state. Pectus carinatum deformity may also be caused by rickets.

Pectus excavatum (funnel chest).   This is a developmental defect in which there is either a localised depression of the lower end of the sternum (Fig. 5.9), or, less commonly, depression of the whole length of the body of the sternum and of the costal cartilages attached to it. Pectus excavatum is usually asymptomatic, but, when there is a very marked degree of depression of the sternum, the heart may be displaced to the left, and the ventilatory capacity of the lungs restricted.

Thoracic operations.   Surgery may result in varying degrees of chest deformity.

Lesions of the chest wall

Abnormalities which may be detected by combined inspection and palpation of the chest wall are shown in Table 5.9. The nature of skin and subcutaneous nodules may have to be determined by aspiration or biopsy.

Subcutaneous emphysema (air in subcutaneous tissues) is recognised by the characteristic crackling sensation elicited by palpation of the air-containing tissues. It may cause diffuse swelling of the chest wall, neck and face. Subcutaneous emphysema is a common complication of intercostal tube drainage of a pneumothorax. In severe asthma air tracks into the mediastinum (*mediastinal emphysema*) via ruptured alveoli or

Table 5.9 Lesions of the chest wall

Cutaneous lesions	Skin eruptions, sarcoid nodules, neurofibromas, purpuric spots (Fig. 3.10), bruises, scars, discharging sinuses
Subcutaneous lesions	Inflammatory swellings, metastatic tumour nodules, sebaceous cysts, sarcoid nodules, neurofibromas (Fig. 3.34), lipomas
Subcutaneous emphysema	
Vascular anomalies	Spider naevi, enlarged vascular channels (arterial in coarctation of the aorta; venous in superior vena caval obstruction)
Localised prominences and deformities	Clavicles, scapulae, sternum, ribs, costochondral junctions, spinous processes
Localised tenderness	Fractured rib, tumour involving chest wall, spinal nerve root disorders
Lesions of breast (p. 80)	
Enlargement of axillary lymph nodes (p. 74)	

bronchioli. The air usually escapes innocuously into the neck, and even when there is marked mediastinal and subcutaneous emphysema it is not in itself dangerous. When air is present in the mediastinum normal heart sounds may be replaced by a churning noise accentuated during cardiac systole.

The observation of respiratory movements

Respiratory frequency. The normal frequency at rest in a healthy adult is about 14 respirations per minute. The rate is increased in a variety of pathological states, including pyrexia, acute pulmonary infections, particularly those accompanied by pleural pain, and conditions in which there is any increase in the work of breathing, e.g. bronchial asthma and acute pulmonary oedema.

Respiratory depth. This is difficult to estimate clinically as the movements of the chest and diaphragm, on which it is dependent, cannot be accurately measured. It is usually possible with practice, however, to recognise marked degrees of overventilation and underventilation. The latter may be of considerable importance in the diagnosis of type II respiratory failure.

In massive pulmonary embolism and in metabolic acidosis, usually due to diabetic ketoacidosis or uraemia, pulmonary ventilation at rest may be considerably raised. This can be recognised by an increase in the depth of respiration (*air hunger*) which may give rise to the subjective sensation of breathlessness. In *periodic* or *Cheyne–Stokes breathing* there is a cyclical variation in the depth of respiration, with overventilation alternating with periods during which breathing ceases (apnoea). It is believed to be caused by a decrease in the sensitivity of the respiratory centre to carbon dioxide. This occurs in certain neurological conditions, particularly those involving the medulla and in some patients with cardiac failure. The cycle usually lasts for less than 2 minutes, and during the phase of overventilation the patient may experience respiratory distress.

Overventilation may also occur in patients who are unconscious as a result of severe brain damage caused by trauma, haemorrhage or infarction.

Maximum chest expansion. There is a considerable degree of observer variation with this measurement and it does not correlate well with vital capacity, probably because in some subjects breathing is predominantly diaphragmatic. A value higher than 5 cm can, however, be regarded as normal, and one of 2 cm or less as definitely abnormal. Chest expansion is diminished in almost every type of diffuse bronchopulmonary disease, e.g. bronchial asthma, emphysema and pulmonary fibrosis, and in conditions which restrict movement of the ribs, such as ankylosing spondylitis.

Mode of breathing. In normal subjects inspiration is effected by contraction of the intercostal muscles and the diaphragm, while expiration is a passive process dependent upon the elastic recoil of the lungs. Women make more use of the intercostal muscles than of the diaphragm and their respiratory movements are predominantly thoracic. Men rely more on the diaphragm and their respiratory movements at rest are mainly abdominal. Babies of both sexes are also diaphragmatic breathers.

If respiratory movements are exclusively thoracic this may indicate that diaphragmatic movement is inhibited by pain caused, for example, by peritoneal irritation, or restricted by increased intra-abdominal pressure in conditions such as ascites, gaseous distension of the bowel, a large ovarian cyst or pregnancy. If respiratory movements are exclusively abdominal, ankylosing spondylitis, intercostal paralysis or pleural pain may be responsible for the lack of chest expansion.

Although breathlessness is a subjective phenomenon, it is usually accompanied by objective evidence of respiratory difficulty or distress. There is often an increase in respiratory frequency, which may be accompanied by dilatation of the alae nasi during inspiration. This may be observed in the absence of breathlessness and is not reliable evidence of respiratory distress. A much more useful criterion is the presence of the following types of abnormal respiratory movements:

- *Abnormal inspiratory movements* produced by contraction of the cervical muscles (principally the sternomastoids, scaleni and trapezii), by which the whole thoracic cage is, in effect, lifted off the diaphragm with every inspiration. Patients breathe in this way if adequate pulmonary ventilation cannot be achieved by normal inspiratory efforts, for example when there is gross overdistension of the lungs in advanced emphysema and severe bronchial asthma. More violent inspiratory movements of a similar character are observed in patients with obstruction of the larynx or trachea. Indrawing of the suprasternal and supraclavicular fossae, the intercostal spaces and the epigastrium with each inspiration invariably accompanies airways obstruction of this type and may also be seen, although it is usually less conspicuous, in chronic bronchitis and asthma.

A much more striking degree of indrawing of the chest wall is seen in patients who have sustained double fractures of a series of ribs or of the sternum. The portion of the thoracic cage between the fractures becomes mobile and, with the overlying soft tissues, is sucked in with every inspiration. *Paradoxical movement* of this type interferes seriously with pulmonary ventilation and may cause grave respiratory distress and hypoxaemia.

• *Abnormal expiratory movements* produced by powerful contractions of the abdominal muscles and latissimus dorsi. These are observed if the elastic recoil of the lungs is insufficient to complete the expulsion of air from the alveoli, as in emphysema, or when expiratory airflow obstruction is present, as in bronchial asthma and some cases of chronic bronchitis. Patients with a severe degree of expiratory obstruction prefer to be upright, grasping a bed table or the back of a chair. This enables them to fix the shoulder girdle so that the latissimus dorsi can be used to augment the expiratory efforts. Many patients, especially those with emphysema and with acute exacerbations of chronic bronchitis, exhale through their mouths with pursed lips (Fig. 5.10). This manoeuvre helps to keep the intrabronchial pressure above that within the surrounding alveoli and delays or prevents collapse of the bronchial wall which would otherwise result from the unopposed pressure of air trapped in the alveoli.

• *Localised impairment of respiratory movement* is usually caused by disease in the underlying lung or pleura, and is almost invariably associated with abnormal findings on percussion and auscultation.

Range of movement of the chest wall

Unless the changes are gross, it is difficult to detect differences in the range of movement on the two sides of the chest. Palpation to assess respiratory expansion of the anterior chest is rarely of value and is technically difficult in obese patients. More reliance should therefore be placed on inspection. Some clinicians believe that palpation is of such limited value that they do not perform it.

The significance of reduced movement. Unilateral reduction of chest wall movement occurs in many types of respiratory disease. In pleural effusion (see Fig. 5.13) and empyema, movement may be absent and, if the lesion has persisted for some weeks, retraction of the ribs and intercostal spaces may produce flattening of the affected side of the chest. This condition is sometimes described as a 'frozen chest'. Less marked reduction of movement occurs in pulmonary consolidation and collapse. In pneumothorax (see Fig. 5.19D) the limitation of movement is related to the amount of air

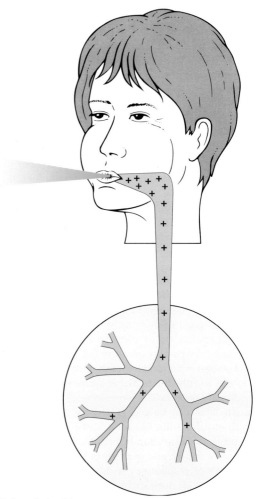

Fig. 5.10 Purse-lip breathing.

in the pleural space; in tension pneumothorax the affected side of the chest may be immobilised in a position of almost full inspiration. In pulmonary tuberculosis even extensive lesions may have little effect on chest wall movement during the early stages of the disease, but later, when fibrosis develops, there may be severe restriction of movement, with flattening of the affected side of the chest.

In bronchial asthma, emphysema and diffuse pulmonary fibrosis movements of the chest wall are symmetrically reduced. In the first two conditions this results from overinflation of the lungs. In diffuse pulmonary fibrosis, on the other hand, inspiratory movement is restricted by the reduced distensibility of the lungs. In severe cases this may bring each inspiration to an abrupt halt and produce the phenomenon of 'doorstop' breathing.

Vocal fremitus

This crude test provides no information that is not obtained using the stethoscope to assess vocal resonance.

Palpable accompaniments

The vibrations from a low-pitched rhonchus or a coarse pleural rub can occasionally be detected by a hand placed on the chest wall. In such cases an unusually loud rhonchus or rub is invariably present on auscultation and there is seldom any difficulty in distinguishing between the two. A palpable rhonchus generally has its origin in a large bronchus and, if persistent and unilateral, suggests partial bronchial obstruction by a tumour or foreign body. A palpable pleural rub, which may be recognised by the patient as a grating sensation within the chest, has no specific significance, but is more often encountered in chronic than in acute pleurisy, and is not always accompanied by pain.

Examination

- ☐ First inspect the chest wall for any abnormality.
- ☐ Surreptitiously count the number of breaths in a full minute by observing the chest movements with the fingers held on the pulse.
- ☐ Note the mode of breathing and the presence of any abnormal inspiratory or expiratory movements.
- ☐ Compare the range of respiratory movements on the two sides during normal and deep breathing.
- ☐ Record with a tape measure the maximum inspiratory/expiratory difference in the lower chest.
- ☐ To compare the range of movement in the infraclavicular regions, position the patient supine, shoulders relaxed and symmetrical with the head resting on a pillow and the head and trunk in a straight line. Then ask the patient to take deep steady breaths while viewing the infraclavicular regions tangentially.
- ☐ Examine breathless patients semirecumbent or sitting if they are made more dyspnoeic when lying flat.
- ☐ Assess lower anterior movements by inspecting the patient semirecumbent and breathing deeply.
- ☐ Assess chest movements posteriorly with the patient sitting erect. Grasp the chest from behind with the two hands. Bring the tip of the outstretched thumbs together in the region of the tenth thoracic spine, ensuring that there is a loose fold of skin between the two thumbs. Now ask the patient to breathe in deeply (Fig. 5.11).

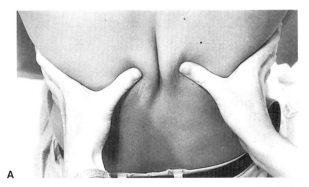

A

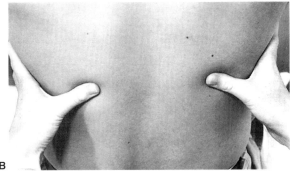

B

Fig. 5.11 Estimation of respiratory movements of the lower ribs posteriorly showing A. the fold of skin on expiration and B. the appearance with full inspiration. Note that this demonstrates an exceptional degree of chest expansion.

- ☐ Palpate the chest wall and determine the site of the cardiac apex and the position of the trachea.

KEY POINTS

- Chest deformity in emphysema is not a reliable guide to the severity of the functional disability.
- Severe kyphoscoliosis may have a profound effect on pulmonary function.
- More reliance should be given to inspection than palpation in detecting differences in the range of movement on the two sides of the chest.
- Localised impairment of respiratory movement is usually caused by underlying lung or pleural disease.

Percussion

The object of percussion is to compare the degree of resonance over equivalent areas on the two sides of the chest, and to map out any area in which the percussion note is abnormal (Table 5.10).

Table 5.10 Percussion note

Type	Lesions by which produced
Tympanitic	Hollow viscus
Hyperresonant	Pneumothorax
Resonant	Normal lung
Impaired	Pulmonary consolidation Pulmonary collapse Pulmonary fibrosis
Dull	Pulmonary consolidation Pulmonary collapse Pulmonary fibrosis
Stony dull	Pleural effusion

Dullness. The percussion note loses its normal resonance whenever aerated lung tissue is separated from the chest wall by pleural fluid or thickening, or when lung tissue is rendered airless by consolidation, collapse or fibrosis. Over such lesions the percussion note is impaired or dull. The most marked degree of dullness on percussion is found over a large pleural effusion.

Hyperresonance. Hyperresonance may be found over a large thin-walled pulmonary cavity, over a pneumothorax, particularly if the pleural pressure is above atmospheric level, and also over lung which is markedly emphysematous. An apparent finding of generalised hyperresonance must, however, be viewed with reserve, since a change in the absolute pitch of a percussion note is difficult to recognise and may depend mainly upon the thickness of the chest wall. It is not usually advisable to attempt to distinguish between normal resonance and hyperresonance when the percussion note is equally resonant on the two sides.

Anatomical considerations

The regions of the thorax over which a resonant percussion note is normally found correspond approximately to the surface marking of the lungs (Fig. 5.12). Percussion over the heart or the liver will elicit a dull note, but the area of dullness is less extensive than would be expected from anatomical surface marking, since aerated lung is interposed between part of the viscus and the chest wall.

When an abnormality of the percussion note is due to pulmonary consolidation or collapse it is usually possible to identify the lobe or lobes involved by reference to the surface marking of the fissures but, unless a lobe is totally consolidated, the area over which the percussion note is impaired is often much smaller than would be expected from its surface marking. This is

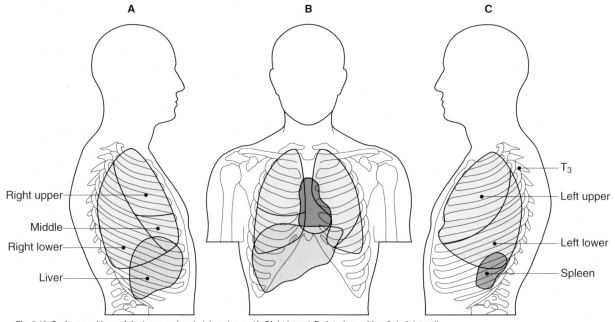

Fig. 5.12 Surface markings of the lungs and underlying viscera (A. Right lateral. B. Arterio-position C. Left lateral).

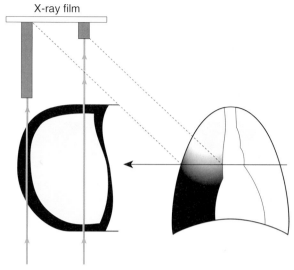

X-ray film

X-ray source

Fig. 5.13 Radiographic appearances of a right pleural effusion. A horizontal section of hemithorax close to the upper margin of the effusion (represented by the horizontal arrow) shows that there is at this site a similar amount of liquid anteriorly, posteriorly and laterally. However, because of the shape of the hemithorax, the x-ray beams traverse more fluid laterally than they do centrally. This produces the characteristic radiographic shape of a pleural effusion shadow with a curved upper margin ascending towards the axilla.

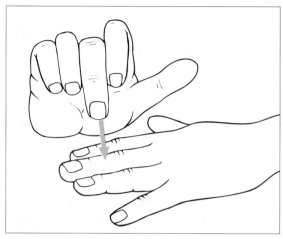

Fig. 5.14 Technique of percussion.

even more striking when a lobe is collapsed. With a pleural effusion the area of dullness on percussion is unrelated to the surface anatomy of the lobes. Except with loculated effusions, it is situated over the lower part of the hemithorax with the patient in the upright position. When there are no pleural adhesions the radiograph shows an effusion to have a curved upper border, which misleadingly suggests more fluid being present laterally (Fig. 5.13).

In localising the position of a pulmonary or pleural lesion the observer should make use of the breath sounds and voice sounds in addition to the percussion note. However, small lesions, such as areas of segmental consolidation or collapse, may not produce any abnormal physical signs. Even with larger lesions the signs may be partly or completely obscured if the lungs are emphysematous.

Technique of percussion

The basic technique of percussion for a right-handed clinician is as follows:

Examination

❑ Place the left hand on the chest wall, palm downwards, fingers slightly separated with the second phalanx of the middle finger over the area to be percussed, usually an intercostal space.
❑ Firmly press the left middle finger against the chest wall.
❑ Strike the centre of the second phalanx with the tip of the right middle finger held at a right angle (to produce a 'hammer' effect) and with the entire movement coming from the wrist joint (Fig. 5.14).
❑ Compare the note obtained from identical sites on the two sides.
❑ Map out any area of impaired resonance (including cardiac and hepatic dullness (p. 181)) by percussing from a resonant to a dull area.

The positions in which the percussion note on the two sides should be compared are as follows:

• *Anterior chest wall* (Fig. 5.15): (a) clavicle; (b) infraclavicular region; (c) second to sixth intercostal spaces.
• *Lateral chest wall* (Fig. 5.15): fourth to seventh intercostal spaces.
• *Posterior chest wall* (Fig. 5.16): (a) trapezius, percussing downwards on lung apex; (b) above the level spine of scapula; (c) at intervals of 4–5 cm from below the level of spine of scapula down to the eleventh rib.

The lung apices are percussed by placing the left middle finger across the anterior border of the trapezius muscle, overlapping the supraclavicular fossa, and directing the percussion downwards (Fig. 5.17). Percussion of the clavicle may be of value in detecting lesions of the upper lobe. The same technique of percussion of the chest wall should be used as direct

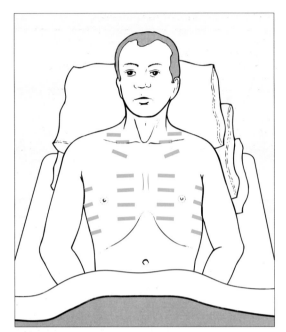

Fig. 5.15 Sites for percussion – anterior and lateral chest wall.

percussion of the clavicle can cause pain. The correct situation for percussion is within the medial third of the clavicle just lateral to its expanded medial end. Percussion more laterally will merely elicit the dullness produced by the muscle masses of the shoulder.

Tidal percussion. A crude impression of the range of diaphragmatic movement can be obtained by measuring

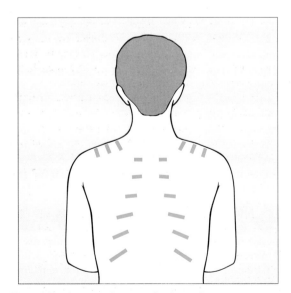

Fig. 5.16 Sites for percussion – posterior chest wall.

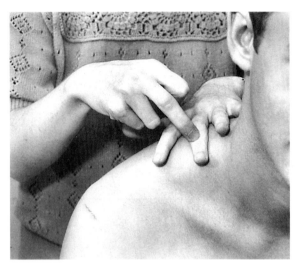

Fig. 5.17 Percussing the right apex from behind.

the distance between the lower borders of pulmonary resonance at the back of the chest in full inspiration and forced expiration, but this procedure is of little practical value.

The terms used to describe different types of percussion note are shown in Table 5.10.

KEY POINTS

- The percussion note is impaired or dull whenever aerated lung is separated from chest wall by pleural fluid or thickening, or when lung tissue is rendered airless by consolidation, collapse or fibrosis.

- Always compare identical sites on the two sides.

- General hyperresonance on both sides is rarely of clinical significance.

- Areas of impaired percussion are often smaller than anticipated from the surface markings.

- Map out areas of impaired resonance by percussing from resonant to dull.

Auscultation

Auscultation of the lungs is important in the diagnosis of certain respiratory diseases, but is of little or no value in others. In bronchial asthma and pleurisy, for example, the stethoscope provides information which cannot be obtained in any other way. In contrast, auscultation is unhelpful in the early diagnosis of pulmonary tuberculosis, which may reach an advanced stage before any abnormality can be detected.

Breath sounds and voice sounds

Breath sounds are produced by vibrations of the vocal cords caused by the turbulent flow of air through the larynx during breathing. The sounds so produced are transmitted along the trachea and bronchi and through the lungs to the chest wall. In their passage through normal lungs the intensity and frequency pattern of the sounds are altered. When they are heard through a stethoscope on the chest wall they have a characteristic rustling quality to which the term *vesicular* is applied. The intensity of the sounds increases steadily during inspiration and then quickly fades away during the first one-third of expiration (Fig. 5.18). Disease of the bronchi, lungs and pleura may alter the breath sounds in two main ways:

- Diminished vesicular breath sounds. If the conduction of the breath sounds to the chest wall is attenuated they remain vesicular but are diminished in amplitude (see Table 5.11). This change in the breath sounds is invariably accompanied by a reduction in the amplitude of the conducted voice sounds.
- Bronchial breath sounds. If the lung tissue through which the breath sounds are transmitted from the air passages to the chest wall has lost its normal spongy consistence and has become firm or solid, e.g. in consolidation or fibrosis, the sounds picked up by the stethoscope resemble more closely those pro-

Table 5.11 Causes of diminished vesicular breathing

Reduced airflow	*Reduced conduction*
Generalised (e.g. emphysema)	Thick chest wall
Localised (e.g. bronchial obstruction by tumour)	Pleural effusion/thickening
	Small pneumothorax

duced at the larynx than those heard over normal lung. Such *bronchial breath sounds* are found whenever (a) normal lung tissue is replaced by a uniform conducting medium, be it consolidation, fibrosis or collapse, and (b) the relevant major bronchus remains patent.

The pathological processes which produce these criteria are detailed in Table 5.15 and some are illustrated in Fig. 5.19.

Bronchial breath sounds (Fig. 5.18) resemble more closely those produced at the larynx than those heard over normal lung. The criteria for the recognition of bronchial breathing must be strict and unambiguous. Four conditions must be satisfied (see Table 5.12)

The pitch of bronchial breath sounds varies according to the nature of the pulmonary changes. As high-frequency sounds are selectively conducted through consolidated lung tissue, high-pitched bronchial breath sounds are heard in lobar or segmental pneumonia (Fig. 5.19B). Fibrotic lung tissue, on the other hand, transmits sounds of lower frequency and thus produces lower pitched bronchial breath sounds. With voice sounds, there is a similar selective conduction of certain frequencies.

When bronchial breath sounds traverse air-containing cavities in their passage to the chest wall, they may occasionally acquire a resonating *amphoric* quality, resembling the sound produced by blowing across the top of a bottle. Breath sounds may be intermediate in type between vesicular and bronchial, for example vesicular with prolonged expiration.

Vocal resonance (voice sounds) conducted through consolidated lung tissue, extensive fibrosis and pulmonary collapse associated with a patent bronchus resemble more closely those produced at the larynx than those heard over normal lungs in that they are louder and more distinct. In some cases a whispered

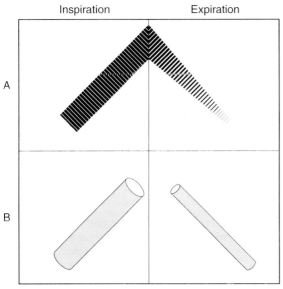

Fig. 5.18 Diagrammatic representation of breath sounds.
A. vesicular; **B.** bronchial.

Table 5.12 Bronchial breath sounds

- Both the inspiratory and expiratory sounds are blowing, sometimes called tubular, in character
- The expiratory sound is as long and as loud as the inspiratory sound
- There is a pause between the end of inspiration and the beginning of the expiratory sound
- Vocal resonance is increased to allow whispering pectoriloquy to be heard

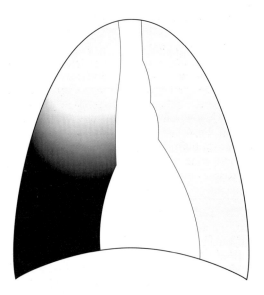

Chest expansion — Reduced
Percussion note — Stony dull
Breath sounds — Absent or decreased
(occasionally bronchial)
Added sounds — None
A **Vocal resonance** — Absent or decreased

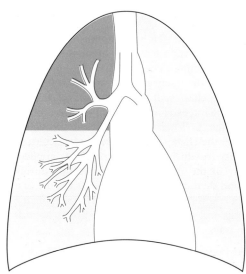

Chest expansion — Reduced
Percussion note — Dull
Breath sounds — Bronchial
Added sounds — Crepitations
Vocal resonance — Increased (whispering
pectoriloquy) B

	Right	Left
Chest expansion	— Reduced	Reduced
Percussion note	— Dull	Dull
Breath sounds	— Absent or decreased	Bronchial
Added sounds	— None	Crepitations ± rhonchi
Vocal resonance	— Absent or decreased	Increasing (whispering pectoriloquy)

C

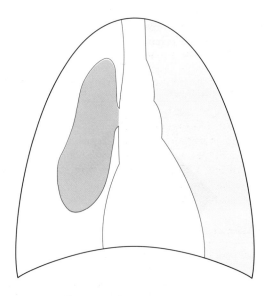

Chest expansion — Reduced
Percussion note — Hyperresonant
Breath sounds — Absent or decreased
Added sounds — Usually none
Vocal resonance — Decreased D

Fig. 5.19 Clinical findings in A. right-sided effusion, B. right-sided consolidation, C. collapse, with bronchial obstruction on the right side and with patent bronchi on the left side, and D. right pneumothorax.

voice may be transmitted almost without distortion so that individual syllables can be clearly recognised (*whispering pectoriloquy*).

Added sounds

Added sounds heard on auscultation of the chest are of three types: rhonchi, crepitations and pleural sounds (Table 5.13).

Rhonchus is a latinised version of the Greek *rhonchos*, meaning wheezing, and its use should be restricted to the musical sounds produced in narrowed bronchi. The word crepitation, derived from the latin *crepitare*, to crack or rattle, is a term which can be appropriately used to describe all non-musical crackling sounds.

It has been suggested that the terms wheezes and crackles should replace rhonchi and crepitations. The word wheeze is, however, also used to describe the sound heard without a stethoscope in patients with generalised expiratory airflow obstruction. The substitution of wheezes for rhonchi may give rise to confusion.

Rhonchi (wheezes). These are musical sounds of high, medium or low pitch produced by the passage of air through narrowed bronchi. Rhonchi caused by mucosal oedema or spasm of the bronchial musculature are usually superimposed upon the expiratory phase of the respiratory noise, which is always prolonged when rhonchi are present. Rhonchi heard during inspiration are more often due to secretions in the large bronchi and may disappear, or at least become less numerous, after coughing. A constant low-pitched rhonchus (fixed rhonchus) usually indicates partial obstruction of a major bronchus by a local lesion, such as a tumour or an inhaled foreign body.

Crepitations (crackles). These are non-musical sounds mainly audible during inspiration. At one time they were attributed to the bubbling of air through secretions in the bronchi and alveoli, but that view is no longer tenable, except when the sounds originate in the

major bronchi, dilated bronchi (bronchiectasis) and pulmonary cavities. In these circumstances the presence of secretions is confirmed by the observation that the crepitations either decrease in number or disappear temporarily after coughing.

A much more frequent cause of crepitations in lung disease is the explosive reopening, during inspiration, of peripheral small airways which have become occluded during expiration. These crepitations are most numerous during the second half of inspiration and in some cases confined to its last part (end-inspiratory crepitations). Such crepitations are not influenced by coughing, and are more conspicuous over the lower parts of the lungs because in the upright position small airway closure is more liable to occur there than in the upper lobes.

Pleural sounds. A *pleural rub* is a leathery or creaking sound produced by movement of the visceral pleura over the parietal pleura, when both surfaces are roughened as by fibrinous exudate. It is usually heard at two separate stages in the respiratory cycle, towards the end of inspiration and just after the beginning of expiration. A pleural rub may be inaudible during normal breathing but can be heard when the patient is asked to breathe deeply.

A *pneumothorax click* is a rhythmical sound, synchronous with cardiac systole, which may be heard with or sometimes without the aid of a stethoscope. It is produced when there is air between the two layers of pleura overlying the heart.

Technique of auscultation

The design of stethoscope recommended for routine clinical use provides the choice of a bell or diaphragm. As most of the sounds reaching the chest wall from the bronchi and lungs are in the low-frequency range, the bell with a rubber rim cover should normally be used in preference to the diaphragm. Another reason for selecting the bell is that stretching of the skin and hairs under the diaphragm during deep breathing is apt to produce sounds which may be difficult to distinguish from a pleural rub and/or crepitations. It is also impossible in some thin patients to achieve full contact between the diaphragm and the skin of the chest wall, and if this is the case nothing may be heard.

It is sometimes difficult to distinguish between a low-pitched rhonchus, coarse crepitations and a pleural rub. If there is any doubt auscultation should be repeated after a forceful cough, when rhonchi or crepitations will usually alter in character or disappear, while a pleural rub will remain unchanged. Patients with pleural pain should not be asked to cough or take

Table 5.13 Added sounds

• Rhonchi (wheezes)	Musical sounds produced by air passing through narrowed airways, e.g. asthma
• Crepitations (crackles)	Non-musical sounds mainly heard during inspiration caused by reopening of occluded small airways or air bubbling through secretions, e.g. pulmonary oedema, fibrosing alveolitis, resolving pneumonia, bronchiectasis
• Pleural friction rub	Leathery or creaking sounds produced by movement of roughened pleural surfaces, e.g. pleurisy caused by pneumonia, pulmonary infarction. Usually associated with pleural pain

deep breaths until an effective analgesic has been given.

Cough may also help when the breath sounds are diminished or absent over a lobe or segment thought to be involved in pneumonia. This may be due to bronchial obstruction by secretions, and bronchial breath sounds may become audible when these secretions are dislodged by coughing.

The technique of auscultation may also have to be modified to meet the needs of individual cases.

Examination

❑ Perform auscultation with the patient relaxed and breathing deeply and fairly rapidly through the mouth.
❑ Avoid prolonged deep breathing, which may cause giddiness or even tetany.
❑ Avoid auscultation within 2–3 cm of the midline.
❑ Auscultate the two sides alternately, comparing findings over a large number of equivalent positions to ensure that small localised lesions are not missed.
❑ Auscultate in two stages; compare first the amplitude of breath sounds and then the vocal resonance.
❑ Auscultate anteriorly from above the clavicle down to the sixth rib, laterally from the axilla to the eighth rib and posteriorly down to the level of the eleventh rib.
❑ In each area listen in turn to the quality and amplitude of the inspiratory phase and then to the expiratory phase. Identify if there is a gap between the two and listen for added sounds.
❑ If necessary, repeat after coughing.
❑ Assess the quality and amplitude of vocal resonance by asking the patient to say 'one, one, one' and, if resonance is increased, ask the patient to whisper.

Special situations

❑ Do not ask a patient with severe pleural pain to take frequent deep breaths. Test the vocal resonance first. If an area is found in which the voice sounds are increased, ask the patient to take one or two deep breaths and bronchial breath sounds will usually be heard in the same area.
❑ When abnormal breath sounds are heard, map out the extent of the lesion by moving the bell of the stethoscope with each breath from the normal towards the abnormal zone and note the level at which the breath sounds change.

The information which should be obtained from auscultation is listed in Table 5.14.

Auscultation within 2–3 cm of the midline, either

Table 5.14 Information obtained from auscultation

- The type and amplitude of breath sounds
- The type and number of any added sounds and their position in the respiratory cycle
- The quality and amplitude of the conducted voice sounds

anteriorly or posteriorly, may give misleading information in regard to the type of breath sounds and voice sounds, particularly in the upper half of the chest, where the stethoscope may pick up sounds transmitted directly from the trachea and main bronchi to the chest wall. Bronchial breath sounds heard in these situations should be disregarded in the absence of other pathological signs.

Examples of common disorders which give rise to abnormal clinical findings which are usually easily detected by inspection, percussion and auscultation are shown diagrammatically in Figure 5.19.

The interpretation of auscultatory findings

Causes of bronchial breath sounds and diminished or absent breath sounds are given in Table 5.15. When bronchial breath sounds are audible the voice sounds are louder than normal and whispering pectoriloquy is usually present. When breath sounds are diminished vocal resonance is decreased in amplitude to the same degree as the breath sounds are diminished.

Rhonchi (wheezes) are heard diffusely over both lungs in bronchial asthma and in most cases of acute and chronic bronchitis. In asthma the rhonchi are medium or high pitched and are mainly heard during expiration, which is prolonged. In bronchitis they are

Table 5.15 Bronchial, diminished or absent breath sounds

Auscultatory findings	Disease process
High-pitched bronchial breath sounds	Pneumonic consolidation (Fig. 5.19B) Large superficial pulmonary cavity Collapsed lung or lobe when large bronchi are patent (Fig. 5.19C) Lung compressed by pleural effusion (sometimes) Tension pneumothorax (sometimes)
Low-pitched bronchial breath sounds	Localised areas of pulmonary fibrosis e.g. chronic pulmonary tuberculosis, chronic suppurative pneumonia
Diminished or absent breath sounds	Pleural effusion (Fig. 5.19A) Marked pleural thickening Collapsed lung or lobe when large bronchi occluded (Fig. 5.19C) Pneumothorax (Fig. 5.19D) Emphysema (symmetrical diminution over both lungs)

usually low or medium pitched and both inspiratory and expiratory. A localised rhonchus may be heard over a partially obstructed large bronchus. If the obstruction is caused by a fixed lesion, such as a tumour or foreign body in a large bronchus, the rhonchus is usually louder during inspiration, is not altered by coughing and is often accompanied by stridor. If due to secretions, these are usually removed by coughing, which causes the rhonchus to disappear.

Forced expiratory time (FET) is measured by placing the chest piece of a stethoscope over the trachea and timing the duration of forced expiration following a full inspiration. This is normally less than 4 seconds. A prolonged FET is indicative of diffuse airflow limitation, and is a feature of chronic bronchitis, emphysema and bronchial asthma.

Crepitations (crackles) caused by secretions within the large bronchi in acute or chronic bronchitis, or in resolving bronchopneumonia, are widespread and bilateral, while those audible over resolving lobar or segmental pneumonic consolidation, dilated bronchi (bronchiectasis), lung abscesses or tuberculous cavities are localised to the site of the lesions. In all these conditions they are audible throughout inspiration, and alter after coughing (p. 155).

Crepitations in other parenchymal lung conditions, such as interstitial pulmonary oedema, allergic and fibrosing alveolitis, and perhaps early pneumonic consolidation and miliary tuberculosis, are in contrast audible mainly during the second half of inspiration, and are uninfluenced by coughing. No useful purpose is served by trying to distinguish between moist and dry and between fine, medium and coarse crepitations. It is much more important to note their timing in the respiratory cycle and whether or not they are affected by coughing.

A *pleural rub* is heard over areas of pleurisy. It disappears as soon as the visceral and parietal pleura are separated by fluid, but often remains audible above an effusion. If pleurisy involves the pleura adjacent to the pericardium, a pleuropericardial rub may also be heard. This is a rather misleading term since the pericardial element in the sound is not due to pericarditis. It is caused merely by roughened pleural surfaces adjacent to the pericardium being moved across one another by cardiac pulsation. A pleuropericardial rub may, in some cases, be impossible to distinguish from a pericardial rub.

Integration of physical signs

Certain groups of physical signs are typically associated with certain pathological changes in the lungs and pleura. Such changes are not necessarily specific for one particular disease. For example, the physical signs of consolidation may occur in pneumonia, pulmonary infarction or tuberculosis, and those of pleural effusion may be present in malignant disease, empyema or cardiac failure. Each group of physical signs therefore gives an indication only of the gross pathology of the lesion, and not of its precise nature, the diagnosis of which depends on an analysis of all the clinical and other evidence. The characteristic physical signs of the more common lesions are shown in Figure 5.19, namely pleural effusion, consolidation, collapse and pneumothorax. It must be emphasised that these signs are not necessarily present in every case. An area of consolidation or collapse may, for example, be too small to give rise to the classical pattern of physical signs. Furthermore, the picture may be confused by the coincidence of two groups of signs, as when consolidation is accompanied by pleural effusion. Difficulties are also apt to arise when the differential diagnosis rests on the observer's estimate of the position of the mediastinum. In patients with pulmonary collapse or pleural effusion mediastinal displacement is an inconstant feature and, even when present, may be difficult to detect since the trachea may be displaced and the apex beat is not always palpable.

KEY POINTS

- Vesicular breathing is diminished if there is reduced airflow or impairment of conduction from the lung to the chest wall.

- Bronchial breathing occurs when the relevant major bronchus remains patent and normal lung tissue is replaced by a uniform conducting medium.

- A fixed low-pitched rhonchus usually indicates partial obstruction of a major bronchus.

- Crepitations are usually caused by explosive reopening of peripheral airways during inspiration. These are more conspicuous over the lower lung fields and are not influenced by coughing.

- Crepitations caused by bronchial secretions may decrease or even disappear on coughing.

- Patients with pleuritic pain should not be asked to cough or take deep breaths until effective analgesia has been given.

- Auscultate the chest using the bell with a rubber rim cover.

- Avoid auscultating within 2–3 cm of the midline.

- It is often helpful to repeat auscultation after asking the patient to cough.

FURTHER INVESTIGATIONS

In many cases it is possible to make a reliable diagnosis from the history and clinical examination. This applies, for example, to conditions such as bronchial asthma, chronic bronchitis and to some cases of pneumonia and pulmonary infarction. At other times clinical examination fails to reveal any abnormality and the diagnosis depends entirely on specialised investigations, particularly radiology.

Pulmonary tuberculosis and bronchial carcinoma are two important diseases which may not give rise to any clinical abnormality in the early stages. It is therefore essential to advise chest radiological examination whenever one of these conditions is suspected from the history. It is not possible to determine accurately the site of most abnormalities visible on posteroanterior or anteroposterior radiographs and a lateral should be used to elucidate any abnormality shown on a PA film (Fig. 5.20). A comparison between current and previous films, if they can be obtained, may provide vital diagnostic information:

- If a pulmonary opacity has not increased in size over a period of a year or longer, a diagnosis of bronchial carcinoma is highly improbable.
- If an opacity has become smaller or less dense in the course of a few days or weeks, pneumonia or pulmonary infarction is its most likely cause.
- If a lesion was not present on an earlier film, or has become larger, it is almost certainly a tumour or an active tuberculous infection.

By means of radiology the precise anatomical position of a lesion can be determined, and from this and other features its pathology may be deduced.

Even when a precise diagnosis has been made, it is usually desirable to measure the effect of the disease on respiratory function. This is useful for the assessment of fitness for work and suitability for certain forms of treatment, such as surgery for bronchial carcinoma.

A full account of all the special methods of investigation cannot be given here, nor is it possible to indicate in any detail the information they can be expected to provide. The summary in Table 5.16 is therefore intended to serve only as a guide to the value of each investigation and the indications for its use.

Finally, the important symptom of haemoptysis (Tables 5.17 to 5.19) is used to illustrate how the nature of the presentation influences the likely diagnosis and hence the choice of investigations.

KEY POINTS

- Groups of physical signs are typically associated with certain pathological changes but are not necessarily specific for any particular disease.

- Tuberculosis and bronchial carcinoma are two conditions in which there may be no abnormal physical signs.

- A chest radiograph is an essential investigation in all patients with suspected pulmonary or pleural disease.

- Comparison of the present and a previous chest radiograph may provide vital information.

- Once a diagnosis has been established it is often important to complete the investigations by assessing respiratory function.

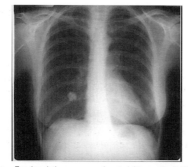 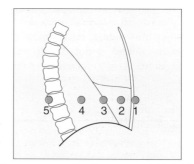

Fig. 5.20 Chest radiographs. For descriptive purposes the straight x-ray is divided into zones – upper, mid and lower – separated by imaginary horizontal lines between the anterior ends of the second and fourth ribs. There is a round shadow in the right lower zone of the straight x-ray. The lateral view shows five possible sites of the abnormality; **1.** anterior chest wall or pleura; **2.** right middle lobe; **3.** fissure between the lobes; **4.** right lower lobe; **5.** posterior chest wall or pleura.

Table 5.16 Summary of respiratory investigations

Sputum	Should be examined in all cases of suspected pulmonary infection and most patients with bronchial infection. Specific requests for examination of separate specimens for tubercle bacilli and fungi (including *Pneumocystis* pneumonia) must be made
Induced sputum	In patients who cannot produce sputum the inhalation of nebulised hypertonic saline can induce sputum production
Skin tests	Tuberculin test: chiefly of value in excluding present or past-tuberculous infection Kveim test: a positive reaction confirms a diagnosis of sarcoidosis Skin sensitivity tests (usually common inhaled allergens, e.g. house dust mite, pollens, animal danders) confirm presence or absence of atopy. Not usually used for diagnostic purposes
Blood tests	Total and differential white cell count is helpful in cases of pulmonary bacterial infection and in diseases in which there is pulmonary radiographic shadowing and a high peripheral blood eosinophil count (pulmonary eosinophilia). Blood culture should be a routine investigation in all cases of acute pneumonia Examination of serum for viral and other antibodies may be of value in determining the cause of 'atypical' pneumonia
Nasal sinus radiograph	Integral part of the investigation of chronic upper respiratory tract infection and of some pulmonary infections
Chest radiograph	Essential in initial investigation of all patients in whom pulmonary or pleural disease suspected
Lateral chest radiograph	Essential to localise the site of an abnormality visible on the posteroanterior (PA) radiograph (Fig. 5. 20)
Previous radiograph	May be invaluable in determining whether a radiographic abnormality is new or old, or increasing or decreasing in size
Tomography	Allows an opacity or part of an opacity to be visualised clearly in different planes or cuts. Can be of help in differentiating between a pulmonary tumour and a tuberculous lesion. Now rarely used if computed tomography is available
Computed tomography	Provides accurate information about single or multiple pulmonary lesions. Allows assessment of structures in the mediastinum including lymph nodes. High-resolution CT is useful in the investigation of diffuse interstitial lung disease. It has replaced bronchography for the diagnosis of bronchiectasis
Screening	Allows diaphragm movement to be observed. Can detect unilateral diaphragmatic paralysis. Ultrasonography is now used more often for this purpose
Ultrasonography	Used in localisation of loculated pleural effusions. Can be used to aid needle aspiration of lesions invading the chest wall. Also can assess diaphragm movement
Pulmonary angiography	Outlines pulmonary vascular bed. Used in the assessment of pulmonary embolism and in some cases of pulmonary hypertension
Radionuclide scanning	Accurate assessment of lung perfusion (Q scan) and ventilation (V scan). Its main use is in the diagnosis of pulmonary embolism/infarction. A Q scan can be used in patients with previously normal lungs and heart. A V/Q scan is necessary in patients with chronic lung disease
Bronchoscopy	Diagnosis and assessment of operability of bronchial carcinoma (biopsy, brushings and bronchial washings) Diagnosis of pulmonary infections (diffuse and localised) in patients who cannot produce sputum (bronchial washings/brushings) Assessment of diffuse interstitial lung diseases, e.g. fibrosing/allergic alveolitis, sarcoids, etc (transbronchial biopsy and differential cell counts of bronchoalveolar lavage fluid)
Pleural aspiration and biopsy	Aspiration of pleural liquid from pleural effusions and 'blind' biopsy of parietal pleura. Diagnosis of malignant and tuberculous pleural effusion usually established in this way
Thoracoscopy	Allows visualisation of pleural space and biopsy of abnormal tissue. Mainly used in the investigation of pleural effusions when diagnosis has not been made by pleural needle aspiration and biopsy. Also allows video-assisted lung biopsy to be performed
Lymph node aspiration/biopsy	Allows cytological/histological examination of supraclavicular lymph glands (carcinoma, sarcoidosis and tuberculosis)
Mediastinoscopy	Allows visualisation of structures in anterior mediastinum and biopsy of lymph glands. Used in the diagnosis and assessment of operability of bronchial carcinoma
Tests of respiratory function	
Arterial blood gas analysis	Essential investigation in all ill patients with respiratory problems. Partial pressure of oxygen (PaO_2) low in severe asthma, pneumonia, pulmonary embolism and oedema (type I respiratory failure). Partial pressure of carbon dioxide also elevated in very severe asthma, severe chronic bronchitis and emphysema (type II respiratory failure). Hydrogen ion concentration or pH allows assessment of degree of respiratory acidosis caused by carbon dioxide retention
Pulmonary function tests	Forced expiratory volume in one second (FEV_1) and forced vital capacity (FVC) measured by spirometry provide an accurate assessment of the degree of airflow obstruction in asthma and chronic bronchitis. The FEV_1/FVC ratio is less than 70–75% in all patients with diffuse airflow obstruction. Serial measurements of peak expiratory flow (PEF) are invaluable in the diagnosis and management of asthma
Lung volumes and transfer factor	Used in the assessment of diffuse interstitial lung diseases (e.g. fibrosing alveolitis) in which lung volumes are decreased (restrictive defect) and transfer factor is often low. Lung volumes are increased in emphysema and transfer factor is decreased

Table 5.17 Causes of haemoptysis

Common causes	Uncommon causes
Pulmonary thromboembolism	Bronchial adenoma
Bronchial carcinoma	Aspergilloma
Tuberculosis	Alveolar haemorrhage
Bronchiectasis	(Goodpasture's syndrome,
Chronic bronchitis	idiopathic pulmonary
Pulmonary oedema	haemosiderosis
Suppurative pneumonia	Anticoagulant therapy
	Blood dyscrasias

With the exception of chronic bronchitis and some cases of bronchiectasis all the common causes usually result in an abnormal chest radiograph at the time of presentation

Table 5.18 Relating the presentation of haemoptysis to the common causes

Nature of presentation	Consider
Massive haemoptysis	Tuberculosis
	Bronchiectasis
	Pulmonary thromboembolism
	Bronchial carcinoma
	Suppurative pneumonia
Scanty haemoptysis	Bronchial carcinoma
	Pulmonary thromboembolism
	Chronic bronchitis
Haemoptysis and purulent sputum	Bronchiectasis
	Chronic bronchitis
	Suppurative pneumonia
Recurrent haemoptysis	Pulmonary thromboembolism
	Bronchial carcinoma
	Bronchiectasis
	Chronic bronchitis

Table 5.19 Relating the investigations to the suspected diagnosis

Suspected diagnosis	Possible further investigations
Pulmonary thromboembolism	Ventilation perfusion lung scan
	Ascending venography
	Pulmonary angiography
Bronchial carcinoma	Sputum examination for malignant cells
	Bronchoscopy
	Transthoracic needle aspiration
Tuberculosis	Sputum examination for tubercle bacilli if no sputum
	Bronchoscopy to obtain bronchial washings
	Tuberculin test
Bronchiectasis	Sputum examination for bacterial pathogens
	CT scan if chest radiography not diagnostic
	Bronchography (rarely necessary if CT available)
Chronic bronchitis	Sputum for malignant cells
	Bronchoscopy may be necessary to exclude bronchial carcinoma
Pulmonary oedema	Electrocardiography
	Echocardiography
Suppurative pneumonia	Sputum examination for bacterial pathogens tubercle bacilli and fungi

M. J. Ford • D. W. Hamer-Hodges

6

The alimentary and genitourinary systems

The diagnosis of intra-abdominal disease is more often dependent upon a careful history than on the presence of physical signs. Pain is prominent among the symptoms encountered in the alimentary and genitourinary systems. When pain is present, interrogation is essential before any investigation is performed. If this is neglected, unnecessary tests may result in the discovery of asymptomatic abnormalities such as hiatus hernia or gall stones, leading to inappropriate management and even unnecessary surgery.

THE HISTORY

ALIMENTARY SYMPTOMS

Disorders of the alimentary tract may present with oral symptoms, e.g. dry mouth or painful mouth, difficulty in swallowing (dysphagia), nausea and vomiting, abdominal pain, heartburn, indigestion (dyspepsia), loss of appetite (anorexia), weight loss, abdominal distension, altered bowel habit, rectal bleeding and jaundice. Sometimes, alimentary disease is suggested only by the occurrence of a secondary feature such as anaemia. Occasionally patients may conceal important symptoms such as rectal bleeding because of embarrassment, a belief that the cause is trivial or fear of serious illness. The clinician must not only listen carefully to the patient's presenting complaints but also enquire systematically about the other principal symptoms of abdominal disease. It is also important to remember that, even in the absence of disease, alimentary symptoms may develop in response to emotional distress.

Painful mouth

Soreness of the lips, tongue or buccal mucosa has a wide variety of causes, including iron, folate or vitamin B_{12} deficiency, dermatological disorders, chemotherapy, aphthous ulceration and infective stomatitis (p. 62). Gastrointestinal disorders particularly associated with mouth ulcers and stomatitis include inflammatory bowel disease and gluten enteropathy. A history of recurrent painful tiny mouth ulcers with its onset at the menarche, exacerbations during menstruation and a family history of mouth ulcers suggests idiopathic aphthous ulceration.

Difficulty in swallowing (dysphagia)

The swallowing mechanism involves the brain stem, the glossopharyngeal and vagal nerves and the enteric

Table 6.1 Common causes of dysphagia

Painful mouth or throat	Aphthous ulceration
	Tonsillitis
	Glandular fever
Neurological	Pseudobulbar palsy
	Bulbar palsy
Neuromuscular	Achalasia
	Myasthenia gravis
Luminal obstruction	Peptic stricture
	Oesophageal carcinoma

nervous system of oesophageal smooth muscle. The swallowing reflex begins with an oral phase which drives the food bolus into the pharynx; the pharyngeal phase ensues with closure of the larynx, relaxation of the upper pharyngeal sphincter (cricopharyngeus) and sequential contraction of the pharyngeal constrictors to propel the bolus into the oesophagus. The oesophageal phase comprises oesophageal peristaltic contractions associated with relaxation of the lower oesophageal sphincter.

Retrosternal chest pain experienced during swallowing, *odynophagia*, is characteristic of inflammatory disorders of the oesophagus, e.g. peptic oesophagitis and herpetic oesophagitis. Food sticking during swallowing is an important symptom of oesophageal disease for which an explanation should always be sought. Some common causes of dysphagia are given in Table 6.1.

Dysphagia is usually first apparent for solids and progresses to affect the swallowing of fluids. Difficulty in initiating swallowing fluids, rather than solids, accompanied by coughing and spluttering suggests a neurological disorder. Dysphagia localised to the level of the cricoid cartilage may result from tumour, stricture, pharyngeal pouch or from a reflex effect resulting from disease in the lower oesophagus. Dysphagia localised to the level of the lower sternum suggests disease of the lower oesophagus, e.g. tumour, achalasia or peptic oesophagitis. Dysphagia may be slowly progressive or intermittent, occurring only with a large food bolus such as meat. Dysphagia may be painful or painless. Food sticking at the level of narrowing may produce severe *impact pain* and suggests an intact sensory innervation. It is relieved when food is either regurgitated or passes through the stricture into the stomach. Painless dysphagia suggests denervation of the oesophagus and is often due to tumour. In patients with a pharyngeal pouch or long-standing oesophageal obstruction, recognisable food may be regurgitated long after it was eaten. Achalasia of the cardia and chronic oesophageal obstruction may produce bouts of nocturnal cough and dyspnoea as a result of the reflux of oesophageal contents into the trachea and major bronchi, sometimes resulting in an aspiration pneumonia.

Dysphagia should not be confused with *globus*, a symptom in which there is a feeling of a lump in the throat often associated with suppressed emotional distress; it is not associated with eating, does not interfere with swallowing and is rapidly relieved by the release of pent-up emotions, e.g. crying.

Nausea and vomiting

The combination of nausea and vomiting usually suggests an upper gastrointestinal disorder but may also be a prominent feature of non-alimentary disorders (Table 6.2). In most instances, vomiting is preceded by nausea, but in some cases, e.g. intracranial tumour, the vomiting can occur without warning. Vomiting may also result from severe pain, as in renal or biliary colic or myocardial infarction, from systemic disease, metabolic disorders and drug therapy. Vomiting may be self-induced in patients with peptic ulceration (for pain relief) or with bulimia nervosa.

Gastric outlet obstruction is associated with the projectile vomiting of large volumes of gastric content, the vomitus also being noteworthy for the absence of bile staining. Obstruction distal to the pylorus produces bile-stained vomiting; the lower the level of intestinal obstruction, the more marked are the accompanying symptoms of abdominal distension and intestinal colic. Vomiting also occurs in other gastrointestinal disorders, such as acute gastroenteritis, acute cholecystitis, acute pancreatitis and hepatitis.

Enquiry should be made about the frequency of vomiting, the time of day at which it occurs and the taste, colour, quantity and smell of the vomitus. A yellow colour and bitter taste indicate the presence of the bile and imply regurgitation of duodenal content into the stomach. If the taste and smell are

Table 6.2 Non-alimentary causes of nausea and vomiting

Neurological	Vasovagal syncope
	Fear, severe pain
	Migraine, labyrinthine disorders
	Cerebral haemorrhage or tumour, meningitis
Psychological	Anorexia nervosa, bulimia
Metabolic	Renal failure, hyperparathyroidism
	Hypoadrenalism, diabetic ketoacidosis
	Pregnancy
Pharmacological	Digoxin, morphine, aminophylline
	Alcohol abuse

Table 6.3 Checklist for the history of haematemesis

- Colour and volume of vomitus and stools
- Violent retching preceding vomiting
- Past history of haematemesis, melaena, peptic ulcer or jaundice
- Recent drug ingestion, especially analgesics and non-steroidal anti-inflammatory drugs
- Alcohol consumption

inconspicuous, this suggests either the presence of achlorhydria or that the vomitus has been regurgitated from the oesophagus. Foul-smelling vomitus suggests pyloric obstruction, carcinoma of the stomach or gastrocolic fistula. Feculent vomiting may occur in distal small bowel or colonic obstruction and in gastrocolic fistula. Special attention should be paid to the presence of blood in the vomit (*haematemesis*) (Table 6.3). Bright red blood usually arises from pharyngeal or oesophageal lesions. Dark red vomitus, sometimes containing liver-like clots of blood, is due to profuse bleeding as may occur from oesophageal varices or peptic ulcer. In less acute upper gastrointestinal bleeding, the vomitus is often blackish or dark brown and can contain sediment like 'coffee grounds' resulting from the conversion of the haemoglobin to acid haematin by gastric acid. Whenever possible, the patient's description should be supplemented by inspection of the vomitus.

Abdominal pain

This is a common symptom. After listening to the patient's history, additional questions should be framed as described on page 29. Pain from unpaired intra-abdominal structures is usually in the midline. The patient should be asked to demonstrate the exact site and also any areas to which the pain may radiate. The character of the pain should be noted, e.g. 'stitch-like'. Frequency, duration and timing of attacks may be of diagnostic significance, as may be the associated features. In Table 6.4 the principal features of four common disorders are listed to illustrate the value of an analytical approach to diagnosis.

Abdominal pain, sometimes of great intensity, may result from disorders outwith the alimentary system. Associated features such as pain aggravated by movement and coughing usually help to indicate the likely origin of the pain. Table 6.5 illustrates some non-alimentary causes of abdominal pain.

Heartburn

Most healthy individuals have experienced heartburn: the sensation of a hot, burning retrosternal discomfort

Table 6.4 The analysis of abdominal pain

	Peptic ulcer	Biliary colic	Acute pancreatitis	Renal colic
Main site	Epigastric	Epigastric Right hypochondrium	Epigastric	From loin to groin
Radiation	Into the back	Beneath right scapula Right shoulder tip	Into the back May become generalised	Into genitalia
Character	Gnawing	Constant	Constant	Constant with small fluctuations
Severity	Mild to moderate	Severe	Severe	Severe
Duration	$\frac{1}{2}$–2 h	4–24 h	> 24 h	4–24 h
Frequency and periodicity	Remission for weeks or months History > 4 years	Unpredictable Patient able to enumerate attacks History < 6 months	Unpredictable	
Special times of occurrence	Nocturnal Between meals		After heavy drinking	Following periods of dehydration
Aggravating factors	Spicy foods Smoking Alcohol Aspirin	Patient unable to eat during pain	Alcohol	
Relieving factors	Food, antacids Vomiting		Eased by sitting upright	
Associated phenomena	Family history GI haemorrhage Perforation	Restlessness Vomiting Jaundice Symptom free between attacks	Gall stones Vomiting Jaundice Paralytic ileus	Restlessness Vomiting Haematuria Dysuria

often accompanied by the reflux of bitter-tasting gastric fluid into the mouth. It commonly occurs after

Table 6.5 Non-alimentary causes of abdominal pain

Condition	Clinical features
Myocardial infarction	Epigastric pain without tenderness Angor animi, hypotension Third heart sound Cardiac arrhythmias
Dissecting aortic aneurysm	Tearing interscapular pain Angor animi, hypotension Asymmetry of femoral pulses
Acute vertebral collapse	Lateralised pain restricting movement
Cord compression	Pain on percussion of thoracic spine Dermatomal hyperaesthesia Spinal cord signs
Pleurisy	Lateralised pain on coughing Chest signs, e.g. pleural rub
Herpes zoster	Dermatomal hyperaesthesia Vesicular eruption
Diabetic ketoacidosis	Cramp-like pain Vomiting, air hunger Tachycardia, ketotic breath
Torsion of the testis/ovary	Lower abdominal pain Nausea, vomiting Localised tenderness

meals or on bending or lying on the left side and is particularly frequent during pregnancy or following recent weight gain. Heartburn is caused by the reflux of acid, pepsin or bile into the oesophagus and may be accompanied by odynophagia and oesophagitis. It results from a combination of relaxation of the lower oesophageal sphincter and increased intra-abdominal pressure. It is commonly experienced by patients with a duodenal ulcer, oesophagitis or both. It may be accompanied by reflex salivation, *waterbrash*, when the mouth fills with tasteless saliva, in contrast to the bitter taste of acid reflux.

Dyspepsia (indigestion)

These vague terms are common complaints. Their use is of value in obtaining a history, but it is essential that the patient explains in detail what is meant. Thus 'indigestion' might describe nausea, heartburn, epigastric discomfort, abdominal pain, belching or a feeling of post-prandial bloating. It may even be used to describe angina pectoris.

Peptic ulcers usually produce characteristic symptoms, as shown in Table 6.4. Differentiation between oesophageal, gastric or duodenal ulcers on the basis of symptoms alone is often unreliable. Persistent dyspepsia,

Table 6.6 Functional dyspepsia: symptom subsets

Reflux-like	Acid reflux and heartburn relieved by antacids
Ulcer-like	Localised epigastric pain, frequent nocturnal pain, relief with food, antacids or vomiting
Dysmotility-like	Hunger, premature satiety, nausea, belching, abdominal pain and bloating When occurring in association with an altered bowel habit, the disorder is synonymous with the irritable bowel syndrome

in the absence of alimentary disease or a previous history of peptic ulcer disease, *functional dyspepsia*, is common and can be classified as in Table 6.6. Many patients with functional dyspepsia have more than one subset of these symptoms.

Anorexia and weight loss

A decrease in weight may be the first indication of disease (p. 36). The significance of weight loss relates to its duration and extent together with the presence or absence of anorexia (loss of appetite) or deliberate reduction in food intake. Weight loss of less than 3 kg in the previous 6 months is rarely of significance. Weight loss accompanied by severe anorexia or other alimentary symptoms may not necessarily be due to intra-abdominal disease; such features may occur, for example, in depression. Weight loss without a major reduction in food intake may occur in diabetes mellitus, hyperthyroidism or malabsorption syndromes.

Wind (flatulence)

Repeated belching, excessive or offensive rectal flatus, abdominal distension and even borborygmi may all be called 'wind' and the patient should therefore be asked for clarification. Belched wind is often swallowed (aerophagy) without the patient's awareness. Belching itself is of no significance and may be a feature of anxiety but sometimes occurs in an attempt to relieve abdominal pain or discomfort. The normal volume of flatus per rectum varies greatly from person to person in the range of 200–2000 ml per day. It consists of a mixture of gases derived principally from swallowed air together with the products of colonic bacterial fermentation of poorly absorbed carbohydrates. Excessive flatus is particularly troublesome in lactase deficiency and intestinal malabsorption. Absence of flatus may be a notable feature of intestinal obstruction. *Borborygmi*, audible bowel sounds, result from the movement of fluid and gas along the bowel; though often no more than a source of embarrassment, they may indicate disordered small bowel motility.

Abdominal distension (bloating)

The principal physical elements contributing to abdominal distension are *fat*, *flatus*, *faeces*, *fluid* and *fetus*. Increasing abdominal girth is usually due to adiposity and should alert the clinician to the possibility of alcohol abuse. Its development in a patient who is otherwise becoming thinner suggests intra-abdominal disease.

Ascites, the accumulation of fluid in the peritoneal cavity, is usually due to cirrhosis of the liver, malignancy, tuberculous peritonitis, cardiac or pericardial disease. The acute development of tense ascites suggests intra-abdominal malignancy, infective peritonitis or the onset of hepatic or portal vein obstruction.

Painless abdominal distension in women may be the presenting symptom of an ovarian cyst or of an undisclosed pregnancy. It is also typical of *pseudo-obstruction* in association with severe constipation in elderly patients taking drugs with anticholinergic effects, e.g. antidepressant therapy.

Painful abdominal distension suggests intestinal obstruction associated with intestinal colic. Chronic simple constipation rarely produces painful distension unless associated with other features of the irritable bowel syndrome. In childhood constipation, the possibility of Hirschsprung's disease must be considered and is suggested by painless abdominal distension and constipation from birth, often in the absence of faecal soiling. Fluctuating abdominal swelling which develops during the day but resolves overnight is particularly common in women and is rarely if ever due to organic disease. It usually occurs with other symptoms of the irritable bowel syndrome, namely abdominal pain relieved by defecation and altered bowel habit.

Altered bowel habit

The normal bowel habit varies between several evacuations per day to one every 3 days or so. Changes in bowel habit may be the first symptom of serious underlying disease. *Constipation* may be used by the patient to describe hard pellety stools, infrequent defecation or excessive straining at stool with difficulty in evacuation (*dyschezia*). Similarly, diarrhoea may be used to describe frequent defecation, loose or fluid stools, urgency of defecation, the persistent desire to defecate or faecal incontinence. *Tenesmus*, the feeling of incomplete rectal evacuation with a persistent desire to defecate, is common in infective colitis, rectal carcinoma, rectal prolapse and the irritable bowel syndrome.

The irritable bowel syndrome is a common cause of altered bowel function developing before the age of 50 years. The principal symptoms include episodic consti-pation and diarrhoea associated with abdominal distension, intermittent abdominal pain relieved by defecation and often accompanied with non-specific symptoms including dyspepsia, urinary frequency, backache and tiredness.

The important questions in the clinical history of diarrhoea include the following:

- Is the diarrhoea acute, chronic or intermittent?
- Is there tenesmus, urgency or incontinence?
- Is the stool watery, unformed or semisolid?
- Is the stool predominantly of large volume and not excessively frequent, suggesting small bowel disease, or small volume and very frequent, suggesting large bowel disease?
- Is blood, mucus or pus associated with the stool?
- Does diarrhoea occur during the night, suggesting organic disease?
- Is there a history of contact with diarrhoea or of travel abroad?
- Does the sexual history provide a clue (gay bowel syndrome, HIV)?
- Is there a history of alcohol abuse or relevant drug therapy?
- Is there a past medical history of GI surgery or relevant disorder?
- Is there a family history of GI disorder, e.g. gluten enteropathy, Crohn's?
- Are there any other GI symptoms, e.g. abdominal pain and vomiting?
- Are there symptoms of systemic disease, e.g. rigors or arthralgia?

The nature of any medication, prescribed or self-administered, should be established. Patients may be unaware of the laxative effects of some agents, e.g. magnesium-containing antacids and mefenamic acid, or the constipating effects of others, e.g. aluminium-containing antacids, codeine phosphate and anti-depressant therapy. Constipation and faecal incon-tinence or soiling may coexist, especially with faecal impaction in children or the elderly. It is important to determine the timing and frequency of defecation, any association with abdominal, rectal or anal pain and any difficulty, urgency or tenesmus experienced during evacuation. In addition, the patient should be asked to describe the appearance, colour, consistency and characteristics of the faeces. Sometimes words like 'stool' or 'faeces' are not understood, especially by children, and if there is doubt it is best to use a colloquial phrase.

Special enquiry should be made about the presence

Table 6.7 Characteristic abnormalities of stool colour

Black	Upper gastrointestinal haemorrhage Iron or colloidal bismuth therapy
Tarry black	Severe upper gastrointestinal haemorrhage
Pale and bulky	Small bowel or pancreatic malabsorption
Silvery pale	Pancreatic carcinoma
Blood and mucus	Ulcerative colitis

of blood and about pus or mucus, often described by the patient as 'slime'. Since many patients do not normally inspect their faeces, only positive observ-ations should be accepted; if necessary, the clinician should confirm the description by inspection of the stools. Abnormalities such as threadworms, round-worms or segments of tapeworms may be also present. Examples of abnormal stools are given in Table 6.7.

Rectal bleeding

The cause of this important symptom should always be determined. Though frequently due to haemorrhoids, these are so commonplace that their presence in a patient with rectal bleeding should not lead to the assumption of cause and effect. The differential diagnosis includes colorectal carcinoma, ulcerative colitis, infective colitis, diverticular disease and anal fissure. Bleeding from the anal canal is bright red; it is usually clearly separate from the faeces and often seen only on the toilet paper. Haemorrhoidal bleeding may be profuse and splash the toilet bowl or drip from the anus following defecation. Bleeding from an anal fissure is usually associated with anal pain which occurs during and after defecation. Colitis is com-monly associated with the symptoms of urgency of defecation and the passage of unformed stools with blood, mucus and pus. Both colonic adenomas and carcinomas may cause excessive mucus production. Bleeding from any site along the gastrointestinal tract may also present with syncope, peripheral circulatory failure or the symptoms of chronic anaemia.

Jaundice

Jaundice may be *haemolytic, hepatocellular* or *obstructive* in origin. A checklist for patients with a history of jaundice is shown in Table 6.8.

Haemolytic jaundice. Unconjugated hyperbilirubinaemia such as occurs in Gilbert's syndrome and haemolytic anaemia occur without either symptoms or urine dis-coloration (hence the term *acholuric jaundice*).

Table 6.8 Checklist for the history of jaundice

- Past medical history and operations
- Previous jaundice or hepatitis
- Blood transfusions
- Family history
- Sexual and contact history
- Travel history and immunisations
- Drug and alcohol history
- Skin tattooing
- Pruritus, dark urine, rigors
- Appetite and weight change
- Abdominal pain, altered bowel habit
- Gastrointestinal bleeding

Hepatocellular jaundice. Characteristic symptoms include anorexia with impairment of taste, nausea, vomiting and upper abdominal pain (often associated with hepatic tenderness). Common causes include viral hepatitis and chemical hepatitis, e.g. alcohol abuse and drug therapy.

Obstructive jaundice. Typical symptoms include itching (*pruritus*), dark urine and pale stools. Obstruction of the biliary tract is usually *extrahepatic* in origin and caused by either gallstones or pancreatic carcinoma. The former is suggested by a history of fever, rigors, biliary colic or previous biliary surgery; in the latter, chronic persistent back pain, aggravated by recumbency, and palpable enlargement of the gall bladder may occur. *Intrahepatic* obstruction is most often due to alcohol abuse, drug therapy and primary biliary cirrhosis (a disorder of middle-aged women often preceded by marked pruritus).

GENITOURINARY SYMPTOMS

All patients, irrespective of the presenting complaint, should be asked about the principal symptoms of genitourinary disorders, which otherwise they may not volunteer because of embarrassment (see Table 6.9).

Sometimes renal disease may only be suspected as a result of non-specific symptoms such as weakness or lethargy due to uraemia or following the finding of oedema, proteinuria or hypertension.

Dysuria, strangury, frequency and urgency

Dysuria is pain experienced prior to, during or following micturition. The term strangury is used when, in addition to dysuria, the patient experiences the repeated and urgent desire to urinate every few minutes without gaining relief of pain; this symptom has also been called 'vesical tenesmus'. Urinary frequency describes an increased frequency of micturition without implying any increase in the total urine volume. Urgency is a strong desire to pass urine which may be followed by incontinence if the opportunity to urinate is not available.

Dysuria, strangury, urgency and frequency are associated with disorders of the bladder, prostate and urethra due to infection, tumour, urinary calculi or urinary tract obstruction. Dysuria alone may be due to infection of the urethra, as in gonorrhoea. Urgency alone may be a feature of anatomical changes consequent upon pregnancy or uterine prolapse or it may be a feature of neurological disease affecting the motor control of the bladder. Frequency alone, particularly in young adults, is often the result of anxiety; in the elderly, it is more often the result of detrusor instability.

Haematuria

Haematuria is a serious symptom which demands explanation. The history often indicates the probable source of bleeding. Painless haematuria in the adult is usually due to bladder papilloma or renal, bladder or prostatic carcinoma. Haematuria associated with severe loin pain indicates a renal or ureteric origin, commonly due to the passage of a calculus. When haematuria is accompanied by frequency or dysuria, its source is usually in the bladder. Haematuria that rapidly clears during micturition is usually urethral in origin. Sometimes urinary discoloration may be confused with haematuria (Table 6.10).

Table 6.9 Checklist for the genitourinary history

General	Dysuria, strangury
	Urinary frequency, polyuria, nocturia
	Oliguria, anuria, haematuria
Males	Hesitancy, impaired force of micturition
	Post-micturition dribbling, incontinence
	Sexual function, impotence
Females	Stress and urge urinary incontinence
	Menstrual and obstetric history
	Sexual function, dyspareunia

Table 6.10 Abnormalities of urine colour

Orange–brown	Rhubarb, senna, bilirubin
Red–brown	Blood, myoglobin, haemoglobin, porphyrins
	Rifampicin, beetroot, blackberries
	Phenolphthalein
Brown–black	Bilirubin, methaemoglobin, melanin
	Homogentisic acid (alkaptonuria), L-dopa

Polyuria

Polyuria, an increased urinary volume, must be distinguished from urinary frequency in which there is the frequent passage of small volumes of urine. It may be the result of increased fluid intake, increased solute load producing an osmotic diuresis, as in diabetes mellitus and chronic renal failure, or impairment of renal concentrating ability due to analgesic nephropathy, hypoadrenalism or the absence of antidiuretic hormone (ADH) effects, e.g. diabetes insipidus or renal tubules non-responsive to ADH (nephrogenic diabetes insipidus).

The patient's assessment of increased urine volume can be misleading and should be confirmed by 24-hour urinary collections. Excessive thirst (*polydipsia*) may be the presenting symptom in severe polyuria.

Nocturia

The need to rise from bed to pass urine may be a life-long habit. When of recent onset, it may reflect insomnia, polyuria or prostatic obstruction. Nocturia is also a common symptom of cardiac failure, the diuresis resulting from the improvement in renal blood flow which occurs with recumbency.

Oliguria and anuria

Oliguria, a reduction in the urine volume, may be a feature of acute renal failure. The minimum urine volume necessary to excrete the daily solute load varies with the diet, physical activity and the metabolic rate as well as with renal function. Thus about 200 ml might be sufficient for a healthy man at rest on a protein-free diet, whereas 2000 ml might be insufficient when renal failure is present. For this reason, non-oliguric renal failure may fail to be recognised by the unwary. Anuria, the total cessation of urine production, is uncommon. The complaint of being unable to pass urine is usually due to urinary retention arising from bladder neck or urethral obstruction; a mechanical or neurological explanation should always be sought.

Pneumaturia

This bizarre and rare symptom describes the sensation of passing air bubbles in the urine. It is almost always caused by a vesicocolic fistula.

Impaired force of micturition

A poor urinary stream in males suggests obstruction due to prostatic hypertrophy in the elderly or, less commonly, a urethral stricture. The force of the stream can be assessed roughly by asking the patient to demonstrate how near he has to stand to an imaginary toilet. Other features of obstructed micturition include *hesitancy* (difficulty in initiating bladder emptying), urinary dribbling after micturition and frequency with nocturia due to incomplete bladder emptying.

Urinary incontinence

This can be a difficult symptom to assess but is usefully categorised as *urge incontinence* when the desire to urinate cannot be forestalled, *stress incontinence* when micturition occurs in response to coughing, sneezing or laughing, or as a combination of both. The information that should be elicited is shown in Table 6.11.

Many multiparous women experience stress incontinence because of the weakness of the anterior wall of the vagina, often accompanied by a degree of uterine prolapse. Incontinence may also arise from neurological disorders of bladder function. In sensory denervation of the bladder, dribbling incontinence results from painless over-distension of the bladder, as in diabetic autonomic neuropathy. Loss of motor control results in urgency. If the desire to urinate is not resolved promptly, because of either immobility or severe urgency, incontinence ensues. Combined motor and sensory damage occurs in spinal cord lesions, e.g. multiple sclerosis. The bladder fills to a certain pressure and then empties reflexly. The patient may be able to control bladder emptying by raising the intravesical pressure at regular intervals by manual compression of the lower abdomen.

Urogenital pain

The renal parenchyma is devoid of pain fibres, and renal pain is usually due to stretching of the renal capsule or renal pelvis. A chronic dull aching discomfort in the loin and renal angle may occur in renal infection and hydronephrosis. Intermittent pain can occur in polycystic disease from spontaneous bleeding into a cyst. In acute pyelonephritis the pain is often accompanied by dysuria and sometimes rigors.

Table 6.11 Checklist in the history of urinary incontinence

- Age at onset
- Occurrence only during sleep (*enuresis*)
- Associated urinary symptoms
- Factors provoking incontinence (coughing, urgency)
- Urine volume passed
- Precautions or protection required

Severe pain is caused by acute distension of the renal pelvis and kidney resulting from obstruction of the ureter by calculus or blood clot. Renal colic is not a true colic; the pain is severe, sustained and unremitting and the patient is restless, nauseated and often vomits. The pain may radiate from the renal angle and loin to iliac fossa, the groin and into the genitalia. Once the stone reaches the bladder, it is usually asymptomatic until it enters the urethra to cause dysuria. In patients with renal colic specific questions should be asked to try and determine the cause (see Fig. 6.22 p. 90).

Conditions causing bladder pain also produce frequency. Perineal and rectal pain with dysuria suggests a prostatic origin and when due to prostatitis may be associated with features of bladder neck obstruction. Testicular and epididymal pain may be felt in the groin and lower abdomen to such an extent that its testicular origin may be obscured. Its occurrence in pubertal boys and young men is most often the result of torsion of the testis and demands urgent intervention. Its onset is frequently at night with pain in the iliac fossa. Tenderness and swelling of the testis may need to be distinguished from a strangulated hernia or acute epididymo-orchitis. Ovarian pain is also felt in the iliac fossa and may be episodic and cyclical, as in endometriosis, or more constant, as in malignant tumours. Uterine pain is felt centrally in the hypogastrium and may radiate to the lumbosacral area, e.g. labour pains and dysmenorrhoea.

Menstrual and obstetric history

The menstrual history should include a note of the age of the *menarche* and menopause (*telarche*) and details of the menstrual cycle including the date of the first day of the last menstrual period (Table 6.12). Secondary amenorrhoea is common and often psychological, but the possibility of an organic cause such as hyperprolactinaemia, androgen excess or post-partum hypopituitarism should be considered. Primary amenorrhoea demands a gynaecological or endocrinological explanation.

The occurrence and the nature of any vaginal discharge requires assessment and note made of its colour,

Table 6.12 Checklist in the menstrual history

- Age of onset of the menarche
- Age of onset of the menopause (telarche)
- Use of the contraceptive pill or hormone replacement therapy
- Date of first day of the last menstrual period
- Frequency, regularity and duration of menstruation
- Amount of blood loss – number of tampons used
- Presence of blood clots (heavy menstrual losses)

consistency and smell. Symptoms of vaginal discharge, intermenstrual, post-coital or post-menopausal bleeding require a gynaecological examination. The obstetric history should include details of any problems with fertility and pregnancies. Useful questions to ask include the following:

- Date of the first day of the last menstrual period?
- Any difficulties in becoming pregnant?
- Number of pregnancies and live births, miscarriages and terminations
- Any health problems during any previous pregnancy or after delivery?
- Any difficulties during previous labours?
- Were the previous deliveries vaginal or caesarean?
- Were forceps or episiotomy used?
- Was there an accidental tear?

Remember to ask about medical disorders complicating pregnancy including dyspepsia, arthritis, colitis, cardiac murmurs, hypertension and diabetes.

The sexual history

Sexual dysfunction and sexually transmitted diseases are common; they are not confined to young adults, the promiscuous or the deviant. It is particularly important to ask about sexual function and activity if there are any conditions which may predispose to sexual dysfunction such as diabetes mellitus, alcohol abuse, marital difficulty or psychological disorder. Similarly, when sexually transmitted diseases are suspected, e.g. HIV, hepatitis or pelvic inflammatory disease, a careful sexual history should be undertaken.

Questions should be asked objectively with tact and sensitivity in a non-judgemental manner using a non-medical vocabulary to facilitate better communication. Useful questions to ask include:

- How many sexual partners have you had in the last 12 months?
- How many of your partners have been male and how many female?
- How many of your partners have been casual relationships?
- Do you use a condom most of the time, all of the time or not at all?
- Have you ever had a sexually transmitted disease?
- Do you experience any problems with libido, erections, ejaculation, penetration or orgasm?

In females, *dyspareunia* (pain related to sexual intercourse) and failure to achieve an orgasm are common and are frequently caused by, or lead to, psychological difficulties. Such topics may be avoided by the patient (or the clinician) because of embarrassment; once rapport has been established, start by asking if sexual intercourse is satisfactory and, if not, why not.

With practice, the clinician will become more competent taking a sexual history and patients should then feel less uncomfortable answering the questions. Even so, a sexual history may prove difficult, and an alternative method of overcoming patients' embarrassment is to ask patients to complete a confidential questionnaire detailing explicitly their sexual history and any problems they may have experienced (Appendix p. 365). This should allow the clinician to identify the main problem and to achieve a better rapport.

KEY POINTS

- Patients may conceal some symptoms, including genitourinary complaints and rectal bleeding, because of embarrassment.

- Haemorrhoids are so common that their presence in a patient with rectal bleeding should not lead to the assumption of cause and effect.

- Dysphagia is a cardinal symptom which requires investigation even when transient.

- Painless dysphagia is often due to tumour.

- Difficulty in swallowing fluids rather than solids, associated with spluttering and coughing, suggests a neurological disorder.

- There are many non-alimentary causes of vomiting and of abdominal pain.

- Bright-red blood in the vomitus is usually caused by a pharyngeal or oesophageal lesion. Dark-red vomitus with clots of blood is an indication of profuse bleeding, usually from the stomach.

- The acute development of tense ascites suggests infective peritonitis, intra-abdominal malignancy or portal vein obstruction.

- Changes in bowel habit may be the first symptom of serious underlying disease.

- Painless haematuria in the adult is usually due to a bladder papilloma or carcinoma.

- The minimum urinary volume necessary to maintain the *milieu interieur* depends upon renal function and the solute load, which is influenced by factors such as trauma, metabolic rate and diet.

- Testicular pain may be referred to the groin and lower abdomen.

- Sexual dysfunction and sexually transmitted diseases are not confined to the young, the promiscuous or the deviant.

- Complete anuria is very uncommon. Most patients who stop passing urine have obstructed bladder emptying.

THE PHYSICAL EXAMINATION

MOUTH AND THROAT

The examination of the mouth and throat is described on page 60. It is important to assess whether the teeth provide an adequate chewing surface or, if the patient is edentulous, to know if dentures fit and are used for eating.

OESOPHAGUS

When there is a complaint of dysphagia it can be helpful to watch the act of swallowing solids and liquids. This may reveal the organic nature and the site of the lesion. If swallowing is immediately followed by a distressing bout of coughing, either a neuromuscular disturbance such as bulbar or pseudobulbar palsy or more rarely a fistula between the trachea and the oesophagus should be suspected.

ABDOMEN

For descriptive purposes it is customary to divide the abdomen into nine regions by the intersection of

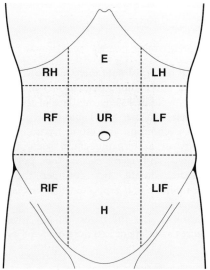

RH	Right hypochondrium	**UR**	Umbilical region
LH	Left hypochondrium	**RIF**	Right iliac fossa
E	Epigastrium	**LIF**	Left iliac fossa
RF	Right flank or lumbar region	**H**	Hypogastrium or supra-pubic region
LF	Left flank or lumbar region		

Fig. 6.1 Regions of the abdomen.

imaginary planes, two horizontal and two sagittal. The upper horizontal plane (transpyloric) lies at the level of the first lumbar vertebra, midway between the suprasternal notch and the symphysis pubis. The lower plane passes through the upper borders of the iliac crests. The sagittal planes are indicated on the surface by lines drawn vertically from the mid-inguinal points to the mid-clavicular points (Fig. 6.1).

The resultant regions are artificial but are helpful in localising most lesions. An alternative description is to refer to the right and left upper and lower quadrants of the abdomen, using vertical and horizontal lines passing through the umbilicus. The contents of the abdomen are illustrated in Figures 6.2 to 6.5.

The examination follows the routine sequence of inspection, palpation, percussion and auscultation.

Examination

General

☐ Whenever possible, examine the patient in good light and in warm surroundings.

☐ Lie the patient comfortably supine with the head resting on one or two pillows in order to relax the muscles of the abdominal wall.

☐ Use extra pillows to prop up a patient with kyphosis

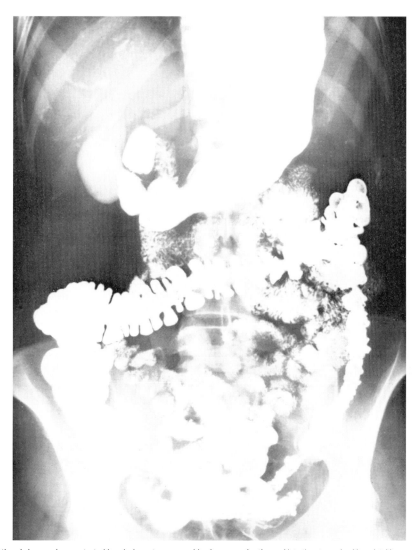

Figure 6.2 Contents of the abdomen demonstrated by cholecystogram and barium examination.   Note the stomach with peristaltic waves most marked in the gastric antrum which is surmounted by the duodenal cap; the feathery jejunal pattern in the left hypochondrium and the ileum in the hypogastrium; the caecum, and colon. Note the gall bladder alongside the duodenal cap and the calcification in the costal cartilages superimposed on the liver shadow. (Courtesy of Dr W A Copeland.)

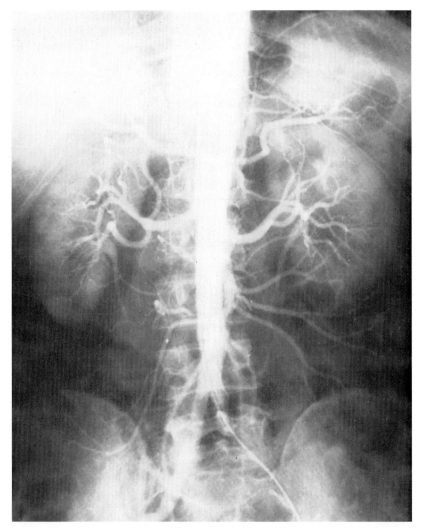

Fig. 6.3 Contents of the abdomen demonstrated by aortography.   Note on the left side, from above downwards, the left phrenic artery immediately below the diaphragm and the translucency from air in the splenic flexure overlying the splenic shadow; the splenic artery; the left renal artery; the left kidney and ureter; the superior mesenteric artery; the catheter in the left iliac artery passing into the aorta. Note, on the right side, the liver; the hepatic artery; the right renal artery; the right kidney and ureter; the psoas muscles; the right iliac artery. (Courtesy of Professor Eric Samuel.)

or with severe breathlessness.

❏ Remove the patient's clothes so that there is complete exposure from the xiphisternum to the pubis, leaving the chest and legs suitably covered.

❏ When examining a patient in bed, pull down all bedclothing except for a sheet and then fold back the sheet to the pubis; draw up the night clothes to the chest.

Inspection

❏ Observe the shape and symmetry of the abdomen, identify scars and note any other abnormalities.

❏ Inspect the abdomen tangentially looking for any movements including the slow waves of gastric peristalsis passing from the rib margin on the left, across the midline and subsiding beneath to the right of the midline.

❏ Attempt to stimulate peristalsis by giving the patient a fizzy drink or flicking the skin over the area.

Skin lesions. In elderly patients seborrhoeic warts, ranging from pink to brown or black, and haemangiomas (*Campbell de Morgan spots*) are so common that they could be considered normal changes. The presence of striae requires explanation (p. 68).

Any abnormality of the skin should be noted, includ-

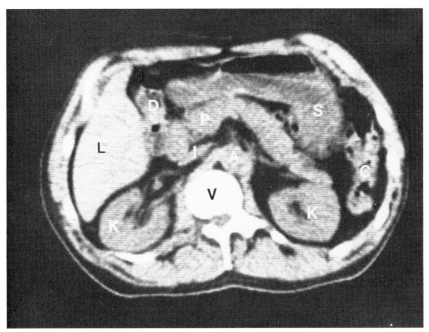

Fig. 6.4 Contents of the abdomen and pelvis shown by CT scan.   A, aorta and renal arteries; C, colon and faeces; D, duodenum; I, inferior vena cava; K, kidney; L, liver; P, pancreas; S, stomach; V, vertebra (the apparent deformity of which is due to the scan passing through the pedicle and lamina on the left side and through the foramen on the right. (Courtesy of Dr Andrew R. Wright.)

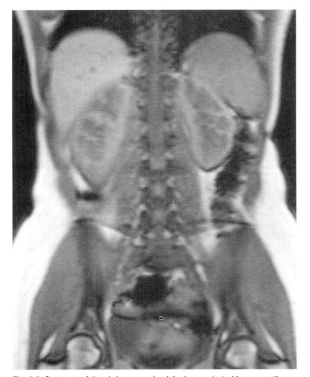

Fig. 6.5 Contents of the abdomen and pelvis demonstrated by magnetic resonance imaging (MRI) scan obtained in an angled coronal-type plane to demonstrate the various structures. (Courtesy of Dr Andrew R. Wright.)

Table 6.13 Surgical incisions

Non-specific incisions	
Vertical incisions	Midline or paramedian
(used for general access)	Upper, lower or full length
Specific incisions	
Subcostal	Gall bladder
Suprapubic	Bladder, prostate, gynaecology
McBurney's point	Appendix
Inguinal	Hernia

ing surgical scars, and the nature of the surgery undertaken should be recorded. Laparoscopic incisions are usually immediately below the umbilicus and may be difficult to see. The common sites of surgical incisions shown in Table 6.13 and illustrated in Figure 6.6.

Other transverse incisions are used for access to the aorta, kidneys, adrenals, ureters, sympathetic chain or stoma closures.

The common types of stoma are illustrated in Figure 6.7. The effluent from a colostomy is solid with a faecal odour; in an ileostomy there is a fluid, odourless, effluent.

Hair. Secondary sexual hair appears at puberty; its absence after this time suggests the possibility of hypopituitarism or hypogonadism (p. 57). Virilism in the female leads to a male distribution of pubic and body

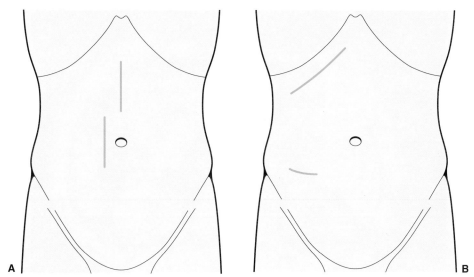

Fig. 6.6 Surgical incision. A. Vertical incisions may be midline or paramedian and are used for general access. **B.** Specific incisions may indicate the nature of operation, e.g. biliary or appendix. Note also that McBurney's point is situated one-third of the distance along a line from the anterior superior iliac spine to the umbilicus.

hair, whereas cirrhosis in the male may produce a female distribution of body hair.

Veins. Collateral veins may be visible if the inferior vena cava is obstructed or if there is portal hypertension. These are usually tortuous dilated superficial epigastric veins; in obstruction of the inferior vena cava, the blood flows upwards in the lower abdomen instead of downwards towards the groins. In cirrhosis, dilated collateral veins may also radiate from the umbilicus (*caput Medusa*), blood flowing away from the umbilicus as the portal vein drains through collateral vessels along the falciform ligament.

Shape. An inverted abdomen (*scaphoid abdomen*) may be due to starvation or wasting diseases. Protuberance may be due to obesity, gaseous distension, ascites, pregnancy or other swellings. In obesity the umbilicus is usually sunken, whereas in the other conditions it is flat or even projecting. Visible enlargement of the bladder, uterus or ovary may be evident as a characteristic shape arising from the pelvis, the swelling being predominantly central in contrast to the bulging of the flanks in ascites. Visible bulges may also be due to gross enlargement of the liver, spleen or kidneys or to large tumours. Distension of the stomach due to pyloric obstruction causes bulging of the upper part of the abdomen.

Movements. Quiet respiration is predominantly diaphragmatic, particularly in males, so that the abdominal wall moves out during inspiration. Respiratory movements of the abdomen usually cease in the presence of acute peritonitis.

Pulsation in the epigastrium is usually transmitted from the abdominal aorta. Less frequently it is caused by the right ventricle, the liver or an abdominal aneurysm. It may sometimes be difficult to distinguish between pulsation of the aorta transmitted through an abdominal mass from an aneurysm. Expansile pulsation favours the latter. The distinction is best confirmed by abdominal ultrasonography.

Peristalsis of the small intestine may be seen through a thin abdominal wall, or if there is divarication of the recti abdominis or an incisional hernia. It may become unduly prominent in small intestinal obstruction. It is recognised as writhing movements in the centre of the abdomen.

Hernias. Hernias are common causes of localised swellings and must be distinguished from divarication of the recti abdominis. Divarication of the recti, common in the multiparous, becomes more obvious as the supine patient attempts to sit upright; the intraabdominal pressure rises and the region of the linea alba bulges between the recti.

An *umbilical hernia* bulges through the navel. It is very common in babies and usually disappears spontaneously.

An *epigastric hernia* is visible as a small swelling usually not more than 1 cm in diameter. It is due to herniation of extraperitoneal fat through a defect in the linea alba. By gentle massage with the fingertip it is often possible to reduce such a hernia and then the small defect can be felt.

An *incisional hernia* may form at the site of any

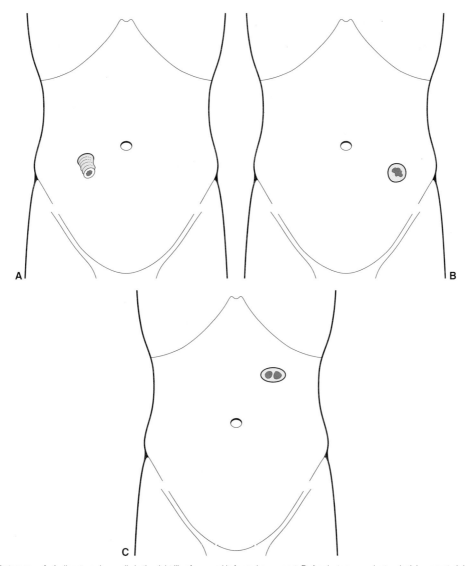

Fig. 6.7 Surgical stomas.   A. An ileostomy is usually in the right iliac fossa and is formed as a spout. **B.** A colostomy may be terminal, i.e. resected distal bowel. It is usually flush and in the left iliac fossa. **C.** A loop colostomy may be created for temporary defunctioning of the distal bowel. It is usually in the transverse colon and has afferent and efferent limbs.

operation on the abdomen, especially if the wound has been complicated by sepsis.

Femoral and *inguinal hernias* and the methods of examination are described on page 183.

Palpation

Palpation can be conveniently divided into three phases: light, deep and palpation during respiration.

Light palpation

The tendency to contract the abdominal muscles may be minimised by ensuring that the patient is warm and comfortable and by gaining the patient's confidence with a gentle approach. Generalised resistance is commonly due to anxiety in a patient unable to relax, a finding which may be confirmed by a reduction in resistance to palpation during the early phase of expiration. Resistance due to increased muscle tone accompanies intra-abdominal disease, particularly when pain is present. It may be restricted to one site according to the organ affected and the extent of the peritoneal involvement, e.g. McBurney's point in appendicitis.

Deep-seated inflammation not causing localised guarding may be revealed by *rebound tenderness*. Although the initial pressure of palpation may fail to elicit a painful response, the abrupt withdrawal may cause the sudden movement of a deeply placed, inflamed organ, resulting in pain. Generalised 'board-like' rigidity implies peritonitis; the abdomen does not move on respiration and bowel sounds are absent. Attempts to elicit other signs such as rebound tenderness are inappropriate.

It should however be remembered that pelvic peritonitis may be advanced before the signs are apparent abdominally and may only be revealed by rectal examination.

The elasticity of the skin provides only a rough index of the degree of hydration and redundant skin folds are evidence of weight loss.

Examination

General

- ☐ Ensure that the examining hands are warm.
- ☐ Position is important; if the patient is in a low bed, sit on, or kneel beside, the bed.
- ☐ Ask the patient to report any tenderness elicited during the examination and to place the arms alongside the body, explaining that this helps to relax the abdomen.
- ☐ During palpation, observe the patient's face for any grimace indicative of local discomfort.
- ☐ Assess obesity and evidence of weight loss by grasping a fold of skin and subcutaneous tissues between the fingers and thumb.

Light palpation

- ☐ Place the examining hand on the abdomen and thereafter maintain continuous contact with the patient's abdominal wall.
- ☐ Test muscle tone by light dipping movements over symmetrical areas commencing at a point remote from the site of any pain.
- ☐ To elicit rebound tenderness, press the examining hand gently but firmly into the abdomen and then swiftly release the pressure.

Deep palpation

In healthy subjects, it may be possible to feel the colon in the left iliac fossa. The caecum and sometimes the transverse colon may also be palpable, especially if the

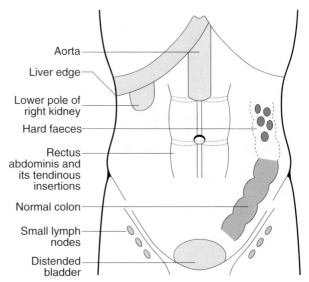

Aorta
Liver edge
Lower pole of right kidney
Hard faeces
Rectus abdominis and its tendinous insertions
Normal colon
Small lymph nodes
Distended bladder

Fig. 6.8 Palpation of the abdomen. Diagrammatic representation of some findings which may be normal and are often misinterpreted.

latter contains hard faeces. The aorta, the liver edge and the lower pole of the right kidney are often palpable (Fig. 6.8). Faeces are commonly palpable in the sigmoid colon but in severe constipation can be felt in any part of the lower bowel. Indentation of a lump by finger pressure is evidence that it is faecal. Sometimes, however, a hard, craggy lump of faeces can only be distinguished from malignancy by re-examination following defecation.

Enlargement of the bladder, ovary or uterus, suspected from inspection, may be confirmed as a dome-shaped swelling rising from the pubis. An upper abdominal mass which does not move on respiration either arises from or has become attached to the abdominal wall. Masses which are situated in the abdominal wall itself continue to be palpable when the muscles are contracted, as for example by raising the head off the pillow. Tightening the abdominal muscles in this way identifies the intersections of the recti abdominis (Fig. 6.8). An intersection may mislead the beginner into believing that a tumour or the liver edge has been felt. Masses situated more deeply within the abdominal cavity are less easily palpable when the muscles are contracted. The characteristics of any mass found should be assessed systematically with respect to its size, position, attachments, surface, edge, consistency, thrills, signs of inflammation and trans-illumination (p. 72) and illustrated diagrammatically, as in Figure 6.9.

Dipping technique. This manoeuvre may be useful in tense ascites, particularly to detect the presence of

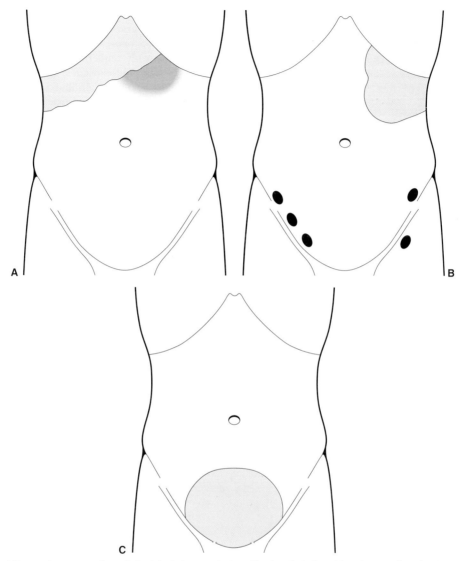

Fig. 6.9 The use of diagrams in case recording.   A. An abdominal mass and enlarged liver in patient with gastric carcinoma and hepatic metastases.
B. Splenomegaly and lymphadenopathy in a patient with Hodgkin's lymphoma. **C.** Tumour arising from the pelvis. This could be a bladder, uterine or ovarian swelling.

hepatic or splenic enlargement. The technique may help to detect and map the outlines of enlarged organs or of tumours that might otherwise have been missed because of the ascites. The sudden displacement of liquid gives a tapping sensation over the surface of the liver or spleen similar to a patellar tap (p. 308).

Examination

❑ Palpate the abdomen more deeply with the flat of the hand.

❑ Examine each region in turn, starting remote from any area of tenderness. The predominant use of fingertips should be avoided as it is apt to induce muscular resistance.
❑ To perform the dipping technique, place the examining hand flat on the abdomen and make quick dipping movements.

Palpation during inspiration

The liver and gall bladder, spleen and kidneys should

Table 6.14 Common causes of hepatomegaly

Disorder	Features
Viral hepatitis	Tender, sharp edge
Acute cardiac failure	Tender, sharp edge, may be pulsatile
Cirrhosis	Hard, rounded or irregular edge
Carcinomatosis	Hard, irregular, sometimes tender

now be examined in turn during deep inspiration. The key to success is to keep the examining hand or hands still and wait for the diaphragm to push the organ down onto the hands.

Palpation of the liver. Two common errors should be avoided: one is to feel for the liver using the side of the forefinger with the hand placed horizontally. In this position the palm of the hand may depress the liver edge, which then escapes detection. The other error is to begin palpation too close to the costal margin, thereby missing the liver edge. As the liver descends 1–3 cm on inspiration, it can normally be palpated in adults below the right costal margin during deep inspiration. Common causes of hepatomegaly in adults in Britain are shown in Table 6.14. Physical signs that may occur in hepatobiliary disorders are illustrated in Figure 6.10.

Palpation of the gall bladder. Gall stones are common with advancing years, especially in women. They are not palpable. Stones, however, may result in acute cholecystitis, with tenderness below the right costal margin in the mid-clavicular line. A palpable gall bladder is an abnormal finding and denotes enlargement. In the absence of jaundice, it is due to obstruction of the cystic duct leading to mucocele or empyema. Obstruction of the common bile duct produces jaundice; if the gall bladder is enlarged, the obstruction is usually due to causes other than gall stones such as carcinoma of the pancreas, since in cholelithiasis the gall bladder wall is diseased and thickened and cannot enlarge (*Courvoisier's law*).

Palpation of the spleen. The normal spleen lies against the posterolateral wall of the abdominal cavity, beneath ribs 9–11, with its anterior border extending to the mid-axillary line. As it enlarges, it expands forwards, downwards and medially, the tip emerging beneath the left costal margin. A palpable spleen is always pathological and a spleen which remains palpable during expiration is grossly enlarged. Common causes of splenomegaly include infections such as glandular fever and malaria, cirrhosis, the leukaemias and the myeloproliferative disorders. Splenomegaly may however be mistaken for an enlarged kidney.

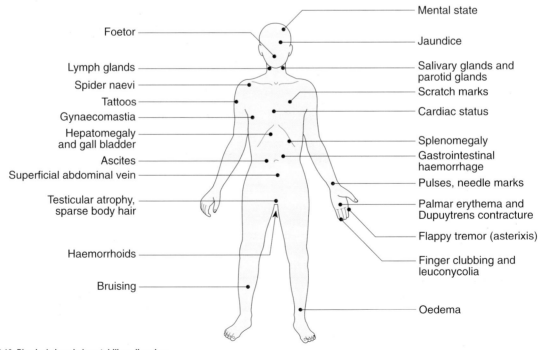

Foetor

Lymph glands

Spider naevi

Tattoos

Gynaecomastia

Hepatomegaly and gall bladder

Ascites

Superficial abdominal vein

Testicular atrophy, sparse body hair

Haemorrhoids

Bruising

Mental state

Jaundice

Salivary glands and parotid glands

Scratch marks

Cardiac status

Splenomegaly

Gastrointestinal haemorrhage

Pulses, needle marks

Palmar erythema and Dupuytrens contracture

Flappy tremor (asterixis)

Finger clubbing and leuconycolia

Oedema

Fig. 6.10 Physical signs in hepatobiliary disorders.

Differentiation can be difficult but is usually possible by asking the following questions:

- Is the mass smooth and regular in shape?
  If so, it probably is the spleen; if not, it is the kidney.
- Does the mass move early in inspiration?
  If it moves early, it may be the spleen; if late, the kidney. If it does not move at all, it may be a colonic or retroperitoneal mass.
- Is it possible to feel above the mass below the costal margin?
  If so, it is not the spleen but could be the kidney.
- Elsewhere, can the fingers be inserted deep to the mass at any point?
  If so, it is the spleen not the kidney
- Is the anterior edge palpably notched?
  If so, it is the spleen.
- Is the mass better appreciated bimanually than with one hand?
  If so, it is the kidney.
- Does the mass extend across the midline towards the right iliac fossa?
  If so, it is the spleen.
- Are masses palpable bilaterally?
  If so, polycystic kidneys are likely.
- Is there resonance to percussion overlying the mass?
  If so, the mass is renal or colonic.

Palpation of the kidneys. A normal kidney has a firm consistency and smooth surface. The lower pole of the normal right kidney is often palpable, especially in thin subjects. The normal left kidney is less often palpable. Owing to the varying thickness of the abdomen, kidney enlargement is difficult for the inexperienced to assess unless there is gross enlargement. Irregularity of the surface or an abnormally hard consistency is more easily appreciated. When the liver is readily palpable, it may be difficult to decide whether the right kidney can also be felt. Tenderness of the kidney is usually greatest posteriorly and readily elicited by tapping the renal angle with the patient sitting forward.

Examination

Liver
- Place the hand flat on the abdomen with the fingers pointing upwards and position the sensing fingers (index and middle) lateral to the rectus muscle so that the fingertips lie on a line parallel to the expected liver edge (Fig. 6.11).
- Press the hand firmly inwards and upwards and keep it steady while the patient takes a deep breath through the mouth.

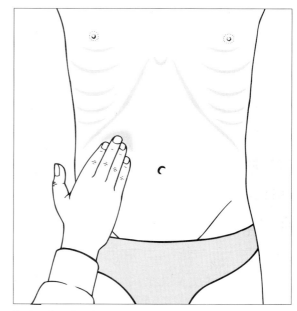

Fig. 6.11 Palpation of the liver.

- At the height of inspiration, release the inward pressure on the hand while maintaining the upward pressure. With this movement, the tips of the fingers should slip over the edge of a palpable liver.
- Note whether the edge is sharp as is normal, or whether it is rounded, firm, irregular or tender.
- Trace the surface and edge of a palpable liver across the abdomen and examine it for irregularities using the fingertips, keeping them steady in a new position each time the patient takes a deep breath. Irregularities may be felt as the liver slides under the fingertips with each respiration.

Gall bladder
- Place the examining fingers over the gall bladder area and ask the patient to take a deep breath. Inspiration may be sharply arrested with tensing of the abdominal muscles because of a sudden accentuation of pain (*Murphy's sign*).

Spleen
- Place the examining hand on the anterior abdominal wall with the fingertips well below the left costal margin, pressing inwards and upwards (Fig. 6.12A).
- Ask the patient to breathe in deeply. If the spleen is significantly enlarged, it will bump against the fingertips.
- At the height of inspiration, release the pressure on the examining hand so that the fingertips slip over

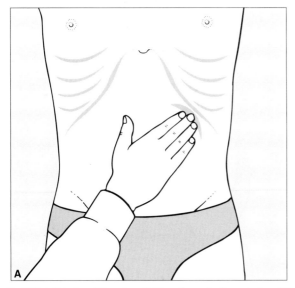

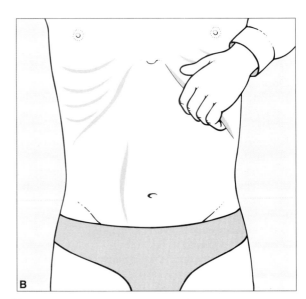

Fig. 6.12 A. Palpation of the spleen. B. Alternative method for palpation of the spleen.

the lower pole of the spleen, confirming its presence and surface characteristics.

❑ If the spleen is not palpable, move the examining hand upwards after each inspiration until the fingertips are under the costal margin.

❑ Repeat this process along the entire rib margin as the position of the enlarging splenic tip is variable.

❑ If still not palpable, position the patient in the right lateral position with the left hip and knee flexed.

❑ Place the other hand posteriorly to support the lower rib cage and repeat the examination.

❑ Alternatively, examine for the spleen from the left side of the patient, curling the fingers of the left hand beneath the costal margin as the patient breathes deeply (Fig. 6.12B).

Kidneys

❑ Use a bimanual technique to palpate the kidneys.

❑ Place one hand posteriorly below the lower rib cage and the other over the upper quadrant.

❑ Push the two hands together firmly but gently as the patient breathes out.

❑ Feel for the lower pole as the patient breathes in deeply.

❑ Try to trap a palpable kidney between the two hands by delaying applying pressure until the end of inspiration. This facilitates palpation of the kidney as it slides upwards on expiration when the pressure between the two hands is reduced.

❑ Confirm that the structure being palpated is the kidney by 'pushing' the kidney between the two

hands (*ballotting*) and by assessing its degree of movement during respiration.

❑ Assess the size, surface and consistency of a palpable kidney.

❑ Examine the left kidney from either side (Fig. 6.13A and B).

Percussion

The distended abdomen. The main value of abdominal percussion is to distinguish between distension due to gas, ascites, cystic or solid tumours. Gaseous distension is resonant. Ovarian cysts, bladder enlargement and solid pelvic masses extend out of the pelvis into the abdomen to produce central abdominal dullness with resonance of the flanks caused by gas in the surrounding displaced gut. In contrast, ascites is suggested by the presence of dullness in the flanks with central abdominal resonance. Ascites is often first suspected from the convexity of the abdomen and flanks on inspection but confirmed by percussion. In the presence of ascites, the gas-containing gut floats uppermost. The liquid gravitates to the dependent part of the peritoneal cavity, namely the flanks and pelvis.

The presence of small quantities of free fluid in the peritoneal cavity is not clinically detectable since minor changes in percussion note may be due to gravitational shift of normal bowel. The presence of tense ascites may be confirmed by demonstrating *shifting dullness* or eliciting a *fluid thrill*, but an enormous ovarian cyst may also produce a fluid thrill.

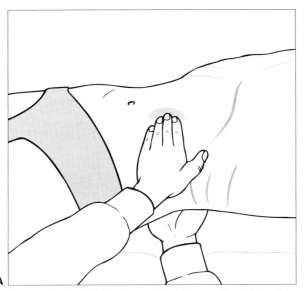 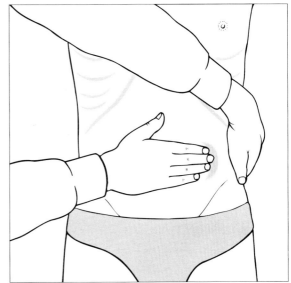

Fig. 6.13 Palpation of the left kidney. **A.** from the same side and **B.** from the opposite side.

The spleen. Percussion is of limited value in determining the size and position of the spleen as this can only be crudely assessed from the percussion note. However, dullness to percussion overlying a palpable mass in the left upper quadrant indicates the mass is likely to be splenic in origin.

The liver. Percussion can give only a rough estimate of the size of the liver, particularly in regard to the upper border. Although this may be raised above the level of the fifth rib by a greatly enlarged liver, the percussion note is largely dependent upon the state of the lung and pleura. The apparent level of the lower border of the liver varies with the amount of gas in the colon, and a palpable lower border may be 3–4 cm below the edge detected by percussion. However, a positive finding on percussion implies that the borders of the liver extend at least as far as the extent of dullness.

Reduced liver dullness may be due to:

- pulmonary hyperinflation, e.g. chronic bronchitis
- a small liver, e.g. cirrhosis
- air beneath the diaphragm, e.g. perforated hollow viscus
- interposition of the colon between the liver and the diaphragm (an unusual but normal anatomical variant).

Examination

General
❑ Percussion from resonance to dull.

❑ Place the percussing finger on the trunk parallel to the anticipated note change (Fig. 6.14 A).
❑ Percuss lightly for superficial structures such as the lower border of the liver, more firmly for deeply placed structures such as the upper border of liver or the bladder.
❑ Examine the spleen with the patient holding the breath during full inspiration; percuss both below and then above the left costal margin.

Shifting dullness
❑ Examine the patient supine and percuss from the centre of the abdomen into the flank until a dull note is obtained (Fig. 6.14B).
❑ Mark the level or keep the finger in place as the patient rolls on to the other side.
❑ Pause for a few seconds. Ascites is suggested if the note becomes resonant and confirmed by obtaining a dull note while percussing back towards the umbilicus (Fig. 6.14).

Fluid thrill
❑ With a detecting hand on the patient's flank, flick the skin of the abdominal wall over the other flank using the thumb or forefinger.
❑ If a fluid thrill or impulse is felt, repeat the procedure with the patient's hand placed on the abdomen along the midline sagittal plane to dampen any possible thrill transmitted via the abdominal wall.

Auscultation

Bowel sounds. Normal activity of the gut creates

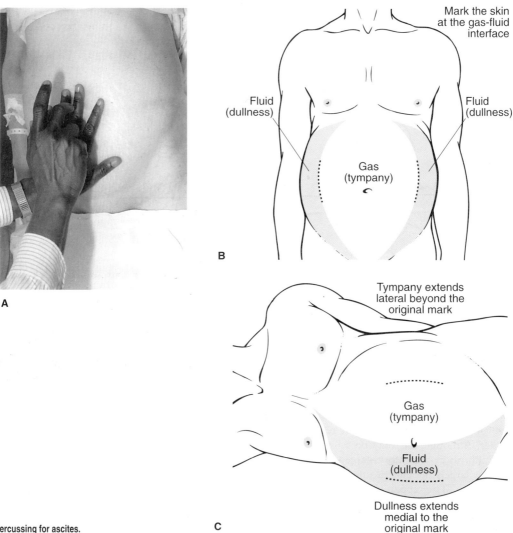

Fig. 6.14 Percussing for ascites.

characteristic gurgling sounds which may be heard from time to time by the unaided ear (*borborygmi*). Through the stethoscope, they can be heard every 5–10 seconds, though the interval varies greatly and has a close relationship to meals. Absent bowel sounds suggest peritonitis and/or paralytic ileus.

Increased frequency and intensity of bowel sounds occur in:

- small bowel malabsorption
- intestinal obstruction (with a tinkling quality)
- severe gastrointestinal bleeding
- the carcinoid syndrome (embarrassingly loud borborygmi).

Arterial bruits. Arterial bruits in the abdomen usually arise from the aorta. A systolic murmur due to stenosis of a mesenteric or renal artery may be audible but, owing to the distracting effects of the bowel sounds, a conscious effort must be made to listen for them. A systolic bruit may be heard over the liver in hepatoma.

Venous hum. A venous hum is occasionally audible between the xiphisternum and the umbilicus due to turbulent blood flow in a well-developed collateral circulation from portal hypertension.

Friction sounds. Friction sounds resembling those of pleurisy may be present over an area of perisplenitis or perihepatitis.

Succussion splash. A sound like shaking a half-filled hot-water bottle is termed a succussion splash. This can be produced from a normal stomach within 2 hours after food or drink. In other circumstances it is a feature of gastric outlet hold-up.

Examination

☐ Auscultate for peristalsis bowel sounds for at least 3 minutes before deciding that they are absent.
☐ Auscultate over the aorta for a bruit.
☐ To elicit a succussion splash, place the hands over the lower ribs and shake the patient quickly but rhythmically from side to side.

KEY POINTS

- Any surgical scar and the nature of the operation should be documented.

- The umbilicus is normally sunken in obesity; in other causes of abdominal protuberance it is usually flat or even projecting.

- A succussion splash is suggestive of gastric outlet obstruction only if it is elicited at least 2 hours after food or drink.

- Rebound tenderness is evidence of peritoneal irritation. Pelvic peritonitis is often best elicited by rectal examination.

- A palpable spleen is always pathological.

- The dipping technique is of value in detecting organomegaly if there is marked ascites.

- Carcinoma of the pancreas is the usual explanation for a palpable gall bladder in the jaundiced patient.

- Important principles of abdominal percussion are

  a. percuss from resonant to dull;

  b. percuss parallel to the anticipated note change;

  c. percuss softly for superficial structures but firmly for deep structures.

- Shifting dullness is a feature of ascites.

HERNIAL ORIFICES AND GENITALIA

The groins should be examined for hernias, femoral pulses (p. 128) and for lymph nodes (p. 74); in health inguinal lymph nodes vary considerably in size and consistency.

Examination of hernias and hernial orifices

Abdominal hernias are protrusions of a viscus through an abnormal opening.

External hernias occur at the site of defects in the abdominal wall, e.g. operation scars and points of anatomical weakness.

Internal hernias occur through defects of the mesentery or into the retroperitoneal fossae.

External hernias of the abdominal wall are more prominent in the erect position, when the pressure within them rises, and during coughing when an impulse can often be felt in the hernia (*cough impulse*). After the identification of a hernia, an attempt should be made to replace the contents by the application of a gentle sustained pressure (*reduction*).

Hernias may be reducible or irreducible. Irreducible hernias may become *obstructed*, when the bowel lumen is occluded. Obstructed hernias may become *strangulated* when the vascular supply of the hernial contents is threatened. A strangulated hernia is tense and tender and shows no impulse on coughing; this is a surgical emergency if bowel infarction is to be avoided.

A *femoral hernia* lies in the femoral canal below the inguinal ligament and is therefore palpable below and lateral to the pubic tubercle (Fig. 6.15).

An *inguinal hernia* emerges from the abdominal wall through the external inguinal ring and is therefore palpable above and medial to the pubic tubercle (Fig. 6.15). It is customary to attempt to differentiate direct from indirect inguinal hernias.

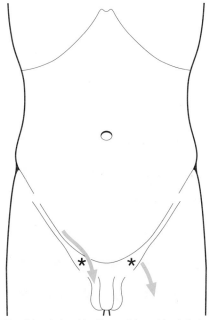

Fig. 6.15 Examining the hernial orifices. A femoral hernia lies below and lateral to the pubic tubercle. An inguinal hernia lies above and medial to the pubic tubercle.

An *indirect inguinal hernia* occurs into a persistent remnant of the processus vaginalis. It occurs in young men and may extend to the testes. Following reduction, control can be achieved by pressure over the internal inguinal ring, just above the mid-point of the inguinal ligament.

A *direct inguinal hernia* occurs directly through the weakened posterior wall of the inguinal canal medial to the inferior epigastric artery and lateral to the rectus muscle. It is more common in older men and does not reach the testes. It will not be controlled by pressure over the internal inguinal ring. By invaginating the skin of the scrotum with the examiner's little finger, the external inguinal ring can be entered to assess the posterior wall of the inguinal canal.

Examination of the male genitalia

The stages of physical sexual development in relation to age are given on page 334. In the male, examination of the genitalia conveniently follows palpation of the groins.

A hydrocele, spermatocele and cyst of the epi-

didymis are differentiated by their relationships to the testis (Fig. 6.16). The possibility that a hydrocele may obscure a testicular tumour must not be overlooked and careful palpation of both testes is therefore necessary. Infections other than syphilis and mumps primarily affect the epididymis; tuberculosis produces a characteristic nodular change within the epididymis accompanied by thickening of the cord. Shortening of the cord is a characteristic of torsion of the testis.

The contents of the male pelvis are shown in Figure 6.17.

Specific considerations

- Patients may sometimes be concerned by mistaking a normal epididymis for a testicular mass.
- The left testis usually lies lower than the right.
- Minor degrees of hypospadias are common (one in 300 males).
- Bilateral testicular atrophy suggests hypogonadism.
- Unilateral atrophy may occur following mumps orchitis.

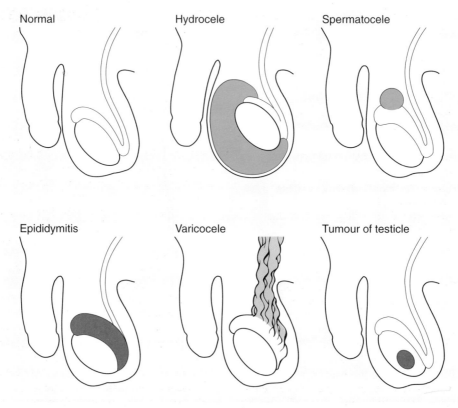

Normal   Hydrocele   Spermatocele

Epididymitis   Varicocele   Tumour of testicle

Fig. 6.16 Swellings of the scrotum.

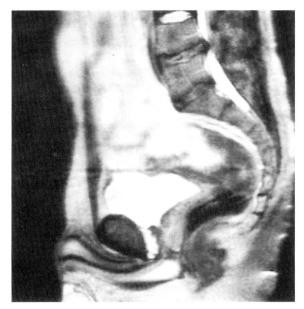

Fig. 6.17 MRI scan showing contents of the male pelvis.
(Courtesy of Dr Andrew R. Wright.)

- Absence of one or both testes from the scrotum should lead to a search for incompletely descended testes in the inguinal canal or for ectopic testes in sites such as the groin.

Examination

- ☐ Examine the penis and scrotum and carefully palpate the testes, epididymes and vasa deferentia.
- ☐ Assess any scrotal swelling using the principles described on page 72.
- ☐ Confirm that any swelling originates in the scrotum and is not an inguinal hernia.
- ☐ Carefully palpate both testes to determine the exact site of any swelling.
- ☐ Perform transillumination to confirm the cystic nature of any swelling.

Examination of the female genitalia

The contents of the female pelvis are illustrated in Figure 6.18. Vaginal examination is not routine. Its intimate nature raises medico-legal considerations necessitating both informed consent and the presence of a chaperone throughout the examination.

The vaginal examination with the introitus is intact should be avoided if possible, particularly as the information sought can often be obtained by digital examination of the rectum. Vaginal examination of a minor requires the consent of a parent or guardian.

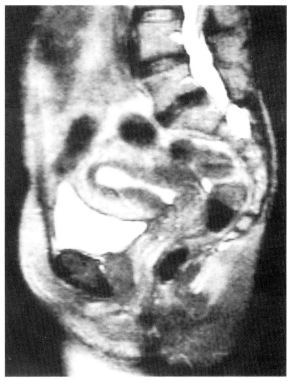

Fig. 6.18 MRI showing the contents of the female pelvis.
(Courtesy of Dr Andrew R. Wright.)

Examination

Vaginal examination
- ☐ Ask the patient to empty the bladder before hand.
- ☐ Position the patient comfortably either on her back or in the left lateral position with her head on a pillow, hips and knees flexed and thighs abducted.
- ☐ Use an angle-poise lamp to illuminate the vulva adequately.
- ☐ Use suitable gloves and lubricate the examining fingers.
- ☐ Separate the labia minora with the forefinger and thumb of the left hand, bringing into view the clitoris anteriorly, then the urethra, the vagina and the anus posteriorly.
- ☐ Look for any evidence of discharge, ulceration or abnormalities of Bartholin's glands.
- ☐ Inspect the vaginal walls for prolapse by asking the patient to strain down and then to cough.
- ☐ Note the position and degree of any vaginal prolapse and the occurrence of any involuntary urinary incontinence on coughing.
- ☐ Insert the index and middle fingers of the right hand into the vagina and rotate palm-upwards

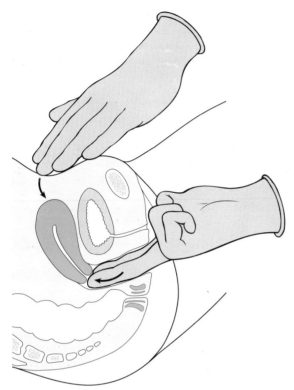

Fig. 6.19 Vaginal examination.

(Fig. 6.19). Use only one finger if vaginismus or atrophic vaginitis makes examination painful.

- ☐ Palpate the cervix; the normal cervix points downwards and slightly backwards and feels like the tip of the nose.
- ☐ Note any tenderness on movement of the cervix (*cervical excitation*).
- ☐ Now perform bimanual palpation; with two fingers in the anterior fornix, place the left hand flat on the abdomen above the pubis.
- ☐ Identify the size, position and surface characteristics of the uterus between the hands.
- ☐ If the uterus is not palpable, palpate with the fingers in the posterior fornix as the uterus may be retroverted.
- ☐ Palpate each lateral fornix in turn bimanually.
- ☐ Note any tenderness or swelling of the fallopian tubes or ovaries (*adnexae*), the bladder anteriorly and the pouch of Douglas posteriorly.
- ☐ Supplement digital examination by inspection of the vagina and uterine cervix using a vaginal speculum.

Using a vaginal speculum
- ☐ Gently insert a lubricated, warmed speculum into the vagina; do not use a lubricant other than water

if a cervical smear is being performed.
- ☐ Rotate the blades through 90 degrees pointing the handles anteriorly if the patient is supine and posteriorly if in the left lateral position
- ☐ Gently open the blades and identify the cervix.
- ☐ Use the notched end of a spatula and rotate through 360 degrees to scrape off a cytological sample from the cervical os.
- ☐ Spread the sample thinly onto a labelled, cleaned glass slide and fix immediately with a 50/50 mixture of alcohol and ether.
- ☐ Swab any discharge from the urethra, vagina and cervix.
- ☐ Send one specimen for culture and smear another on to a glass slide for direct microscopy; unstained smears are helpful to confirm trichomonal infection and stained smears to confirm gonorrhoea or thrush.

RECTUM

Digital rectal examination

Digital examination of the rectum is a part of the general medical examination and the student must become familiar with the feel of the normal structures. Because this simple procedure is disagreeable to the patient, it is often inappropriately omitted. It is recommended that a third person should be present to act as chaperone.

Rectal examination should be routine in the following circumstances:

1. *Alimentary problems*
   All 'acute abdomens', suspected appendicitis, pelvic abscess, peritonitis and lower abdominal pain. Diarrhoea or constipation; mucus or blood in stools. Anal irritation or pain; tenesmus or rectal pain. Bimanual examination of a lower abdominal mass. In the search for tumours or transperitoneal metastases either diagnostically or in making a decision about treatment.
2. *Genitourinary problems*
   Dysuria; haematuria; haematospermia; epididymo-orchitis. In lieu of gynaecological examination if the introitus is intact.
3. *Miscellaneous problems*
   In the search for a cause of backache, root pain in the legs, unexplained bone pain or iron deficiency anaemia. In all cases of pyrexia of unknown origin or unexplained weight loss.

Spasm of the external anal sphincter is commonly due to anxiety, but when associated with local pain, it is likely to be due to an anal fissure and a local anaesthetic suppository should be used before taking the examination.

The upper end of the anal canal is marked by the pubo-rectalis muscle which is readily palpable and which contracts reflexly on coughing or under voluntary control. Beyond the anal canal, the rectum passes upwards and backwards along the curve of the coccyx and the sacrum. The normal rectum is usually empty and smooth-walled. The coccyx and sacrum lie posteriorly. Anteriorly in the male, from below upwards, lie the membranous urethra, the prostate and base of the bladder; in the female, the vagina and cervix. The presence of a vaginal tampon can confuse the inexperienced examiner.

Haemorrhoids are not palpable unless thrombosed; similarly, normal seminal vesicles cannot be felt. In patients with chronic constipation the rectum is often loaded with faeces. An obstructing carcinoma of the upper rectum may produce ballooning of the empty rectal cavity below. Faecal masses are commonly palpable; they should be movable and can be indented. Metastases or colonic tumours within the pelvis may be mistaken for faeces and vice versa.

The prostate gland. The normal prostate is smooth and has a firm consistency with lateral lobes and a median groove between them. Prostatic hyperplasia in the adult male often produces a palpable symmetrical enlargement but may not do so if the hyperplasia is confined to the median lobe. A hard, irregular gland suggests prostatic carcinoma; the rectal mucosa may be tethered implying extra-capsular spread and often the median groove is undetectable. The prostate is abnormally small in hypogonadism. Tenderness accompanied by a change in the consistency of the gland may be due to prostatitis or an abscess.

Examination

⬜ Position the patient in the left lateral position with the buttocks at the edge of the couch, the knees drawn up to the chest and the heels clear of the perineum.

⬜ Reassure the patient and explain that the examination may be uncomfortable but should not be painful.

⬜ Lubricate the examining index finger, protected by a suitable glove.

⬜ Examine the perianal skin in a good light looking for evidence of skin lesions, external haemorrhoids or fistulae.

⬜ Place the tip of the forefinger on the anal margin and with steady pressure on the sphincter pass the

finger gently through the anal canal into the rectum (Fig. 6.20). If anal spasm is encountered, ask the patient to breathe out and relax.

⬜ Ask the patient to squeeze the examining forefinger with the anal sphincter.

⬜ Note any weakness of sphincter contraction.

⬜ Palpate around the entire rectum.

⬜ Note any abnormality and examine any mass systematically (p. 72).

⬜ Note the percentage of the rectal circumference involved by disease and the distance of the upper and lower edges of disease from the anal canal.

⬜ Perform bimanual examination if necessary, using the other hand laid flat over the lower abdomen.

⬜ Repeat the examination after the patient has defecated if in doubt about palpable masses.

⬜ After withdrawal, examine the finger for stool colour and the presence of blood and mucus.

⬜ Test the stool sample for blood using a 'Haemoccult' card.

Proctoscopy

Visual examination of the rectum and anal canal complements digital examination but should always be preceded by digital examination. Only by proctoscopy can the anorectum be adequately examined for haemorrhoids, anal fissures (tears in the mucosa), rectal prolapse and mucosal disease.

The appearance of normal rectal mucosa is similar to buccal mucosa with the exception of the presence of prominent submucosal veins. On straining, haemorrhoids, if present, distend with blood and may prolapse. If the degree of protrusion is more than 3–4 cm, the possibility of a full thickness rectal prolapse should be considered.

Examination

⬜ Position the patient in the left lateral position with the buttocks at the edge of the couch, the knees drawn up to the chest and the heels clear of the perineum.

⬜ Separate the buttocks with the forefinger and thumb of one hand and with the other hand gently insert a well-lubricated proctoscope with its obturator into the anal canal and rectum in the direction of the umbilicus.

⬜ Remove the obturator and examine the rectal mucosa carefully under good illumination, noting any abnormality seen.

⬜ Ask the patient to strain down as the instrument is slowly withdrawn to detect any degree of rectal prolapse and the severity of any haemorrhoids.

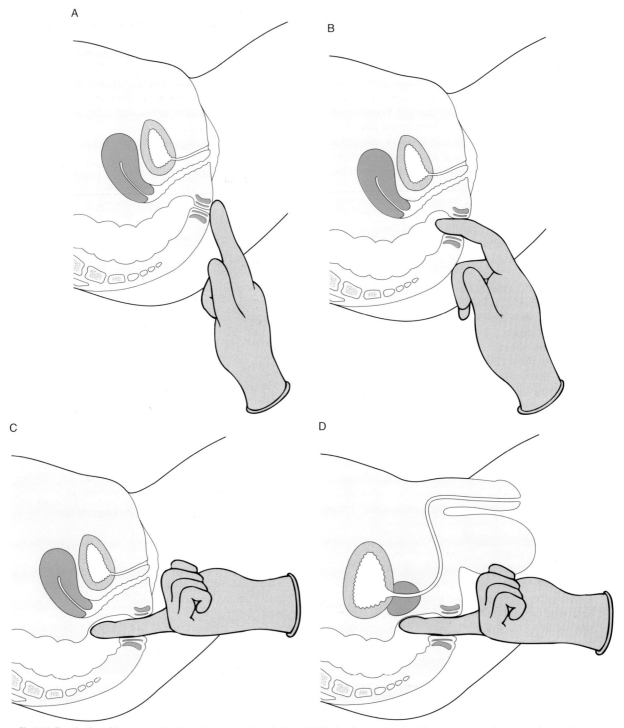

Fig. 6.20 Examination of the rectum. The finger is inserted as shown in **A.** and **B.** The hand is then rotated and the most prominent features are the cervix in the female **C.** and the prostate in the male **D.**

❑ Carefully examine the anal canal for fissures, particularly if the patient has experienced pain during the procedure.

Rigid sigmoidoscopy and rectal biopsy

Satisfactory visualisation of the bowel lumen is essential during sigmoidoscopy and the instrument should never be advanced if vision is obscured. Preparation of the bowel prior to the procedure may therefore be necessary and is best achieved by the use of a phosphate enema given 30 minutes beforehand. Proctoscopy should always be undertaken before sigmoidoscopy. Because of the increased risk of bowel perforation during a barium enema examination, rigid sigmoidoscopy and biopsy should be avoided for seven days prior to a barium enema.

Rectal biopsy should only be performed under direct vision and with adequate illumination. Since the upper rectum is intraperitoneal above 12 cm from the anal margin, rectal biopsies should not be undertaken beyond 12 cm to avoid intra-peritoneal perforation. Only biopsy forceps and never grasping (toothed) forceps should be used to obtain the biopsy. The patient should be warned to expect transient, minor rectal bleeding following rectal biopsy and to report promptly if bleeding is profuse.

Indications for sigmoidoscopy and rectal biopsy include:

- investigation of rectal bleeding and altered bowel habit
- assessment of colitis and colorectal neoplasms
- assessment of rectal histology.

Examination

❑ Explain the procedure to the patient and reassure them that though it may be uncomfortable, it should not be painful.

❑ Position the patient in the left lateral position with the buttocks at the edge of the couch, the knees drawn up to the chest and the heels clear of the perineum.

❑ Gently insert a well-lubricated sigmoidoscope with its obturator into the anal canal and rectum.

❑ Remove the obturator and attach the light source and air insufflator.

❑ Advance the scope under direct vision posteriorly towards the sacrum.

❑ Insufflate only to identify the lumen if progress cannot otherwise be achieved and never advance the instrument if the lumen cannot be visualised.

❑ Identify the rectosigmoid junction 12–15 cm from the anal margin where the bowel enters the pelvis at 90 degrees to the long axis of the rectum.

❑ Advance the scope anteriorly and to the patient's left to enter the sigmoid colon.

❑ Note the total distance travelled from the anus and carefully examine the mucosa, noting its vascular pattern and friability as well as the presence of blood, mucous and ulceration.

Rectal biopsy

❑ Using biopsy forceps, pinch the mucosa and pull into the lumen, checking that only the mucosa, not the rectal wall, moves.

❑ Firmly bite, twist then sharply retract the forceps to detach the biopsy specimen.

❑ Place the biopsy into buffered formalin for routine histology.

❑ Inspect the mucosal damage at the biopsy site before withdrawing the scope.

❑ If bleeding is brisk, apply a dry swab to the bleeding point for five minutes. Alternatively, use a swab soaked in 1:100,000 adrenaline. If profuse bleeding persists or recurs, seek surgical advice urgently.

KEY POINTS

- Absence of one or both testes from the scrotum should promote a search for an incompletely descended or ectopic testis.

- Vaginal examination should be avoided if the introitus is intact.

- Always obtain informed consent before performing a rectal or vaginal examination.

- Haemorrhoids are not normally palpable on rectal examination.

- A hard craggy gland and loss of the median sulcus are features of a carcinoma of the prostate.

- Avoid performing a barium enema within 7 days following rigid sigmoidoscopy with rectal biopsy.

- In children it is best to defer rectal examination to the senior clinician making the management decisions.

THE METHODS IN PRACTICE

The history and physical examination will often provide the diagnosis in a patient with an abdominal complaint. It is important to relate the general examin-

Ask about:

Past history	Dyspeptic symptoms
Family history	Vomiting/diarrhoea
Bleeding tendency	Anorexia/weight
Drug/alcohol use	Dizziness or fainting

- Mental state
- Fundal haemorrhage
- Pallor
- Spider naevi etc.
- Heart rate
- Blood pressure
- Liver
- Spleen
- Bowel sounds
- Rectal examination
- Bruising

Fig. 6.21 Checklist for upper gastrointestinal tract haemorrhage.

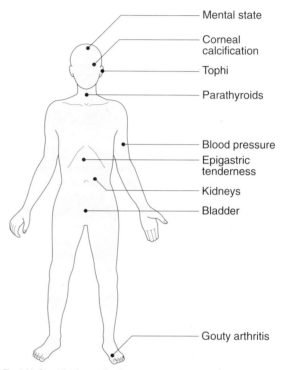

Ask about:

Family history	Intake of Vit. D,
Occupational history	milk, antacids
Previous urinary	Associated renal
infections	symptoms
Intake of analgesics	Bone and joint pain,
(NSAIDS) and diuretics	dyspepsia
	Immobilisation,
	dehydration and tremor

- Mental state
- Corneal calcification
- Tophi
- Parathyroids
- Blood pressure
- Epigastric tenderness
- Kidneys
- Bladder
- Gouty arthritis

Fig. 6.22 Checklist for renal colic.

ation to the specific problem. This has been illustrated in the instance of hepatobiliary disease (Fig. 6.10). Other examples include gastrointestinal haemorrhage (Fig. 6.21) and the approach to the patient with renal colic (Fig. 6.22).

The acute abdomen

The term 'acute abdomen' is generally applied to conditions in which the patient presents with acute distress related to an abdominal complaint. Usually the patient or relatives expect an immediate diagnosis and often a surgical cure. Many such situations are neither acute nor amenable to surgery, and it is important not to get swept along by the apparent urgency into a premature or unnecessary operation.

Although in some patients the physical evidence of disease indicates that the 'acute abdomen' has occurred in the context of pre-existing ill-health, in others

underlying disease may be obscured by the acute complications. Corticosteroids, non-steroidal analgesics, alcohol abuse and previous surgery are examples of factors that may cause the 'acute abdomen' or modify its presentation.

The conventional principles of history and examination are perhaps even more important in the acute abdomen than in non-acute situations when omissions or errors can be corrected at subsequent consultations. However, severe pain, shock and poor physical condition may make it difficult for a patient to concentrate and talk at length. For these reasons, the standard sequence of history, examination, diagnosis and therapy may need to be put aside and treatment commenced before a detailed history and examination are possible.

Important points in the history

- The patient's own history is the most valuable, and this should be obtained whenever possible.
- When patients are too ill to give their own account, the history must be obtained from observers.
- It is very important that the first history should be as accurate and as detailed as possible; ill patients may be disinclined to repeat their accounts of the illness.
- If, however, doubt remains as to the cause of the problem, the patient should be encouraged to recount the story again because histories relayed through other clinicians may be erroneous.
- Since abdominal pain may arise from disease outwith the alimentary tract, a thorough and systematic history is vital.
- The most recent and severe symptoms may occupy the patient's attention to such an extent that important but apparently unrelated details of the history are forgotten until questioned directly.
- The onset of symptoms can be clarified by specific questions such as 'When were you last at work?' or, in the more elderly, 'How were you feeling at Christmas time?'.
- The history may appear to change as it is taken at different times by different clinicians; the patient's symptoms may also change as the disease progresses.
- Where appropriate, remember to pay specific attention to the:
  - reproductive, contraceptive and menstrual history
  - possibility of pregnancy and its complications
  - drug history including self-administered remedies and alcohol consumption
  - past medical history and previous surgical operations.

Patterns of presentation

Site of pain. Visceral abdominal pain results from distension of hollow organs, mesenteric traction or excessive smooth muscle contraction. Pain from embryonic foregut structures is perceived in the epigastrium, from midgut structures around the umbilicus and from hindgut structures the hypogastrium (Fig. 6.1) (p. 170). The sympathetic innervation of the abdominal viscera (spinal cord segments T5–L2) is responsible for the conduction of visceral pain; parasympathetic afferents do not convey pain sensation. Accurate localisation of somatic pain due to irritation of the parietal peritoneum is provided by intercostal (spinal) nerves, which innervate the parietal peritoneum and the overlying abdominal wall.

Some acute disorders are rarely if ever bilateral while others are usually if not always bilateral. In young males, when unilateral acute epididymo-orchitis is suspected, torsion of the testis should always be the first diagnosis to be excluded. In young females, when unilateral salpingitis is suspected, an ectopic pregnancy is often the more likely diagnosis. Similarly, in patients with acute right iliac fossa pain, appendicitis should never be ranked less than second in the differential diagnosis.

Speed of onset. The sudden onset of severe abdominal pain which progresses rapidly, becomes generalised in site and constant in nature in a previously asymptomatic patient suggests either perforation of a hollow viscus, ruptured aortic aneurysm or mesenteric arterial occlusion. Any prior symptoms may usefully contribute to the differential diagnosis; preceding constipation suggests colonic carcinoma or diverticular disease as the cause of perforation and preceding dyspepsia suggests perforated peptic ulceration. Coexisting peripheral vascular disease, hypertension, cardiac failure and atrial fibrillation suggest vascular disorders, e.g. mesenteric ischaemia and aortic aneurysm. The sudden onset of peripheral circulatory failure (shock) contemporaneous with the onset of pain, strongly suggests intra-abdominal bleeding, e.g. ruptured ectopic pregnancy or aortic aneurysm.

The rapid onset of abdominal pain may also occur if an organ twists, occluding its vascular supply. Torsion of the testis or ovary produces severe abdominal pain and often nausea. Torsion of the caecum or sigmoid colon (volvulus) commonly presents with sudden abdominal pain associated with the development of acute intestinal obstruction. A slower onset and progression of abdominal pain over hours or days suggests inflammatory disorders such as acute cholecystitis, appendicitis and diverticulitis.

Symptom progression. The development of shoulder tip pain is confirmation of infradiaphragmatic peritoneal inflammation. In some patients seen within the first hour or two of the onset of perforation, a 'silent interval' may be apparent when abdominal pain resolves transiently. This is due to the initial chemical peritonitis, which begins to subside before bacterial contamination and peritonitis ensues.

In appendicitis, pain is initially localised around the umbilicus (visceral pain) and is vague; as the inflammatory response progresses to involve the parietal peritoneum, the main site of pain shifts to the right iliac fossa (parietal or somatic pain). If rupture of the appendix occurs, generalised peritonitis may then develop. If not, the patient may develop a localised abscess which may subsequently rupture to produce generalised peritonitis.

A change in the pattern of symptoms should alert the clinician to the possibility that either the initial diagnosis was wrong or that complications have developed. In a patient with acute small bowel obstruction, a change in the pain from typical intestinal colic to persistent pain with abdominal tenderness suggests intestinal ischaemia, as for example in a strangulated hernia, and is an indication for urgent surgical intervention.

Symptom patterns. The typical pattern of specific symptoms in many gastrointestinal disorders occurs in only a minority of instances; for the most part, the constellation of symptoms encountered often represents a limited subset of the possible symptoms known to occur in a specific disorder. Clusters of specific symptoms and signs can however prove particularly useful diagnostic aids in patients with an 'acute abdomen' and examples are illustrated in Figures 6.24 and 6.25.

Important points in the clinical examination

* The examination may begin with the abdomen but should then proceed to other systems since the disorder may be non-alimentary in origin.
* The hernial orifices, scrotal contents and rectum are important components of the examination.
* In children, rectal examination is upsetting and should be deferred to the senior clinician making the therapeutic decisions.

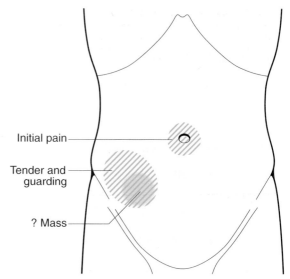

Fig. 6.24 Acute appendicitis.

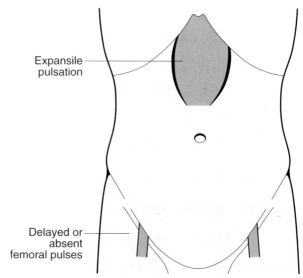

Fig. 6.25 Ruptured aortic aneurysm.

* Tenderness elicited by rectal and vaginal examination may be the sole sign of inflammation of the pelvic peritoneum in acute appendicitis and salpingitis respectively.
* Bimanual rectal and vaginal examination can be useful in assessing pelvic masses.
* Palpation of the abdominal wall overlying an inflamed organ may produce localised pain. In acute cholecystitis, Murphy's sign will be present.
* Localised peritonitis may be revealed by eliciting rebound tenderness on palpation.
* Attempts to elicit rebound are unnecessary and

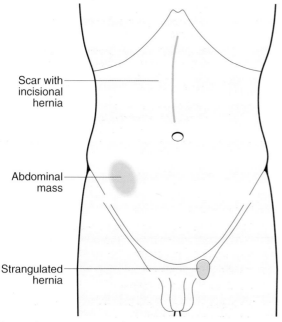

Fig. 6.23 Intestinal obstruction. Some signs which indicate the likely cause.

Table 6.15 Features in various causes of the acute abdomen

Condition	History	Examination
Intestinal obstruction (Fig 6.23)	Colicky, central abdominal pain Nausea and vomiting Constipation	Surgical scars Hernias Abdominal mass Abdominal distension Visible peristalis Increased, tinkling bowel sounds
Acute appendicitis (Fig. 6.24)	Nausea and anorexia; vomiting in children > adults Gradual onset of central abdominal pain Abdominal pain which shifts to the right iliac fossa	Fever Tenderness and guarding in the right iliac fossa Palpable mass in the right iliac fossa Signs of pelvic peritonitis on examination
Ruptured ectopic pregnancy	Premenopausal female Delayed or missed menstrual period Fainting or feeling faint; circulatory collapse Unilateral right or left iliac fossa, cramp-like pain Shoulder tip pleuritic pain Onset of a 'late period' vaginal discharge like prune juice	Suprapubic tenderness Periumbilical bruising (Cullen's sign) Pain/tenderness on vaginal examination (cervical excitation) Swelling/fullness in the fornix on vaginal examination
Pelvic inflammatory disease	Age < 40 with previous history of sexually transmitted disease or pelvic inflammatory disease Recent gynaecological procedure, pregnancy or use of an intrauterine contraceptive device Irregular menstrual bleeding Dysuria and deep dyspareunia Bilateral lower abdominal pain and backache Pleuritic right hypochondrial pain (Fitz Hugh Curtis syndrome)	Fever and vaginal discharge Signs of pelvic peritonitis on rectal examination Right hypochondrial tenderness (perihepatitis) Paint/tenderness on vaginal examination (cervical excitation) Swelling/fullness in the fornix on vaginal examination
Acute pancreatitis	Anorexia, nausea and vomiting Constant severe epigastric pain radiating to the back Excessive alcohol consumption Previous cholelithiasis	Fever Periumbilical bruising (Cullen's sign) Bruising in the loin (Grey–Turner's sign) Epigastric tenderness and guarding less than would be expected Absent or reduced bowel sounds
Acute mesenteric ischaemia	Elderly patient with history of cardiovascular disease Anorexia, nausea and vomiting Watery or bloody diarrhoea Constant severe abdominal pain > 8–12 hours	Atrial fibrillation and/or cardiac failure Absent or asymmetrical peripheral pulses Absent bowel sounds Tenderness and guarding often minimal unless advanced
Acute peritonitis	Vomiting at onset diminishing later Sudden, acute abdominal pain Previous dyspepsia NSAID or corticosteriod therapy	Shallow breathing without abdominal movement Abdominal tenderness, guarding, board-like rigidity Abdominal distension Absent bowel sounds
Ruptured aortic aneurysm (Fig. 6.25)	Elderly aged > 60 years Recent onset of back or loin pain Severe central, lower abdominal pain	Circulatory collapse and shock Pulsatile, midline abdominal mass with bruit Asymmetrical or absent femoral pulses

should not be made when evidence of peritonitis has already been established.

• Inflammation of the parietal peritoneum causes reflex contraction of the overlying abdominal muscles to produce guarding. Generalised peritonitis may produce 'board-like' rigidity when even light percussion may elicit pain.

These principles are now applied to a number of specific conditions (see Table 6.15).

KEY POINTS

• The first history should be as detailed as possible because acutely ill patients tire easily and accuracy may be lost on repetition.

• Speed of onset may be of greater diagnostic significance than site of pain.

• Symptom progression and symptom patterns are often of diagnostic value.

ILLUSTRATIVE CASE STUDIES

Patient A

A 49-year-old woman presented with severe left-sided loin pain associated with vomiting. The pain radiated into the groin and was sustained, suggesting renal colic. The past medical history revealed a previous right nephrectomy for 'chronic pyelonephritis' and 'migraine' for which she had been taking NSAIDs on a daily basis for over 10 years. Her last menstrual period had been 2 weeks ago and for the last 6 hours she had been anuric, suggesting complete urinary tract obstruction.

Physical examination revealed a restless woman distressed by pain necessitating intravenous opiate therapy before clinical examination could proceed further. Tenderness was noted in the renal angle and left iliac fossa and the bladder was impalpable. Both rectal and vaginal examination were normal, excluding cervical or pelvic malignancy as the cause of anuria.

An intravenous pyelogram was undertaken immediately and revealed complete obstruction of the left ureter at the pelvic brim. A urological opinion was sought and ureteric cannulation performed with the retrieval of a large fleshy 'stone'. Urine flow was rapidly re-established; pathological examination of the 'stone' revealed this to be a necrotic renal papilla confirming the diagnosis of necrotising papillitis due to analgesic nephropathy.

Patient B

An 86-year-old man presented with central abdominal pain of 12 hours' duration associated with vomiting and constipation. The history strongly suggested small intestinal obstruction as the pain occurred every 5–10 minutes, in waves lasting 2–3 minutes, yet there was no previous history of abdominal surgery. On physical examination, the patient was pyrexial and the abdomen was distended and tympanitic to percussion but without localising tenderness on palpation.

Treatment with intravenous fluid replacement was instituted and plain abdominal radiographs confirmed obstruction of the distal small bowel with gaseous distension and no air visible in the colon. Abdominal examination was repeated and a rectal examination performed; a more careful examination of the hernial orifices revealed a small mass lying below and medial to the mid-inguinal point. The mass was irreducible with no discernible cough impulse. At laparotomy, a strangulated femoral hernia containing ischaemic small bowel was found, necessitating small bowel resection.

EXAMINATION OF THE URINE

Useful diagnostic information can be obtained from analysis of the urine as significant renal involvement in disease may develop without specific symptoms or signs and is usually accompanied by urinary abnormalities. Their presence may be the first indication of renal disease or of disorders which do not primarily affect the kidneys; for example, glycosuria may be the sole manifestation of diabetes mellitus.

Urine analysis should therefore be performed routinely and is best undertaken on a fresh sample either before or immediately after the physical examination. The components of urine analysis are given in Table 6.16.

The principal uses of urine analysis are shown in Table 6.17. Urine analysis is particularly important in patients presenting with the symptoms shown in Table 6.18.

Table 6.16 Components of urine testing

Macroscopic	Biochemical
Colour	Specific gravity
Clarity	pH
Odour	Protein
Volume/24 h	Blood
	Glucose
Microscopic	Ketones
Erythrocytes	Bilirubin
Leucocytes	Urobilinogen
Casts	Nitrite
Crystals	Hormones
Bacteria	
	Microbiological
	Culture

Table 6.17 Principal uses of urine analysis with examples

Screening	Random	Diabetes mellitus
		Asymptomatic bacteriuria
	Selective	Antenatal care
		Hypertension
Diagnosis	Primary renal	Glomerulonephritis
	Secondary renal	Infective endocarditis
	Non-renal disease	Diabetes mellitus
		Porphyria
Monitoring	Disease progress	Nephrotic syndrome
	Drug toxicity	Penicillamine or gold

Table 6.18 Symptoms for which urine analysis is vital

• Fever	• Weight loss
• Thirst	• Jaundice
• Urinary symptoms	• Abdominal pain

Macroscopic examination

Appearance. Normal fresh urine is clear, though its colour varies greatly. Cloudy urine is characteristically milky after meals in *chyluria* and discoloured in the presence of pus (*pyuria*). Urine that is brownish and cloudy (*smokey urine*) owing to the presence of blood suggests proliferative glomerulonephritis. Other typical colour changes suggest the presence of blood, drugs or chemicals (Table 6.10, p. 167).

Odour. Most people are aware of the peculiar smell of concentrated urine. The typical ammoniacal smell of babies' nappies is due to bacterial decomposition. Foods such as asparagus impart a characteristic smell to the urine. A fishy smell suggests urinary infection with *Escherichia coli*.

Volume. Measurement of the urine volume during 24 hours is important in many clinical situations and can confirm the presence of oliguria or polyuria. In states of shock, the hourly urine flow is achieved by bladder catheterisation and can provide a useful dynamic indicator of 'core perfusion'.

24-hour urine volume. The procedure for collection is important.

* Ask the patient to empty the bladder on waking, e.g. 8 a.m.
* Collect all urine passed in the next 24 hours.
* Remind the patient to collect the final sample at 8 a.m. the following morning.

Biochemical examination

For most clinical purposes, commercially available *reagent strip tests* such as N-Multistix SG are all that are required to obtain the necessary diagnostic information.

* Mix a fresh urine sample thoroughly.
* Completely immerse the reagent strip in urine then remove immediately, remove any excess by tapping the strip on the side of the bottle.
* Read the strip at the time specified for accurate results.
* Hold the strip horizontally while assessing colour changes so that urine does not run down the strip from square to square.

Urinary specific gravity. Urinary specific gravity, like osmolality, is an index of the solute concentration and varies in health between 1002 and 1035. Specific gravity depends upon the gram molecular weight of each solute present, but the osmolality depends on the total solute concentration. In normal urine, they correlate closely in the absence of glycosuria.

The concentrating ability of the kidneys is best assessed by an overnight fluid deprivation test. During this procedure, urinary specific gravity should rise above 1022, corresponding to a urinary osmolality of greater than 800 mosmol/l in healthy subjects, though this value decreases with advancing age.

Urinary pH. Urinary pH varies in health between 8.0 and 4.5 and is usually lowest after an overnight fast. On a normal diet, the healthy subject excretes 40–80 mmol of acid, the majority of which is buffered by phosphates. In renal tubular acidosis, either congenital or acquired in origin, urinary acidification is impaired and urinary pH never falls below 5.3 even after an oral challenge with ammonium chloride.

Proteinuria. Urine testing for protein should be performed on fresh concentrated urine, and an early morning sample in therefore the most suitable. Proteinuria of less than 300 mg/l is a normal finding and values in excess of this may occur transiently in the absence of renal disease (Table 6.19). Proteinuria of less than 1 g/l is an occasional finding in healthy young subjects and disappears on lying supine (*orthostatic proteinuria*).

Proteinuria may be glomerular or tubular in origin; proteinuria greater than 2 g per day suggests glomerular disease. It is important to remember that significant proteinuria may be absent in major renal disease, including polycystic renal disease, chronic pyelonephritis and obstructive uropathy. The reagent strip is impregnated with tetrabromophenol blue and false-positive and false-negative results may occur (Table 6.20).

Haematuria. Haematuria is detected by the peroxidase-like activity of the haem moiety oxidising otolidine and other chemicals in the reagent strip test. A positive finding may occur as a result of conditions outwith the renal tract (see Table 6.21). The presence of haematuria should be confirmed by urine microscopy.

Glycosuria and ketonuria. Both glucose and ketones are small molecules and pass across the glomerulus to be reabsorbed in the proximal tubule. They will appear in the urine if the maximal tubular reabsorption rate is exceeded, either because their concentrations are high or because the glomerular filtrate is increased or both.

Reagent strip tests are glucose specific and false-

Table 6.19 Causes of incidental proteinuria

• Cold exposure	• Adrenaline administration
• Strenuous exercise	• Postural proteinuria
• Abdominal surgery	• Congestive cardiac failure
• Febrile illness	• Severe skin disease and burns

Table 6.20 Misleading reagent strip tests for proteinuria

False positive	Phenothiazine therapy
	Contamination with alkalis or detergents
False negative	Contamination with acid preservatives

Table 6.21 Misleading reagent strip tests for haematuria

False-positive test	Potassium iodide therapy
	Contamination with bleach
	Skin contamination with povidone iodine
	Stale urine (bacterial peroxidase)
Non-urinary origin	Menstruation
	Haemoglobinuria
	Myoglobinuria

Table 6.22 Misleading reagent strip tests for glycosuria and ketonuria

	Glycosuria	Ketonuria
False positive	Bleach and detergents	L-dopa therapy
		Phenolphthalein
False negative	Vitamin C therapy	
	L-dopa therapy	
	Salicylate therapy	

Table 6.23 Misleading reagent strip tests for bilirubinuria and urobilinogenuria

	Bilirubinuria	Urobilinogenuria
False positive	Phenothiazine therapy	Rifampicin therapy
		p-Aminosalicylates
		Azo dye metabolites
False negative	Stale urine	Stale urine
	Rifampicin therapy	
	Azo dye metabolites	

Streptococcus faecalis. The reagent strip contains an alpha-naphthylamine which is converted to an azo dye by the nitrite formed by bacteria from urinary nitrates. The test requires a fresh, early morning urine having incubated within the bladder overnight. False-positive results are rare. False-negative results occur if bladder emptying is frequent, (leaving too little time for in vivo incubation) if dietary nitrogen is insufficient or if the infecting organism is a non-nitrite producer such as *Staphylococcus albus*.

Microscopic examination

Urine microscopy is the only reliable method of establishing the presence of erythrocytes, leucocytes, abnormal cells, casts or crystals. These structures rapidly disintegrate if urine is left standing. Bacillary but not coccal bacteriuria can readily be discerned on an unstained wet film on low-power magnification. High-power magnification is necessary to distinguish erythrocytes from leucocytes, yeasts and small crystals. Phase-contrast and polarised-light microscopy are necessary to best identify casts and crystals respectively.

Cells. *Red blood cells* from the glomeruli are irregular in size and shape; those from the renal pelvis, ureter or bladder are of uniform morphology. *White blood cells* have lobed nuclei and have granular cytoplasm (Fig. 6.26). They are different from renal tubular cells, which are larger in size and have oval nuclei. Leuco-cyturia is marked in urinary infection but also occurs to a lesser degree in chronic pyelonephritis and some forms of glomerulonephritis. *Epithelial cells* are nucleated and three times the size of red cells.

Urinary casts. *Hyaline casts* are best seen on low illumination and consist of Tamm–Horsfall muco-protein. It is unusual to see more than one per low-power field in health; they are numerous in the following situations:

- severe exercise
- febrile illnesses
- severe essential hypertension
- chronic renal disease.

positive results are rare; the test involves glucose oxidase conversion of glucose to gluconic acid, which reacts with a peroxidase to produce a colour change. Acetoacetate alone and not beta-hydroxybutyrate is detected by a nitroprusside reaction in reagent strip tests for ketones.

Causes of false-positive and false-negative test results are shown in Table 6.22.

Bilirubinuria and urobilinogenuria. Unconjugated bilirubin is bound to albumin and does not appear in the urine in haemolytic jaundice (*acholuric jaundice*). However urobilinogen production in the small bowel in greatly increased and appears in the urine as a colourless compound detectable using a reagent strip test.

Conjugated hyperbilirubinaemia results in both hepatocellular and obstructive jaundice. Conjugated bilirubin is not protein-bound and the excess is excreted in the urine. It produces brown urine with a yellow froth (when shaken) and is easily detected by a reagent strip test. The absence of urobilinogen on testing dark-brown urine containing excess bilirubin is characteristic of complete biliary obstruction and its reappearance indicates resolving obstruction.

Causes of false-positive and false-negative results for bilirubinuria and urobilinogenuria are shown in Table 6.23.

Urinary nitrite. Nitrite-producing bacteria represent over 90% of urinary pathogens, particularly *E. coli* and

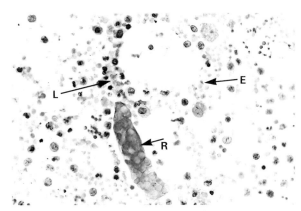

Fig. 6.26 Urine microscopy (magnification × 640). Red cell cast surrounded by red cells and white blood cells with lobed nuclei; E. erythrocytes; L, leucocytes; R, red cell cast. (Courtesy of Dr M. A. McIntyre)

Densely granular casts are always pathological, occasionally confused with red cell casts and comprise hyaline casts containing granules of albumin and immunoglobulins. They are typically found in the following disorders:

• glomerulonephritis except minimal change
• accelerated hypertension
• amyloidosis
• diabetic nephropathy.

Cellular casts are hyaline or granular casts with tubular epithelial cells on their surface. They are characteristic in the following conditions:

• acute tubular necrosis
• proliferative glomerulonephritis.

Red cell casts contain erythrocytes and are always accompanied by biochemical evidence of haematuria on urine testing. They are pathognomonic of glomerular bleeding as seen in proliferative glomerulonephritis.

White cell casts are uncommon and are seen in acute pyelonephritis.

Urine microscopy. This requires to be performed with attention to detail.

• Centrifuge 10 ml of fresh urine for 5 minutes at 3000 r.p.m.
• Remove the supernatant, leaving 0.5 ml of urine and the deposit.
• Mix the sediment gently and place one drop on a clean slide.
• Overlay a cover slip and examine under the microscope with low illumination and low-power magnification.

• Examine under high-power magnification if abnormalities seen require further elucidation.

Microbiological examination

For the detection of tubercle bacilli, several early morning urine samples should be sent to the laboratory. For all other suspected bacterial infections, a fresh, clean-voided, mid-stream urine sample is required; detailed attention must be paid to the collection technique.

• Collect the urine by placing the sterile container (wide-mouthed for females) in the urine stream once micturition is well under way.
• Label the urine sample with the time, date and patient's name.
• Despatch to the laboratory without delay. If a delay is unavoidable, place the sample in an ordinary fridge (not freezer) until transport arrives.

FURTHER INVESTIGATIONS

In most instances, the diagnosis is made clinically but requires confirmation by further investigation. When investigation involves any degree of hazard, including ionising irradiation, the risks and benefits require careful consideration.

Radiological investigations

The effects of ionising irradiation depend upon the dose rate, the tissue distribution and the type of radiation: photon (gamma-rays and X-rays) or particulate (alpha- and beta-particles). Absorbed dosages are measured in Grays (1 Gy = 1 joule/kg or 100 rads).

Table 6.24 Relative radiation dosages of common investigations

Exposure	Effective dose equivalents (μSv)
Background irradiation/year	2000
Chest radiograph	20
Abdominal radiograph	1500
Lumbar spine radiograph	2400
Barium meal	5000
Barium enema	9000
Intravenous urography	4600
Isotope lung scan	1200
Isotope bone scan	3800
Isotope renal scan	700
Isotope liver scan	700
CT brain	2000
CT chest or abdomen	8000

Table 6.25 Special investigations in alimentary and genitourinary disease

Investigation	Indications	Possible findings and comments
Chest radiograph	Acute abdomen	Pneumonia (*or* incidental diagnosis)
	Perforated viscus	Air beneath diaphragm
	Subphrenic abscess	Pleural effusion
		Elevated diaphragm
Abdominal radiograph	Intestinal obstruction	Fluid levels
	Intestinal perforation	Air above the liver
	Renal colic	Calculus in the urinary tract
Intravenous urography	Haematuria	Renal, ureteric or
	Renal colic	bladder disease/stones
Barium meal	Dysphagia	Oesophageal obstruction
	Dyspepsia	Not routinely indicated in patients aged < 45 or post gastric surgery
Small bowel barium examination	Malabsorption	Duodenal diverticuli
	Subacute obstruction	Crohn's disease
	Unexplained GI bleeding	Tumour
Large bowel barium examination	Altered bowel habit	Colonic carcinoma
	Rectal bleeding	Colitis
		Diverticulitis
Upper abdominal ultrasound	Biliary colic	Gall stones
	Malignancy	Hepatic metastases
	Jaundice	Extrahepatic cholestasis
	Pancreatitis	Gall stones/pancreatic calcification
	Abdominal sepsis	Subphrenic abscess
	Aortic aneurysm	CT if leaking suspected
Pelvic ultrasound	Pelvic and abdominal masses	
	Pelvic inflammatory disease	
	Ectopic pregnancy	
	Polycystic ovary syndrome	
Urinary tract ultrasound	Renal failure	Differentiating renal from post-renal causes
	Renal mass	Cystic or solid
	Prostatism	Pre and post voiding bladder residual volume
	Scrotal mass or pain	Unhelpful in torsion

Table 6.25 *Cont'd*

Investigation	Indications	Possible findings and comments
Upper GI endoscopy	GI bleeding	Ideally within 24 hours
	Dysphagia	Even if barium negative
	Dyspepsia	Especially if aged > 45
	Gastric ulcer	Biopsy for ?malignancy
	Malabsorption	Duodenal biopsy. ?Coeliac
Lower GI endoscopy	Rectal bleeding	Even if barium enema negative
	Ulcerative colitis	Biopsy confirmation and exclusion of dysplasia
Endoscopic retrograde cholangio-pancreatography	Obstructive jaundice	Diagnosis
	Pancreatitis	Stenting strictures
Abdominal CT	Renal or pancreatic mass	Tumour
	Lymphadenopathy	Lymphoma
	Tumour staging	Extent of disease
	Abdominal aneurysm	If leaking is suspected, surgery is urgent
Laparoscopy	Acute abdomen	Appendicitis
		Ectopic pregnancy
		Acute salpingitis
		Endometriosis
		Acute pancreatitis
	Tumour staging	Extent of disease
Aspiration cytology	Hepatic metastases	Perform under ultrasound guidance
	Intra-abdominal masses	
	Retroperitoneal masses	
Liver biopsy	Diffuse parenchymal disease	
Renal biopsy	Glomerulonephritis	Perform under ultrasound guidance
Pancreatic stimulation tests	Pancreatic failure	Reduced bicarbonate and enzyme secretion

Since different types of radiation have different effects on different tissues, the effective dose equivalent, measured in Sieverts (1 Sv = 100 rems), is used to express the equivalent dose of uniform whole-body irradiation. Typical radiation dosages incurred during various investigations are shown in Table 6.24. Irradiation of any area between the diaphragm and the knees should be avoided in pregnancy unless there are overriding clinical considerations. Some indications for preferring special investigations are shown in Table 6.25.

KEY POINTS

- Microscopy provides the only reliable method of detecting cells and casts in the urine.
- Red cell casts are an indication of glomerular bleeding.
- It should be possible to justify any investigation performed.

RECOMMENDED READING

Ford M J, Robertson C E, Munro J F 1987 Manual of
   medical procedures. Churchill Livingstone, Edinburgh
Gazzard B, Theodossi A (eds) 1985 Symptoms in
   gastroenterology. Clinics in gastroenterology, 14:3.
   W B Saunders, London

Shearman D J C, Finlayson N D C 1990 Diseases of the
   gastrointestinal tract and liver 2E. Churchill Livingstone,
   Edinburgh
Sweny P, Farrington K, Moorhead J F 1989 The kidney and
   its disorders. Blackwell Scientific Publications, Oxford

R. E. Cull • I. R. Whittle

7

The nervous system

More than any other aspect of clinical medicine, examination of the nervous system is founded on well-established principles of anatomy and physiology. In many instances, the taking of a detailed history and execution of a careful clinical examination will enable the clinician to localise the site of the neurological lesion and to establish a precise or differential diagnosis. When disease processes affect the *structure* of neural tissue (e.g. vascular disease, multiple sclerosis, tumours), changes in neurological function are often found during clinical examination. Disorders of neural *function* (e.g. epilepsy, migraine) may produce no abnormal signs on examination; it is here that careful history taking is of paramount importance.

The important point in neurological examination is to be systematic, irrespective of the order in which the different parts of the nervous system are examined. As experience is gained in clinical practice, aspects of the examination can be either abridged or focused depending upon the history, general observations of the patient's level of cognitive and sensorimotor function and preliminary examination findings.

THE HISTORY

In many instances the diagnosis of a neurological illness can be based on details given from the patient's history. The general principles of history-taking apply as outlined in Chapter 1, but emphasis should be placed on the following special aspects relating to the nervous system:

Time relationships

- When did the symptoms start/stop?
- How long do they last?
- Do they occur at certain times of the day/week/month?
- Do symptoms evolve over seconds, hours, days, weeks or months?

Localisation

- Which part of the body is affected?
- Can the patient localise the problem to one limb or part of it?
- If more widespread, is the problem symmetrical?

Precipitating factors

- Are symptoms triggered by any specific activity, e.g. exercise, sleep, posture, reading, eating, coughing, micturition, sexual activity; or by external stimuli, e.g. light, sound, smell, heat or cold?

Associated symptoms

- Are the presenting symptoms accompanied by other features of neurological disease?
  — numbness, paraesthesiae, cold, warmth (sensory system)
  — weakness, clumsiness, stiffness, unsteady gait (motor system)
  — headache
  — nausea, vomiting
  — loss or alteration of consciousness
  — visual disturbances
  — psychological changes, e.g. depression or elation, weeping, agitation, sleep and appetite disturbance, change in energy and libido.

Past history

Some neurological disorders (e.g. epilepsy, hydrocephalus) present many years after the causative event. It is therefore important to ask about:

— pregnancy (full term; intrauterine problems)
— delivery (normal, assisted or operative)
— neonatal health (severe jaundice, respiratory difficulty, infections and convulsions)
— infancy (infections, convulsions, injuries)
— childhood and early adult life (head and spinal injury, serious infections, particularly meningitis, encephalitis, surgical operations and drug therapy).

Family history

Many neurological disorders have a genetic basis or predisposition. Some may be strictly genetic disorders (e.g. muscular dystrophy, spinocerebellar degeneration, Huntington's chorea). In others, genetic factors appear to influence the development of the condition (e.g. epilepsy, migraine, multiple sclerosis, vascular disease).

Social history

The patient's *occupation* may be relevant in the causation or triggering of neurological disorders, e.g.:

- exposure to toxic chemicals (neuropathies and encephalopathy)
- recurrent overuse of certain joints predisposing to entrapment neuropathy in manual workers (carpal tunnel syndrome).

- prolonged visual work, particularly with visual display units or under artificial light (tension headache and migraine).

Marital status and household dynamics and any change of lifestyle should be ascertained. Marriage, divorce, bereavement and change of occupation are all important factors in emotionally based symptoms, particularly tension headache, migraine and depression, but also may trigger attacks of multiple sclerosis and epilepsy. Smoking habits both past and present should be elicited, as should the use and possible abuse of alcohol or other drugs. It may be appropriate to ask about the patient's sexual orientation and any possibility of exposure to sexually transmitted diseases or HIV.

A summary of the information that should be obtained from patients presenting with neurological symptoms is given in Table 7.1.

KEY POINTS

- Disorders of neural function may produce no abnormal signs. The diagnosis is often dependent on the history.

- Some neurological disorders may present many years after the causative event.

- Stress may induce neurological symptoms.

NEUROLOGICAL EXAMINATION

GENERAL OBSERVATION

Before starting the formal neurological examination it is often possible to obtain useful information by observing the patient before and during history-taking (see Table 7.2).

Gait

The patient should be observed on entering the consulting room. Patients in the hospital ward should be asked to walk if possible. Abnormalities such as hemiparesis and Parkinsonism cause specific types of gait disturbance (see Table 7.3).

Balance mechanisms relying on cerebellar, vestibular and proprioceptive systems can be tested by heel–toe (tandem) walking and by carrying out *Romberg's test*. Patients with cerebellar deficits will often have difficulty standing in this position even with the eyes open.

Table 7.1 Summary of neurological history-taking

Presenting complaint	Time relationships Localisation Trigger factors Associated features
Past medical history	Birth/pregnancy Head/spine injury Infections (meningitis/encephalitis) Surgical procedures Drug therapy
Family history	Epilepsy, migraine, multiple sclerosis, stroke, cerebral aneurysm, muscle disorders, dementia, spinocerebellar degenerations and neuropathies
Social history	Occupation Marital status Smoking habits Alcohol consumption Use of recreational drugs Sexual orientation and habits

Table 7.2 The nervous system: general observations

- Gait
- Romberg's test
- Speech
- Handwriting
- Mental state
- Facial appearance
- Involuntary movements
- Movements of the neck and spine

Table 7.3 Disorders of gait

Hemiparesis	Patient drags affected leg stiffly, foot inverted, arm flexed at the side
Bilateral leg spasticity	Patient leans forward, legs adducted, and walks stiffly on toes (equinus)
Footdrop	Patient flexes the hip, lifting the foot off the ground. The foot slaps down noisily
Parkinsonism	Patient is slow to start walking and takes small strides. There is a tendency to walk faster or to suddenly freeze, failure to swing one or both arms and loss of postural reflexes if pushed from standing position
Cerebellar deficit (ataxia)	The gait is broad based. The patient may sway from side to side and may fall or have to hold on to furniture or walls
Apraxia (e.g. hydrocephalus or multi-infarct states)	Patient has a broad-based, small-stepping, unsteady gait and difficulty in turning

Examination

❏ To perform Romberg's test ask the patient to stand with feet together and eyes open initially (Fig. 7.1A).
❏ Then ask the patient to close the eyes (Fig. 7.1B).

Where there is a proprioceptive or vestibular deficit, balance is impaired only when the eyes are closed, and the patient may fall if not caught.

Speech

Much may be learned about the patient's speech and language function during history-taking. If a deficit of speech is evident a more thorough examination of these functions should be undertaken. By analysing speech and language carefully it is often possible to localise the causative lesion. Speech disorders may be divided into two main groups:

1. Disorders of articulation (*dysarthria*) and phonation (*dysphonia*).

2. Disorders of language areas in the dominant hemisphere (*dysphasia*).

Dysarthria

Dysarthria may be caused by purely mechanical factors such as ill-fitting dentures, but it is usually due to weakness or impaired coordination of the orolingual muscles concerned with the production of consonants (see Table 7.4). Dysarthric speech is indistinct and difficult for the listener to discern. However, its grammatical construction is normal, and the patient's comprehension of spoken and written language is retained. With cerebellar deficits the dysarthria has a slurred quality with imprecise control of word length and tonal inflection, giving it a drawling, 'sing-song' quality. Dysarthria is often evident during conversation with the patient during history-taking. If there is doubt the patient can be asked to enunciate specific phrases which require precise articulation, e.g. 'West Register Street'.

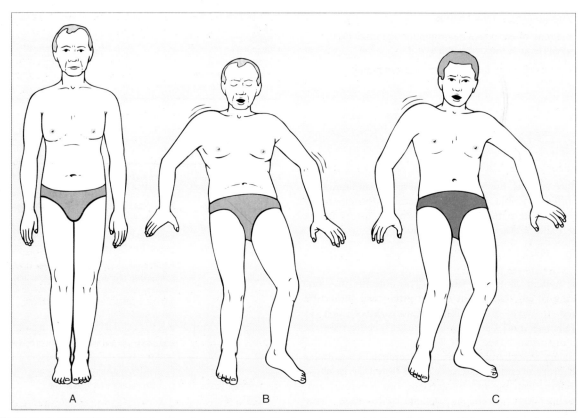

A   B   C

Fig. 7.1 Romberg's test for position sense.   The patient can stand with feet together and eyes open **A.** but falls with eyes closed **B.** In contrast, the patient with a cerebellar lesion cannot stand with feet together and eyes open **C.**

Table 7.4 Causes of dysarthria and dysphonia

Mechanism	Example
Weakness of facial and tongue muscles	Myasthenia gravis
Lesions of lower brain stem (bulbar palsy)	Motor neurone disease
Bilateral corticospinal tract lesions above the pons	Multiple lacunar infarcts
Impaired control of phonation and articulation	Parkinsonism
Imprecise motor control systems	Cerebellar lesions
Impaired larynx function	Recurrent laryngeal nerve palsy

Elevation of the soft palate is used to close off the nasopharynx for the production of explosive consonants ('b' and 'g'). Palatal weakness or anatomical defects in the palate cause 'nasal' speech with failure to produce these sounds correctly. For example, when such a patient tries to say the word 'egg' it is pronounced as 'eng'.

Dysphonia

The production of tones in speech is achieved by movement of expired air through the larynx. Vibration of the vocal cords produces the frequency changes used in speech and singing. Poor respiratory function may cause dysphonia, but more typically it is the result of laryngeal problems, causing hoarseness of the voice, often with reduced speech volume.

Dysphasia

Difficulty with language function is called dysphasia and is due to lesions in the language areas of the dominant cerebral hemisphere. In the vast majority of right-handed people the left hemisphere is dominant. About a third of left handers have a dominant right hemisphere; the others have either left-sided or bilateral language localisation. The main language areas are shown in Figure 7.2.

Broca's area (the inferior frontal region) is concerned with the generation of motor programmes for the production of words or parts of words (phonemes). Damage to this area causes:

- reduced number of words used
- poorly articulated and non-fluent speech
- errors of grammar and syntax.

Such speech has a telegrammatic quality, but if the lesion is relatively localised comprehension of spoken and written language is usually preserved.

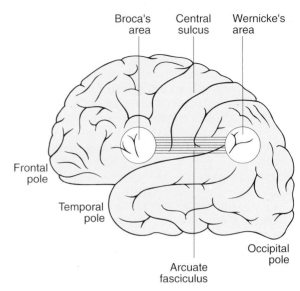

Fig. 7.2 The main language areas.

Wernicke's area, the posterior temporal lobe and the adjoining parietal region are concerned with the comprehension of language and the selection of words to convey meaning. With dysfunction in this area, the output of spontaneous speech may be normal or increased, the speech fluent and the articulation of phonemes is usually intact. However, the speech may contain:

- incorrect words (verbal paraphasias)
- incorrect letters (literal paraphasias)
- nonsense words (neologisms).

Conduction dysphasia. In this disorder the striking defect is inability of the patient to repeat phrases or words spoken by the examiner. The causative lesion lies in the perisylvian area with damage to the arcuate fasciculus of fibres.

Global dysphasia. In this condition there are marked elements of both anterior (Broca) and posterior (Wernicke) dysphasias. This results from large lesions in the middle cerebral artery territory. It may be so marked as to abolish speech completely (aphasia).

Language functions may be examined formally in order to bring out the various elements.

Examination (Table 7.5)

☐ *Spontaneous speech*: Assess the output of spontaneous speech, fluency and use of inappropriate words, paraphasias and neologisms during conversation.

❑ *Naming of objects*: Ask the patient to name a shown object (e.g. a comb or a pen). The test can be made more difficult by asking the patient to name an object or a concept that is described but not shown.

❑ *Comprehension of spoken speech*: Assess comprehension of spoken speech by asking the patient to carry out commands. Staged commands (e.g. 'pick up the blue card, fold it in half and put it under the white card') help bring out subtle defects. A collection of coins can provide suitable objects for similar arrangement tasks. It is important to avoid giving visual clues.

❑ *Repetition of spoken word:* Ask the patient to say simple sentences such as 'Today is Tuesday'. This is often sufficient to detect repetition failure due to conduction dysphasia.

❑ *Reading aloud:* Ask the patient to read aloud from a book or paper. This may reveal an associated dyslexia.

❑ *Handwriting:* Examine the patient's handwriting. This cannot be assessed if there is a motor deficit affecting the writing hand. Errors of form, grammar and syntax may be found in association with dysphasia, indicating a disorder not only of speech but more globally affecting language function.

Involuntary movements

The presence of involuntary movement is often detected during history-taking. The various types of involuntary movements are shown in Table 7.6.

Examination of the neck and spine

Neck movements. Degenerative arthrosis is a frequent cause of neurological disorders in middle-aged and elderly patients. Passive movement of the neck should be tested to assess the mobility or limitation of move-

Table 7.5 Examination of speech and language

Spontaneous speech	Naming objects, concepts
Articulation	Comprehension of spoken commands
Fluency	Repetition of spoken phrases
Paraphasias	Reading aloud
Grammar	Handwriting
Syntax	

ment, particularly for rotation to either side, which may produce neck pain or radicular symptoms in one upper limb. Flexion and extension movements should also be tested (p. 284). Flexion of the neck sometimes evokes electric shock-like sensations which shoot into the limbs, when the cervical spinal cord sensory tracts are diseased (Lhermitte's sign). This phenomenon is particularly common in multiple sclerosis but is also seen in syringomyelia, cervical cord tumours and spondylotic myelopathy.

Meningeal irritation. Inflammation of the meninges due to infection or blood evokes reflex spasm in the paravertebral muscles. In the cervical area this manifests itself as neck stiffness. Normally the chin can be flexed passively to touch the chest. If neck stiffness is present this is not possible, indeed attempted neck flexion may cause the trunk to rise from the bed (Fig. 7.3A). In the lumbar region, meningeal irritation also causes spasm and this can be demonstrated by passive movements of the lower limbs (Kernig's sign). When positive, attempts to extend the knee joint when the hip joint is flexed are resisted and the other limb may flex at the hip (Fig. 7.3B).

Evidence of meningeal irritation should be looked for in any patient in whom meningitis or subarachnoid haemorrhage is a possibility. The signs, however, may be absent in the early evolution of a subarachnoid haemorrhage or in the deeply comatose patient.

Table 7.6 Involuntary movements

Movement	Description	Sites affected
Tremor	Rhythmical oscillations 4–10/s	Hands, arms, legs, head/neck
Chorea	Jerks, rapid, semipurposive, changing in site and variable	Head, arms, hands, legs, trunk
Athetosis	Slow, writhing, distal	Hands, feet
Dystonia	Slow, sustained, turning or postural	Head, neck, arms, legs, trunk
Myoclonus	Sudden shock-like non-purposive, affecting muscles, groups of muscles or whole body	Limbs, trunk, whole body
Hemiballismus	Proximal, flailing, continuous and of wide amplitude	Arm and leg on one side
Orofacial–lingual dyskinesias	Grimacing, chewing tongue, writhing	Face, mouth, tongue
Tics	Repetitive, purposive, stereotyped, jerky	Face, limbs, respiratory muscles, trunk, voice

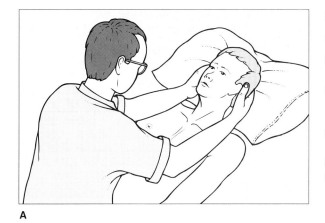

A

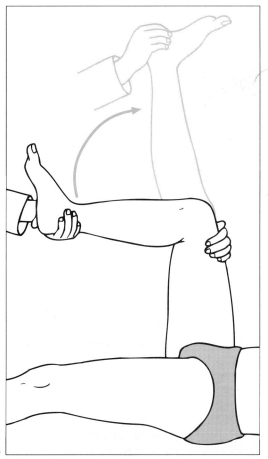

B

Fig. 7.3 Testing for meningeal irritation. A. neck rigidity B. Kernig's test.

Examination

Neck stiffness

❏ Ask the patient to lie supine and to relax the head onto a single pillow.

❏ Support the occiput with both hands and gently flex the neck until the chin touches the chest – *Kernig's test*.

❏ Ask the patient to lie supine with both legs exposed and fully extended.

❏ Passively flex one leg at the hip and the knee.

❏ Then extend the knee while maintaining the hip in flexion and observe the other limb for reflex flexion at the hip.

Palpation of the supraclavicular fossae. Palpation for lymph nodes, cervical ribs or tenderness should be carried out in patients with arm and hand symptoms. Brachial plexus compression at the thoracic outlet is usually associated with tenderness, and sometimes sensory symptoms are evoked by firm pressure over the plexus.

Auscultation for bruits. Vascular disease is the commonest cause of brain dysfunction in the middle-aged and elderly. Although part of the cardiovascular examination, auscultation for cranial and cervical bruits should also be included with the nervous system assessment. Evidence of stenoses in the carotid and vertebral systems may be found by listening for a systolic bruit over the affected vessel (Fig. 7.4), but the absence of a bruit does not exclude a significant stenotic lesion.

Carotid artery stenosis occurs most often at its cervical bifurcation at the angle of the jaw, whereas bruits due to vertebral or subclavian artery stenosis are best heard at the supraclavicular fossa. It is best to also auscultate between the two sites for bruits arising from a common carotid lesion.

Bruits arising from cerebral arteriovenous malformations may be heard over the cranium but, because the orbit acts as an acoustic window, are better heard by listening with the stethoscope bell placed over a gently closed eyelid. The precordium should always be auscultated to ensure that cardiac murmurs are not being transmitted to cranial vessels.

KEY POINTS

• Dysarthria may be caused by purely mechanical factors such as ill-fitting dentures, but it is usually due to weakness or impaired coordination of orolingual muscles.

• Absence of vascular bruit does not exclude a significant stenotic lesion.

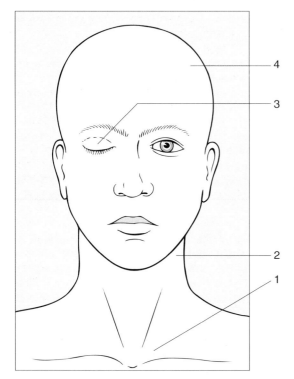

Fig. 7.4 Auscultation for cervical and cranial bruits.   1. Supraclavicular fossa. **2.** Carotid bifurcation. **3.** Over closed eyelid. **4.** Over cranium.

EXAMINATION OF THE CRANIAL NERVES

An understanding of the applied anatomy is essential for correct interpretation of clinical findings. It is prudent to be familiar with the functions, locations and major connections of the cranial nerve nuclei.

The olfactory (I) nerve

The olfactory nerve subserves the sense of smell. Smell receptors are situated high in the nasal cavity, and these bipolar olfactory cells project axons through the cribriform plate of the ethmoid bone to the olfactory bulb. Second-order neurones (mitral cells) then project centrally together with the pyramidal cells of the olfactory nucleus down the olfactory tracts and stria to the primary olfactory cortex (medial temporal lobe) and the ipsilateral amygdaloid body, the anterior perforated substance and the septal area. The primary olfactory cortex has numerous connections with the hypothalamus, reticular system and the limbic lobe.

Testing the sense of smell

Commonly used test substances include vials of peppermint, vanilla, coffee, almond oil or even stronger odours such as whisky or isopropyl alcohol used for skin cleaning.

Examination

- ❏ Check that the nasal passages are clear.
- ❏ Test the sense of smell for each nostril separately.
- ❏ Occlude one nostril by digital pressure.
- ❏ Ask the patient, with eyes closed, to sniff and identify in turn the test substances.

Interpretation

The commonest cause of anosmia is obstruction of the nasal passages. The commonest neurological cause of anosmia is a previous head injury causing shearing damage to the olfactory filaments as they pass through the cribriform plate to the olfactory bulbs. Nasofrontal tumours such as olfactory groove meningiomas and carcinomas arising from the paranasal air sinus are less common causes.

Perversion of smell (parosmia) is sometimes of psychological origin but may occur following partial recovery of the olfactory nerves after trauma. Certain drugs and sinus infection also cause this phenomenon. Olfactory hallucinations, usually of an unpleasant nature, are a characteristic of seizures arising from the primary olfactory cortex. These olfactory hallucinations are often associated with smacking movements of the lips and unusual feelings in the epigastrium.

The optic (II) nerve

The optic nerve transmits the axons of the retinal ganglion cells. It begins at the back of the globe and passes through the optic canal of the sphenoid bone into the cranium, where it joins with the contralateral nerve to form the optic chiasma. The optic tract then passes posteriorly to the lateral geniculate bodies of the thalamus and then to the primary visual cortex (area 17) in the occipital lobe. This tract is termed the geniculocalcarine tract or the optic radiation. The visual association cortex and areas 18 and 19 are in close proximity in the occipital lobe.

General examination

Examination of the optic nerve involves testing:

- visual acuity (see p. 269)
- pupillary reflexes
- visual fields

- colour vision (see p. 270)
- fundoscopy (see p. 263).

Much of the examination of the optic nerve is described in Chapter 8. This section deals with the pupillary reflexes and with the visual fields.

Pupillary reflexes

If a light is directed at one eye, both pupils will normally constrict. The reaction of the pupil on the side stimulated is called the direct light reflex, and the constriction of the other pupil the consensual light reflex. The afferent limb of the reflex involves the retina, optic nerve, chiasma and tract. These fibres terminate in both sides of the midbrain pretectum. The axons then pass to the accessory oculomotor nuclei of Edinger–Westphal. The efferent limbs of the reflex arc are preganglionic parasympathetic fibres in the III nerve, the ciliary ganglion and post-ganglionic fibres that innervate the constrictor muscle of the iris.

When a near object (e.g. at 10 cm) is viewed convergence of the eyes is accompanied by bilateral pupillary constriction referred to as the accommodation reflex.

Examination

☐ Examine the pupils in a dimly lit room for size and symmetry.

☐ Check the direct and consensual reflex in each eye in turn by shining a bright pen torch from the side and from below with the patient looking into the distance in order to avoid an accommodation response.

☐ To test the reaction to accommodation ask the patient first to look into the distance and then at an object held close to the face; observe any change in the pupil size.

Interpretation

Abnormal pupillary reflexes. Impairment or absence of the pupillary reaction to light may be due to damage to either the afferent or efferent sides of the reflex arc. Since both pupils constrict in response to light directed into one eye, afferent lesions can easily be distinguished from damage to the efferent pathway.

With afferent pupillary defect, a pupil does not have a direct light reflex but constricts when light is shone into the opposite eye (i.e. the consensual reflex is preserved). It follows that the dysfunction is on the afferent limb of the reflex arc (retina or optic nerve).

With efferent pupillary defect, one pupil is fixed and dilated and does not respond to light directly, but the contralateral pupil responds consensually. The lesion is on the efferent limb of the unreactive eye (ocular motor nerve, ciliary ganglion).

Other abnormalities of pupillary reflexes are shown in Table 8.2. In the Holmes-Adie syndrome absence of ankle jerks and other deep tendon reflexes are seen in association with myotonic pupils.

Other conditions with abnormalities of either the light or near reflexes are the Parinaud syndrome, oculomotor paresis (see p. 213) and following structural damage to the iris.

Abnormalities of pupillary size. Some abnormalities in pupil size are shown in Table 8.2. Symmetrically small or dilated pupils are commonly drug induced (see Table 7.7).

Pontine haemorrhage causes bilateral pupil constriction, and in anxiety the pupils are symmetrically dilated.

In Horner's syndrome (Fig. 3.16A, p. 59) unilateral miosis is associated with ptosis, impaired sweating and enophthalmos (recession of the globe in the orbital fossa). Paresis of the light reflex and accommodation as a result of a lesion in the ciliary ganglion is termed an internal ophthalmoplegia.

Visual fields

Testing fields assesses the function of the peripheral and central retina, the optic pathways and the cortex. Visual fields can be estimated quickly by the method of confrontation or measured accurately using perimeters. Both methods require a cooperative patient. The normal field extends 160° horizontally and 130° vertically with the physiological blind spot 15° from fixation in the temporal field.

The field for red colour vision is much smaller than that for monochrome. Since colour vision tends to fail early in many disorders of the retina and optic nerve, a red hat-pin is a particularly useful test object for detecting scotomas.

If a patient is unable to cooperate (because of an impaired conscious state or dysphasia) a crude test of visual field integrity can be made by moving the hand

Table 7.7 Drugs affecting the pupil

Dilated (mydriasis)	
Atropine/homatropine	Anticholinergic
Amphetamine and derivatives	Sympathomimetic
Constricted (miosis)	
Neostigmine, morphine and derivatives	Parasympathomimetic

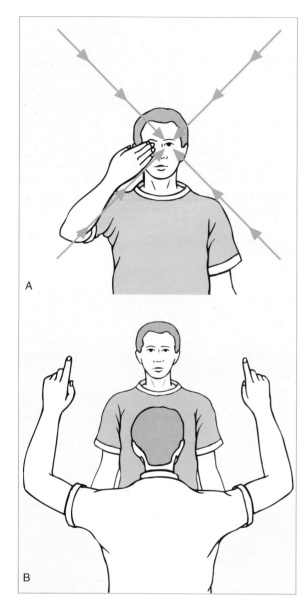

A

B

Fig. 7.5 Testing the visual fields.

quickly towards the patient's face. This menacing stimulus will usually evoke reflex blinking if the incoming stimulus is detected.

When performing confrontation it is convenient to also test for visual inattention by presenting bilateral stimuli. When inattention is present the patient will be able to detect single targets but will ignore objects when two fields are stimulated.

Examination

❏ Sit directly opposite and facing the patient.
❏ Examine each eye separately first.
❏ Ask the patient to cover one eye and look at the examiner's opposing eye (Fig. 7.5).
❏ Examine the outer aspects of the visual fields with a waggling finger or preferably a fine probe with a large red or white head (e.g. a hat pin).
❏ Bring the test object into the field of vision in a curve, not a straight line. Approach from the periphery at several points on the circumference of the upper and lower, nasal and temporal quadrants of the visual fields.
❏ Ask the patient to respond as soon as the movement of the test object is observed.
❏ Map out central field defects by moving the test object across the visual field (Fig. 7.6).
❏ When using a red test object instruct the patient to tell the examiner when it is seen as a red object.
❏ Test for visual inattention by asking the patient to report when the fingertip is moved on one or both sides simultaneously (Fig. 7.7).

Interpretation

Impaired visual acuity can be due to lesions of the cornea, lens, vitreous retina or optic nerve and the more distal visual pathway. Characteristics of optic nerve lesions are shown in Table 7.8.

The common patterns of visual defect are illustrated in Figure 7.8. Lesions proximal to the optic chiasma cause monocular dysfunction. Lesions of the optic chiasma and distal visual pathways will produce binocular visual field defects. Lesions of the optic tract and LGB region are frequently vascular in origin. Common lesions in the optic radiation and occipital cortex are vascular (e.g. posterior cerebral artery infarction), inflammatory (e.g. multiple sclerosis) or neoplastic (e.g. glioma, metastatic neoplasia).

Visual field defects are termed homonymous if the same part of the visual field is affected in each eye. Homonymous defects are due to lesions distal to the optic chiasma (see Fig. 7.8). The field defect can be hemianopic (i.e. if half of the visual field is lost) or

Table 7.8 Common features in optic nerve lesions

Abnormalities	Causes
Abnormal pupillary response	Multiple sclerosis, optic neuritis
Enlargement of blind spot	Vascular disease
Scotomas	Retrobulbar and parasellar neoplasms
Impaired visual acuity	(e.g. pituitary adenomas, craniopharyngioma
Impaired colour vision	and meningioma)
Abnormal fundoscopy	

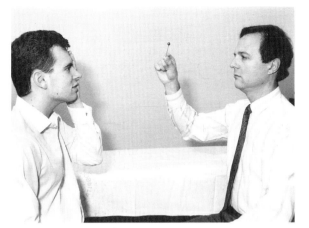

Fig. 7.6 Testing for a central field defect using a red hat-pin.

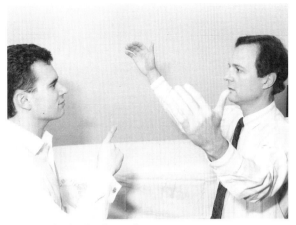

Fig. 7.7 Testing for visual inattention.

quadrantinopic (i.e. only one quarter of the visual field is lost). Furthermore, the field defect can be called upper or lower depending upon which part of the

visual field is impaired. If the visual field loss is not identical in both eyes it is termed incongruous; this type of defect is seen in lesions of the optic tract.

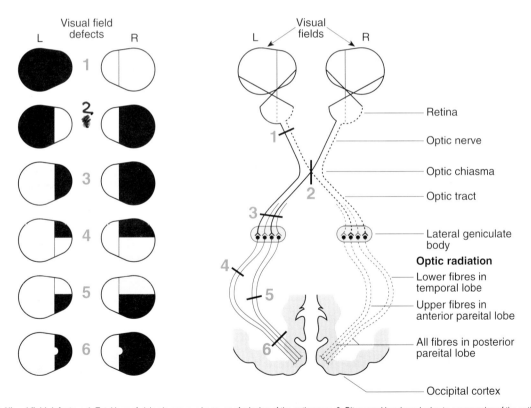

Fig. 7.8 Visual field defects.   1. Total loss of vision in one eye because of a lesion of the optic nerve. 2. Bitemporal hemianopia due to compression of the optic nerve.
3. Right homonymous hemianopia from a lesion of the optic tract. 4. Upper right quadrant hemianopia from a lesion of the lower fibres of the optic radiation in the temporal lobe. 5. Less commonly a lower quadrantic hemanopia occurs from a lesion of the upper fibres of the optic radiation in the anterior part of the parietal lobe.
6. Right homonymous hemianopia with sparing of the macula due to lesion of the optic radiation in the posterior part of the parietal lobe.

Homonymous hemianopia due to occipital cortical lesions tends not to involve the central part of vision (macular sparing).

The oculomotor, trochlear and abducent (III, IV and VI) nerves

These three cranial nerves innervate the muscles controlling eye movement and pupillary size. Although the nerves subserve discrete actions they are examined together because of their close functional inter-relationships.

- The *oculomotor (III)* nerve has its nucleus in the ventral midbrain just anterior to the periaqueductal grey matter. The nerve fibres pass between the cerebral peduncles into the interpeduncular CSF cistern. They pass just below the free edge of the tentorium in relation to the posterior communicating artery and enter the dura surrounding the cavernous sinus. They pass forward and enter the orbital fossa through the superior oblique fissure, where the nerve subdivides into its terminal branches. The oculomotor nerve innervates the superior (SR), medial (MR) and inferior (IR) recti, the inferior oblique (IO) and levator palpebrae superioris (LPS) muscles. These muscles open the upper lid (LPS) and move the globe upwards (SR, IO), downwards (IR) and medially (MR). Through the para-sympathetic fibres it also indirectly innervates the sphincter muscles of the iris, which cause constriction of the pupil. Parasympathetic fibres also pass to the ciliary muscle, which is responsible for focusing the lens for near vision.
- The *trochlear (IV)* nerve arises from a nucleus in the caudal midbrain. The fibres of the IV nerve decussate before leaving the midbrain just below the inferior colliculus. The nerve then passes forward and laterally in relation to the rostral pons and the free edge of the tentorium. It pierces the dura of the tentorial edge and passes through the cavernous sinus and superior orbital fissure. In the orbit it innervates the superior oblique (SO) muscle, contraction of which causes downward movement of the globe when the eye is adducted.
- The *abducent (VI)* nerve originates from a nucleus located near the midline of the caudal pons, where it forms part of the facial colliculus. The fibres emerge from the ventral pontomedullary junction just lateral to the pyramid, pass through the prepontine CSF cistern and pierce the basal dura to enter Dorello's canal and then traverse the cavernous sinus. Here the nerve is in direct relation to the internal carotid

artery before it passes through the superior orbital fissure to the lateral rectus (LR) muscle. Contraction of the LR causes abduction of the eye.

Ocular motility is dependent not only on the integrity of the III, IV and VI nerves but also on the medial longitudinal fasciculus (MLF) which in a central brainstem tract interconnects the nuclei. The MLF also receives direct and indirect input from the vestibular nuclei, cerebellar flocculus and the para-abducens nucleus, also called the nucleus of the paramedian pontine reticular formation (PPRF). This group of neurones is important for lateral gaze. The MLF provides a mechanism by which the optical axes remain parallel or conjugate when the eyes are turned to one side or when there is movement of the head. There are also sypranuclear connections that are important for conjugate eye movements. In area 8 of the frontal lobe there is the frontal eye field (FEF). When this area is stimulated the eyes turn conjugately away from the side of stimulation. There is also an occipital cortical fixation centre, which together with the MLF is important for conjugate eye movements and maintaining visual fixation on a moving target (pursuit movement). The visual cortex is also important for the accommodation-convergence reaction.

The six external ocular muscles move the eyeball in the directions as shown in Figure 7.9.

While the MR and LR subserve horizontal eye movements, vertical eye movement is more complex and mediated both by the IO and SR (upgaze) and the SO and IR (downgaze). Because of the different long axes of the various ocular muscles, the superior oblique is mainly responsible for downgaze and the inferior

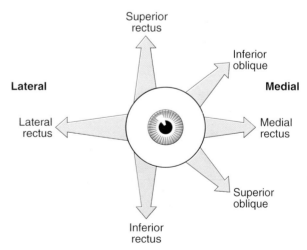

Fig. 7.9 External ocular muscle function.

oblique mainly responsible for upgaze in the adducted eye. The appropriate recti are responsible for vertical gaze in the abducted eye (see Fig. 7.9).

As already mentioned, the parasympathetic fibres derived from the Edinger–Westphal nucleus constrict the pupil. Sympathetic fibres dilate the pupil and also innervate part of the LPS. The preganglionic sympathetic fibres have a very complex course. From their origin in the posterior hypothalamus they emerge through the ventral roots of the first two or three segments of the thoracic spinal cord and ascend through the sympathetic chain to the superior cervical ganglion. Post-ganglionic fibres ascend in the carotid neural plexus and into the orbit with the ophthalmic artery to terminate in the radial muscle of the iris (dilator of the pupil). A lesion of the sympathetic pathway gives rise to Horner's syndrome (Fig. 3.16A, p. 59).

Examination

❏ Inspect the eyes for any abnormality.
❏ With both eyes open, test for ocular movements with the patient's head in the neutral position and, if necessary, held there by one of the examiner's hands on the crown of the head.
❏ Examine carefully for any squint (strabismus) or other abnormality, including nystagmus.
❏ First test by asking the patient to look up and down, and to the right and the left.
❏ Then ask the patient to fix the gaze on the examiner's finger and to report if double vision occurs while following the movement of the finger held 60 cm away.
❏ Move the finger up and down, then to the right and up and down, and then to the left and up and down. If necessary, repeat the examination, one eye at a time, to distinguish between muscle and gaze palsies.
❏ Record the direction in which double vision is present and where maximal separation of the images occurs.
❏ If diplopia is reported ask the patient to close one eye at a time to identify which eye is producing the false image.
❏ To test convergence, ask the patient to focus on the finger as it is brought from a distance towards the tip of the nose.
❏ Look for nystagmus while examining eye movements.
❏ Record the presence of vertical, horizontal or rotatory nystagmus and the direction of gaze in which it is most marked.
❏ Note the direction of the fast component of nystagmus, whether it changes direction with the direction of gaze and whether the degree of nystagmus is different in each eye.

Disorders of ocular movements. On inspection the palpebral fissures should be symmetrical. Abnormalities to note include ptosis (drooping of an eyelid), widening of the palpebral fissures, inequality in pupillary size (anisocoria), abnormal eye movements at rest (nystagmus, opsoclonus and square wave jerks), asymmetrical blinking, conjunctival injection and orbital pulsation.

There are many non-neurological causes of disordered eye movements. These include disorders of the ocular muscles (myopathies) and the neuromuscular junction (e.g. myasthenia gravis) and metabolic encephalopathy (e.g. toxic levels of phenytoin, carbamazepine).

Cranial neuropathies that involve III, IV and VI cause characteristic patterns of eye movement disorders with diplopia (double vision).

A complete unilateral lesion of III causes ptosis, weakness of superior, medial and inferior eye movements, pupillary dilation and an absent or sluggish light reflex. Common causes of an isolated III palsy are diabetic mononeuropathy, carotid-posterior communicating artery aneurysms, pituitary or other tumours, trauma and vascular disease. The III palsy associated with a contralateral hemiplegia (Weber syndrome) is due to a midbrain stroke. III nerve lesions may be incomplete depending on the location and type of lesion. Lesions due to diabetes or vascular disease tend not to involve the pupil, whereas compressive lesions (e.g. aneurysms) do.

Isolated lesions of the IV nerve are not common. The patient usually complains of diplopia, particularly when looking down and reading. The patient will often adopt a compensatory head tilt. Causes of an isolated IV lesion are ischaemic mononeuropathy (diabetes, hypertension) and head trauma, in which the associated intracranial damage to the IV nerve is sometimes bilateral. Damage to the trochlear through which the SO tendon passes, may be responsible for the IV palsy after head injury, ENT surgery and in patients with rheumatoid arthritis.

Isolated lesions of the VI nerve are common. They cause diplopia worse on gaze towards the side of the paretic LR. The paralysis may be complete or partial. In many cases, particularly following head injury and in patients with lesions causing raised intracranial pressure, it is a 'false localising' sign (i.e. the VI nerve is affected by intracranial pathology elsewhere). Abducent paresis may be associated with diabetes and with suppurative otitis media (Gradenigo's syndrome).

Lesions of the cavernous sinus (aneurysms, pituitary adenoma, meningioma) quite commonly cause VI nerve paresis. In general, however, cavernous sinus lesions produce a constellation of cranial neuropathies. Lesions of the VI nerve are occasionally found in conjunction with ipsilateral V and VII paresis and contralateral hemiplegia in unilateral pontine stroke.

Paresis of conjugate upgaze and downgaze may be seen with mass lesions around the pineal gland and tectal region and in patients with aqueductal stenosis and hydrocephalus. This apparent paradox can be explained by the presence of a centre for vertical gaze at the mesodiencephalic junction with medial and lateral neuronal pools subserving downgaze and upgaze respectively. Failure of upgaze, together with loss of the pupillary light response but preservation of miosis to accommodation, is termed Parinaud's syndrome or the pretectal syndrome. This is usually due to a lesion of the pineal gland or ventral midbrain.

Lateral gaze paresis may be due to a lesion in the FEF. If the lesion is destructive (e.g. intracerebral haemorrhage), the eyes are deviated towards the side of the damaged frontal lobe. In most cases the paresis lasts only a few days and eye movements return to normal. If the FEF lesion is irritative (e.g. epileptic) the eyes and head may be deviated to the side opposite the lesion. If there is a lesion in the PPRF the eyes are deviated away from the side of the lesion. This is most commonly caused by a pontine stroke and therefore associated with a plethora of other brain-stem signs. Resolution of the paresis in such cases is much slower than that following damage to the FEF.

Internuclear ophthalmoplegia (INO) occurs when there is a lesion of the MLF. The ipsilateral eye is unable to adduct and there is nystagmus in the contralateral abducting eye. INO is most commonly seen in multiple sclerosis but can also occur with vascular disorders and neoplasms of the brain stem. Supranuclear ophthalmoplegia occurs when the corticonuclear fibres are damaged. Spontaneous eye movements and doll's eye elicitation of ocular movements are preserved, but there is paresis of voluntary eye movements (usually downgaze and sometimes upgaze). The phenomenon may be associated with parkinsonian and dystonic clinical signs in the Steele–Richardson–Olzewski syndrome.

Nystagmus. Minor degrees of nystagmus occur in normal subjects at extremes of lateral gaze, particularly if maintained for more than 10 seconds. *Pendular nystagmus* occurs when the amplitude of the two phases of movement are equal and is often due to poor vision. It is thought to be an exaggeration of the normal tiny movements made by the eye to prevent fatigue of the retinal photoreceptors. Congenital blindness and ocular albinism are often associated with coarse pendular nystagmus.

Horizontal phasic (jerk) nystagmus is usually due to labyrinthine, cerebellar or brain-stem dysfunction. The direction of nystagmus is defined by the direction of the fast phase and its amplitude is usually increased by gaze to that side. It is termed first degree if present only on lateral gaze, second degree if present when looking straight ahead and third degree if still present on gaze in the opposite direction.

- Nystagmus due to lesions of the brain stem is usually multidirectional. Common causes are Wernicke's encephalopathy, multiple sclerosis, anticonvulsant toxicity and brain-stem ischaemia.
- Labyrinthine nystagmus is horizontal or rotary.
- Lesions of the cerebellar hemisphere cause horizontal nystagmus to the side of the diseased hemisphere. *Downbeat nystagmus* (usually due to a lesion of the cervicomedullary junction), *see-saw nystagmus* (due to parasellar lesions) and *convergence-retraction nystagmus* (due to lesions of the tectal and pineal region) are rare forms of disturbance.

Other jerky abnormalities of eye movement which mimic nystagmus are *ocular bobbing* (usually due to a pontine haemorrhage), which is characterised by spontaneous downward jerks of both eyes followed by a slow return to rest position, and *opsoclonus*. The latter is characterised by chaotic rapid eye movements and is seen in children with metastatic neuroblastoma or adults with bronchogenic carcinoma.

The trigeminal (V) nerve

The trigeminal nerve has both sensory and motor functions.

Sensory function

It transmits sensation from the face, mouth, lips, eyes, forehead and anterior part of the scalp as well as the dura of the anterior cranial and middle fossae.

The three sensory nuclei of V are:

- the principal nucleus of the trigeminal nerve (touch, joint position sense and two-point discrimination)
- the mesencephalic nucleus (unconscious proprioceptive information from periodontal membrane, palate, masticatory muscles and the temporomandibular joint)
- the spinal trigeminal nucleus (pain and temperature).

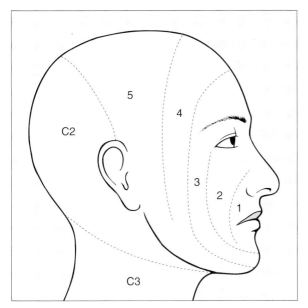

Fig. 7.10 Pain fibres to the head. Areas marked 1 to 5 indicate the central distribution within the spinal tract of the V cranial nerve. 1 is represented in the pons, 2 the pontomedullary region, 3 the lower medulla, 4 and 5 the upper cervical cord. The areas labelled C2 and C3 derive from the spinal segments directly.

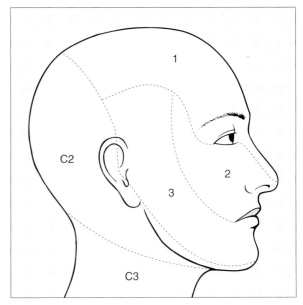

Fig. 7.11 Cutaneous distribution of the trigeminal nerve. 1. Ophthalmic division. **2.** Maxillary division. **3.** Mandibular division. **C2.** Second cervical root. **C3.** Third cervical root.

The spinal trigeminal nucleus extends from the pons to the C2 segment of the spinal cord. Owing to inversion of the fibres going into this nucleus, the upper part of the face is paradoxically represented in the caudal part of the spinal trigeminal nucleus (see Fig. 7.10). The sensory nuclei have multiple connections to the thalamus, particularly the activating system and limbic nuclei.

The V nerve fibres emerge from the anterolateral surface of the pons as several rootlets. The nerve rootlets then traverse the prepontine CSF cistern and enter the Gasserian ganglion, which sits in Meckel's cave in the petrous temporal dura. The three divisions of the V nerve arise from the ganglion:

- *The ophthalmic branch (V₁)* passes forward in the dura mater on the lateral wall of the cavernous sinus and then subdivides into the frontal, lacrimal and nasociliary branches as it passes through the superior orbital fissure. These supply sensation to the skin of the upper nose and eyelid, forehead and scalp (see Fig. 7.10) as well as the cornea, conjunctiva, intraocular structures, parts of the mucosa of the frontal, sphenoidal and ethmoidal sinuses, the upper part of the nasal cavity and dura of the anterior and middle cranial fossae. The afferent part of the corneal reflex is the nasociliary branch of V_1 and the

efferent limb is the facial nerve. Touching the cornea, which is very sensitive, evokes a brisk contraction of the orbicularis oculi (i.e. blinking). Because of the presence of interneurones, a corneal stimulus produces a bilateral reflex blink, i.e. the reflex has direct and consensual responses.

- *The maxillary nerve (V₂)* arises from the Gasserian ganglion and exits the skull base through the foramen rotundum into the pterygopalatine fossa. It innervates the dura of the middle cranial fossa, lower eyelids, skin of the temple, upper cheek and adjacent areas of nose and upper lip, the mucous membranes of the upper mouth, nose, roof of the pharynx and parts of the maxillary, ethmoid and sphenoidal sinuses as well as the gums, teeth and palate of the upper jaw (see Fig. 7.11).

- *The mandibular division (V₃)* of the trigeminal nerve passes from the Gasserian ganglion and exits the skull base through the foramen ovale into the infratemporal fossa. There it subdivides and its lingual branch receives preganglionic fibres from the chorda tympani of the VII nerve. These parasympathetic fibres enter the submandibular ganglion and control saliva secretion. The branches of V_3 supply the dura mater of the middle and anterior cranial fossa, teeth and gums of the lower jaw, mucosa of the cheek and floor of the mouth, the epithelium of the anterior two-thirds of the tongue, the temporomandibular joint, external and internal ear and the skin of the lower lip and jaw region.

Motor functions

The motor branch of V is conveyed in V_3 and innervates muscle of mastication (the masseters, temporalis, medial and lateral ptyergoids, the anterior belly of the diagastric). It also supplies the mylohyoid, tensor veli palatini and tensor tympani muscles. These muscles are responsible for various movements of the jaw, initiation and coordination of swallowing and dampening the amplitude of vibration of the tympanic membrane.

Unilateral pterygoid weakness causes the jaw to deviate to the weak side when the mouth is opened. When the patient tries to move the jaw from side to side there is difficulty in moving it to the contralateral side. Facial asymmetry resulting from a VII nerve lesion may give rise to an apparent deviation of the jaw.

The jaw jerk is analogous to the tendon reflexes in the limbs. The afferent and efferent pathways are subserved by the V cranial nerve. The reflex response is a brisk contraction of the jaw muscles, producing closure of the jaw. This is often not visible in young people but is commonly seen above the age of 50.

Examination

Sensory functions

❏ Test light touch and pain sensation in the territory of the three sensory regions using cotton wool and pin prick respectively. (Temperature sensation may also be tested.)
❏ Test two-point discrimination (see p. 243–4) on the upper and lower lips using calipers. Normally a separation of 3–4 mm can be detected.
❏ Check sensation in each division of the trigeminal nerve independently and compare the right with the left.
❏ Test the corneal reflex by very lightly touching the cornea, not the conjunctiva, with a wisp of damp cotton wool (Fig. 7.12); approach from the side as the patient looks in the opposite direction.
❏ Observe the presence of both direct and consensual corneal reflexes.

Motor functions
❏ Inspect the muscles of mastication for wasting, most easily seen in the temporalis muscle above the zygomatic arch.

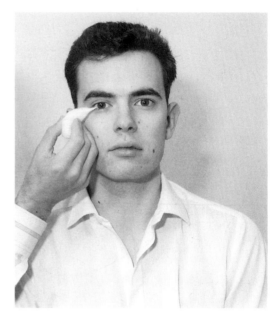

Fig. 7.12 Testing the corneal reflex.

❏ Ask the patient to open the jaw against resistance (pterygoids, mylohyoid, anterior belly of the diagastric).
❏ Palpate the masseters and estimate their bulk and symmetry as the patient clenches the teeth.

Jaw jerk
❏ Place the thumb or forefinger in the midline over the tip of the patient's mandible, with the mouth slightly open.
❏ Tap the examiner's finger downwards with a tendon hammer (see Fig. 7.13).

Interpretation

Unilateral loss of sensory modalities from the distribution of one or more of the branches of the trigeminal nerve is an important finding.

• Lesions within the cavernous sinus commonly cause loss or reduction in corneal reflex as well as diminished forehead sensation (V_1 lesion). This is frequently associated with dysfunction in III, IV or VI.
• Neoplasms of the base of middle cranial fossa (e.g. meningioma, squamous carcinoma from the air sinuses, nasopharyngeal carcinoma, trigeminal neuroma) will lead to sensory impairment in one or more branches of the V nerve.

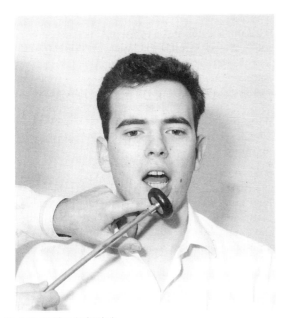

Fig. 7.13 Eliciting the jaw jerk.

• Patchy sensory loss such as on the cheek, certain teeth or forehead may result from direct injury or laceration to peripheral branches of the V (e.g. infraorbital nerve damage with fractures of the zygoma, alveolar nerve damage with fractures of the mandible or maxilla and supraorbital or supratrochlear nerve damage with eyebrow lacerations).

• Large tumours in the cerebellopontine angle region (e.g. acoustic neuroma, petrous meningioma, epidermoid) also may impair V function, as well as VII and VIII.

Detection of paresis or atrophy in the muscles of mastication is very difficult. Even when there are obvious signs of sensory V nerve dysfunction, clinical examination may reveal relatively normal trigeminal motor function. These muscles may be involved in various myopathies, myasthenia gravis or progressive bulbar palsy.

Hyperactivity of the jaw jerk occurs in anxious patients and in bilateral diseases of the upper motor neurone above the level of the pons (e.g. multiple sclerosis or motor neurone disease). Determination of whether a jaw jerk is abnormally brisk can often be very difficult.

The facial (VII) nerve

This nerve has various functions:

• It innervates facial movements.

• It is the efferent limb of the corneal reflex (see p. 215) and also the palmomental reflex (a contraction of the ipsilateral mentalis muscle in response to scratching the thenar eminence), the pout or snout reflex (a bilateral pursing of the lips following a brisk tap on the lips), the nasopalpebral reflex (glabellar tap) and the efferent limb of the stapedius reflex.

• Through the nervus intermedius (sensory and parasympathetic fibres) it supplies parasympathetic secretomotor fibres to the lacrimal gland (producing tears) and submandibular gland (producing saliva).

• It supplies taste sensation to the anterior two-thirds of the tongue through the chorda tympani branch.

The motor nucleus of VII lies in the lower pons and its fibres initially pass posteriorly and medially to loop around the VI nucleus before turning forwards and emerging from the lateral pontomedullary junction (see Fig. 7.14).

The nervus intermedius contains parasympathetic fibres from the superior salivatory nucleus and taste fibres, which have their cell bodies in the geniculate ganglion and synapse centrally in the gustatory or nucleus solitarius. It emerges from the pons in close proximity to VII, and the two nerves pass through the pontomedullary CSF cistern in close relationship to

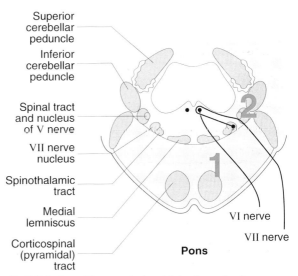

Fig. 7.14 Lesions of the pons. Lesions at **1.** (e.g. haemorrhage), cause ipsilateral VI and/or VII nerve palsies and contralateral pyramidal signs. Lesions at **2.** (e.g. basilar thrombosis), cause ataxia on the side of the lesion (damage to the cerebellar peduncles). There may also be impaired sensation on the ipsilateral side of the face (spinal tract and nucleus of V nerve) and on the contralateral side of the body (spinothalamic tract) and occasionally a VII nerve lesion. Lesions in the pons often cause internuclear ophthalmoplegia (p. 214) and ataxic nystagmus.

the vestibular and cochlear (VIII) nerves. All these nerves enter the internal acoustic meatus. The facial nerve then passes through the facial canal of the temporal bone and emerges from the stylomastoid foramen. It passes through the parotid gland and subdivides into several branches which innervate the muscles of the face. The VII is also the efferent limb of several reflexes. The most important of these is the corneal reflex. Within the temporal bone and distal to the geniculate ganglion the facial nerve has branches to the stapedius muscle (which dampens down tympanic vibrations), to the ptyerogopalatine ganglion (from which arises the greater petrosal nerve, which is secretomotor to the lacrimal gland) and to the tongue (chorda tympani which conveys taste).

Taste sensation is rarely tested in clinical practice; electrical stimulation of the tongue with a small current is more reliable and practical (electrogustometry). Secretomotor function of the lacrimal gland is usually only tested by ophthalmologists doing a Schirmer test.

Testing for decreased saliva production owing to denervation of the submandibular gland is not performed in clinical practice.

Examination

Inspection

❑ Observe the face for any asymmetry which may be related to paresis of the facial muscles.
❑ Observe the symmetry of blinking and eye closure and the presence of any tics or spasms of the facial musculature.
❑ Observe spontaneous movement of the face, particularly the upper and lower facial musculature during such actions as smiling.

Motor function

❑ Test the facial muscles by asking the patient to raise the eyebrows, wrinkle the forehead (this can be achieved by asking the patient to look upwards at the examiner's hand), close the eyes as strongly as possible, to show the teeth (even if these are false), to blow out the cheeks against the closed mouth, to purse the mouth and to whistle (Fig. 7.15A–D).
❑ Check the strength of eye closure for paresis or asymmetry.

Taste sensation

❑ Instruct the patient not to speak during the test because this will cause the tongue to retract and dissipate the substance into the contralateral side of the tongue as well as its posterior one-third.
❑ Gently hold the protruded tongue with a swab.
❑ Place a test substance (e.g. sweet, salt, bitter or sour substances) on the anterior two-thirds of each side of the tongue in turn.
❑ Ask the patient to identify the substance by pointing to the appropriate word written on a card.

Schirmer's test

❑ Put a piece of special blotting paper under the lower eyelid and remove it after 5 minutes. Normally at least 10 mm of the blotting paper will be dampened by evoked tear secretion.

Interpretation

Lesions of corticonuclear fibres (i.e. upper motor neurone type lesion) to the facial nucleus will cause facial paresis that is worse in the lower facial muscles with relative sparing of the upper face (because of bilateral cortical innervation of the upper facial

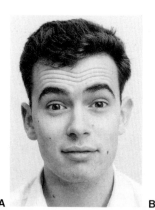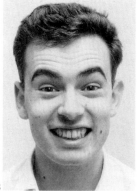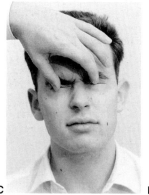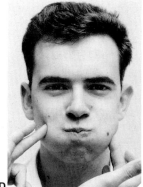

A   B   C   D

Fig. 7.15 Testing the motor function of the facial nerve: Ask the patient to **A.** raise the eyebrows, **B.** show the teeth, **C.** close the eyes against resistance and **D.** blow out the cheeks.

muscles). In such patients the corner of the mouth will droop and saliva may dribble, the nasolabial fold will be flattened, but eye closure, although paretic, is usually well preserved. Smiling may also be preserved because emotional facial movements employ additional neural pathways. Taste is normal. The commonest cause of this type of unilateral facial dysfunction is a vascular lesion involving the contralateral rolandic cortex or its subcortical pathways. Usually there will also be weakness of the ipsilateral upper limb (faciobrachial paresis).

When the facial nucleus or its nerve is damaged there is unilateral paresis of both upper and lower facial muscles with inability to close the eye and impaired blinking, loss of the nasolabial fold and forehead wrinkles (Fig. 7.16). Taste to the anterior two-thirds of the tongue is impaired if the chorda tympani is also damaged. The commonest cause of this condition is idiopathic Bell's palsy (see Table 7.9). A frequent observation in such patients is Bell's phenomenon. This is an upward rotation of the eye on attempted forced contraction of the paretic orbicularis oculi.

The location of the VII lesion along the path of the nerve can be deduced from the clinical findings. Taste and lacrimation will be preserved in those lesions distal to the stylomastoid foramen. The greater petrosal, nerve to stapedius and chorda tympani branches arise sequentially along the facial nerve in the petrous bone. A lesion involving the nerve to the stapedius will cause

Table 7.9 Common causes of VII nerve palsies

Unilateral	Bilateral
Upper motor neurone type weakness	
Usually vascular	Often vascular
Cerebral tumour	Consider motor neurone disease
Multiple sclerosis	
Lower motor neurone type weakness	
Usually Bell's palsy	Neurosarcoidosis
Consider parotid tumour,	Myasthenia gravis
head injuries,	Generalised polyneuropathies
skull base tumours	(Guillain–Barré syndrome)
	Some myopathies (e.g. myotonic dystrophy)

hyperacusis (e.g. sounds appearing louder than normal). A lesion involving the greater petrosal nerve will cause a dry eye.

Bilateral facial weakness can be due to lesions of the upper or lower motor neurone as well as disorders of the muscles and neuromuscular junctions. Progressive supranuclear paresis will cause a bilateral facial paresis associated with a liability of emotional expression and a disassociation between emotional (well preserved) and voluntary (poorly preserved) movement. Such patients may exhibit an obvious snout reflex. Causes of bilateral lower motor neurone facial type paresis (Table 7.9) are relatively uncommon but may be difficult to detect.

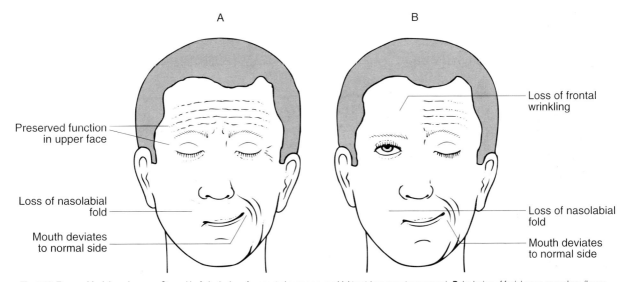

Fig. 7.16 Types of facial weakness.   Caused in **A.** by lesion of precentral area or pyramidal tract (upper motor neurone). **B.** by lesion of facial nerve or nucleus (lower motor neurone).

The vestibulocochlear (VIII) nerve

The VIII cranial nerve has two functional parts, the vestibular and the cochlear components.

The central connections of the four vestibular nuclei are complex. Through fibres in the MLF they interconnect with the III, IV and VI cranial nuclei. Other fibres project to the cerebellar vermis and flocculus, while others descend in the vestibulospinal tracts. Ascending fibres relay through the MGB to the posterior temporal lobe. These central vestibular pathways are very important in the maintenance of the correct body posture, eye coordination and movement.

The vestibular part of the VIII is the afferent limb of both the oculocephalic (doll's eye reflex) and oculovestibular (caloric) reflexes. The oculocephalic reflex involves conjugate movements of the eyes in response to changes in head position. The oculovestibular reflex involves elicitation of eye movements following irrigation of the external ear canal by either cold or warm water.

The cochlear branch subserves hearing, while the inferior and superior vestibular branches are important for balance, posture and equilibrium. Their fibres arise from the respective end organs in the inner ear and have their cells of origin in their respective ganglia. They then pass centrally along the internal acoustic meatus and cross the cerebellopontine CSF cistern to enter the lateral brain stem at the pontomedullary junction. The fibres then synapse in the cochlear (dorsal, ventral) and vestibular (inferior, superior, lateral and medial) nuclear complexes. From the cochlear nucleus second-order fibres ascend to the superior olivary and trapezoid nuclei. Central fibres then ascend up the lateral lemniscus, and synapse in the inferior colliculus and medial geniculate body (MGB) before entering the primary auditory cortex in the superior temporal gyrus (areas 41 and 42). The ascending auditory pathways decussate at several levels so that each cortical region receives impulses from both ears.

Whispering tests hearing for higher frequencies in particular. The volume of the auditory test can be altered so that some deductions as to whether the hearing is normal, abnormal or asymmetrical can be obtained. Rinne's test determines whether air conduction is better than bone conduction. Normally the air-conducted sound is perceived as louder. Weber's lateralising test provides supplementary information about the nature of any hearing impairment. Normally, the sound appears to arise in the midline (Fig. 7.17). A patient with sensorineural deafness will perceive the sound as arising from the better ear. In conduction deafness, however, the sound appears to arise from the

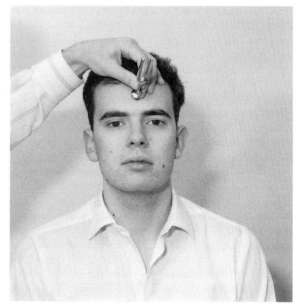

Fig. 7.17 Weber's test.

deaf side; this is because of the improved efficiency of bone conduction in the presence of middle ear damage.

In clinical practice deafness or impaired hearing is best studied using audiometry and brain-stem evoked potentials to determine their precise aetiology.

Examination

Hearing

❑ Mask hearing in the non-tested ear by either rubbing the forefinger and thumb together over the external acoustic meatus or gently massaging the patient's external acoustic meatus with examiner's forefinger.

❑ Test hearing roughly in each ear by asking the patient to repeat whispered numbers or words.

❑ Perform Rinne's test by placing a vibrating tuning fork (256 or 512 Hz) on the mastoid process (to assess bone conduction of sound) then just lateral to the external ear (Fig. 7.18).

❑ Ask the patient which of the two sounds appears louder.

❑ Perform Weber's test by placing the strongly vibrating tuning fork to the middle of the forehead. Ask the patient whether the sound is heard loudest in the midline or preferentially to one side.

❑ Examine the external acoustic canal using an auroscope (p. 59). Visualise the tympanic

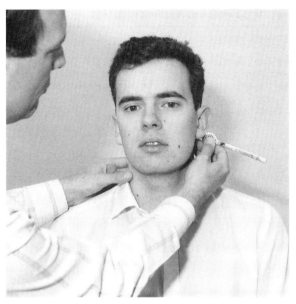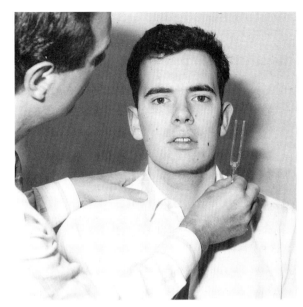

Fig. 7.18 Rinne's test.   **A.** Testing bone conduction. **B.** Testing air conduction.

membranes and note any abnormal vascularity of the membrane or retrotympanic fluid level.

Vestibular function

❑ Perform the oculocephalic reflex or doll's eye manoeuvre with the patient lying down.
❑ Stand above and behind the patient at the head of the bed.
❑ Slightly flex and support the patient's head.
❑ Briskly rotate the head from one side to the other and note lateral movements of the eyes.

The normal response is for the patient's eyes to deviate to the left as the patient's head is turned to the right and vice versa on contralateral forced head turning. If the patient's head is briskly extended the patient's eyes should move downwards.

Another test of labyrinthine and vestibular function involves *induction of positional nystagmus.*

Examination

❑ Support the patient's head, with eyes open, and lower it briskly below the horizontal plane of the couch, turning the head to one side.
❑ Sit the patient up again, and repeat the test, turning the head to the other side.
❑ Note the response of the eyes to head movement (Fig. 7.19).

Nystagmus will not be seen in normal people. If

there is a disorder of the labyrinth or its vestibular connection, the patient may complain of vertigo and develop nystagmus within 10 seconds of head movement.

There are two main types of positional vertigo and nystagmus:

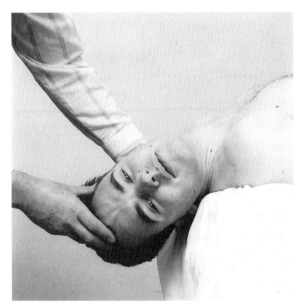

Fig. 7.19 Testing for positional nystagmus.

- Peripheral lesions (usually calcific deposits in the otolith organ) cause vertigo and nystagmus after a latent period of a few seconds; the nystagmus declines if the position is maintained.
- Nystagmus due to rare 'central' type lesions has no latency, does not show fatigue and is less likely to cause vertigo.

Usually caloric vestibular tests are carried out in a special laboratory set up to record eye movement electronically. The *oculovestibular or caloric reflex test* can be performed at the bedside.

Examination

☐ Inspect the canal to ensure the tympanic membranes are visualised.
☐ If necessary, remove any impacted wax.
☐ Gently irrigate the canal with patient's eyes open using water at either 30°C or 44°C and observe the response.

The normal response to unilateral irrigation with cool water is for the patient to develop nystagmus towards the contralateral side. If the ear is irrigated with warm water the patient will have nystagmus towards the side of the irrigated ear. If the patient is unconscious there will be no nystagmus but on irrigation of one ear with cool water the eyes deviate to the irrigated side. Conversely, if the ear of the unconscious patient is irrigated with warm water, the eyes will deviate to the contralateral side. Bilateral irrigation with either cool or warm water induces vertical eye movements. All the reflexes are absent in the presence of brain death (p. 248).

Interpretation

If impaired hearing is unilateral it should be determined whether it is either conductive (i.e. due to disease of the tympanic membrane or ossicular chain) or sensorineural (e.g. involving the organ of Corti or the cochlear nerve) in origin. Common causes of deafness are shown in Table 7.10.

Abnormalities of the vestibular nerves and labyrinth will usually evoke first-degree nystagmus, positional nystagmus or impairment of the caloric response.

- Following acute labyrinthine damage or vestibular nerve lesions (fractured petrous temporal bone after head injury, acute vestibular neuronitis, etc.) the patient will complain of severe nausea, vertigo or dizziness and disturbance of balance. These symptoms are all aggravated by head movements. In such

Table 7.10 Common causes of deafness

Conduction deafness	Effect
Wax in the external canal Damage to tympanic membranes Fluid in inner ear Ossicular chain disruption (head injury) Otosclerosis (degenerative)	Diminished hearing on affected side Rinne's test: bone conduction louder Weber's test: to affected side
Sensorineural deafness	Effect

Damage to cochlear nerve and organ
  of Corti
Acoustic neuroma
Transverse fracture of petrous
  temporal bone
	Diminished hearing on affected side
	Rinne's test: air conduction louder
	Weber's test: to unaffected side

cases there is frequently nystagmus with the fast phase towards the side of the lesion.
- Chronic lesions of the vestibular nerve (e.g. acoustic neuroma) are not normally accompanied by vertigo or nystagmus.

Many patients who complain of vertigo and *tinnitus* (a subjective awareness of noise such as hissing in the ear) may have entirely normal clinical examinations, and require detailed audiometry and vestibular tests for diagnosis.

The glossopharyngeal (IX) and vagus (X) nerves

Since these nerves are intimately related anatomically, functionally and in terms of clinical examination, they will be considered together.

Both nerves arise as a series of rootlets from the post-olivary sulcus of the lateral medulla. They pass anterolaterally across the cerebellomedullary CSF cistern and exit the skull through the jugular foramen. As they traverse the CSF cistern they are in close relationship to the vertebral artery and posterior inferior cerebellar artery. The motor component of both of these nerves arises from the nucleus ambiguus in the medulla.

- The motor component of the glossopharyngeal nerve is small and innervates the stylopharyngeus muscles but sometimes contributes to the innervation of the palatal and upper pharyngeal muscles.
- The IX nerve contains a large sensory component which transmits sensation from part of the lining of the tympanic cavity and the Eustachian tube, and more importantly innervates the mucosa of the pharynx and tonsillar region and conveys taste from the posterior third of the tongue. The latter fibres terminate in the caudal solitary nucleus.

- The IX nerve also contains parasympathetic fibres that are secretomotor to the parotid gland.
- The predominant innervation of the muscles of the upper pharynx and soft palate, as well as the innervation of intrinsic muscles of the larynx and the cricothyroid, is the vagus nerve.
- The vagus nerve conveys sensory sensation from the dura mater of the posterior cranial fossa and from part of the skin of the external auditory meatus.
- The vagus also has extensive afferent and efferent connections with the heart, lungs and intestines.

The IX and X are also involved in several reflexes:

- The gag reflex involves constriction and elevation of the pharynx and palate (X efferent limb) in response to tactile stimulation of the upper pharynx and tonsils (IX afferent limb).
- The oculocardiac reflex (slowing of the heart rate after orbital compression).
- The carotid reflex (slowing of the heart rate and decreased blood pressure following stretch of the carotid sinus).

Lesions of IX and X cause *dysphagia* (difficulty in swallowing due to palatal and pharyngeal paresis), loss of the gag reflex and *dysphonia* (altered voice quality, usually hoarseness, resulting from weakness of the muscles moving the vocal cords and palate).

Examination

❏ Observe movements of the palate and uvula by asking the patient to say 'aah'.
❏ Assess tonsillar, palatal and upper pharyngeal tactile sensation using a dampened swab stick and tongue depressor.
❏ Elicit the **gag** reflex by touching either the tonsil or pharynx. This will cause reflex elevation of the palate and the pharynx and be very similar to the motions seen at the beginning of vomiting. Test each side separately.
❏ Assess the volume and quality of the patient's speech, noting if the voice is hoarse or has a nasal quality.
❏ Ask the patient to cough to determine whether this is more nasal or bovine than normal.
❏ Ask the patient to puff out the cheeks.

Normally both sides of the palate elevate in a symmetrical fashion and the uvula remains in the midline. In order to puff out the cheeks the palate must elevate and occlude the nasopharynx. If palatal movement is weak, air will escape audibly through the nose.

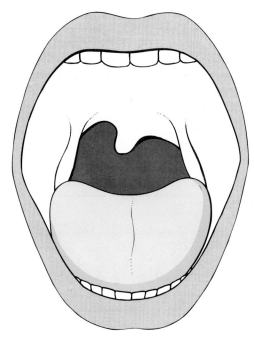

Fig. 7.20 Left X nerve palsy; note the uvula is pulled over to the right side.

Neither the oculocardiac or carotid reflexes nor taste in the posterior one-third of the tongue are routinely tested in clinical practice.

Interpretation

- IX nerve dysfunction is usually seen with other signs of cranial nerve or brain-stem dysfunction.
- A IX nerve lesion is suggested by unilateral loss of palatal, tonsillar or pharyngeal sensation, together with an absent or depressed gag reflex; in isolation such an occurrence is extremely unusual.
- Disorders of the X nerve will cause asymmetrical elevation of the soft palate with deviation of the uvula away from the side of the lesion (Fig. 7.20). The voice may have a nasal quality.
- With lesions to the recurrent laryngeal branch of the vagus nerve, the voice will sound hoarse and the cough 'bovine'.

Some clinical conditions causing IX and X nerve lesions are shown in Table 7.11.

The accessory (XI) nerve

This motor cranial nerve has two nuclei, one which is intimately related to that of X in the caudal part of the nucleus ambiguus (innervates the intrinsic muscles of

Table 7.11 Common causes of IX and X nerve lesions

Unilateral of IX and X
    Skull base neoplasms (including meningioma)
    Skull base fracture

Recurrent laryngeal
    Bronchial carcinoma
    Mediastinal lymphoma
    Aortic arch aneurysms

Bilateral X
    Progressive bulbar palsy (motor neurone disease)
    Bilateral supranuclear lesions (pseudobulbar palsy)
        Cerebrovascular disease
        Multiple sclerosis

the larynx. The much larger spinal element is derived from segments C1–C5. This arises as an extensive series of rootlets from the lateral medulla and spinal cord. Its fibres ascend through the foramen magnum then merge to exit the skull base through the jugular foramen, where the bulbar component rejoins the vagus nerve (see X). The spinal component descends to supply the sternomastoid and the upper half of the trapezius muscle.

Wasting of the trapezius muscle will produce a flaring of the vertebral border of the scapula, which will be displaced away from the spine in its upper part and rotated towards the spine at its lower end. The point of the shoulder will appear dropped and the arm will appear lower.

Examination

❏ Inspect the trapezius muscle from behind.
❏ Ask the patient to shrug the shoulders and maintain them in elevation then apply downward pressure to the shoulders to check for paresis of the trapezius muscle (Fig. 7.21A).
❏ Inspect the sternomastoids for hypertrophy or atrophy and palpate to assess tone and bulk.
❏ Test the left sternomastoid by asking the patient to rotate the head to right side with a hand placed against the right side of the chin in an effort to stop this rotatory movement. (Fig. 7.21B).
❏ Examine the right sternomastoid during rotation to the left.

Interpretation

• Isolated XI lesions are unusual.
• Isolated paresis of the trapezius can occur if branches of the spinal accessory nerve are cut during surgery in the posterior triangle of the neck.

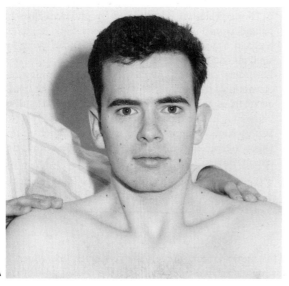

A

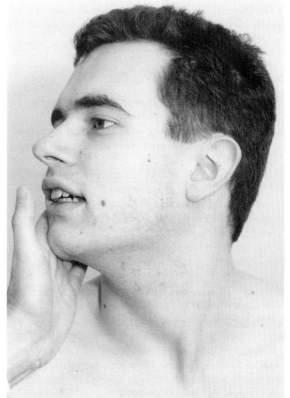

B

Fig. 7.21 Testing A. the trapezius muscle and B. the left sternomastoid.

- The nerve may be involved with other lower cranial nerves in basal skull tumours or following penetrating injury.
- Upper motor neurone lesions involving the spinal accessory nerve or damage to corticobulbar fibres may produce little in the way of clinical signs.
- Lower motor neurone lesions may occur as part of a progressive bulbar palsy.
- Paresis of the sternomastoid muscle occurs in a range of myopathic disorders, especially dystrophia myotonia.

Involuntary turning movements of the head that involve the sternomastoid and other neck muscles are a feature of spasmodic torticollis and other dystonic conditions. If dystonia is long-standing the sternomastoid may be hypertrophic and the mobility of the neck very restricted.

The hypoglossal (XII) nerve

The XII nerve arises from a motor nucleus located beneath the floor of the fourth ventricle. Its rootlets arise from the preolivary sulcus and pass anterolaterally in front of the vertebral and posterior inferior cerebellar arteries. It exits the skull base through the hypoglossal canal in the occipital bone. It then passes to the root of the tongue, where it divides into branches that innervate the various intrinsic and extrinsic tongue muscles. Normal tongue movement is essential for articulation, adequate chewing and the onset of swallowing.

Examination

- ❑ Ask the patient to protrude the tongue; observe the symmetry of movement, bulk and look for wasting and fasciculation.
- ❑ Assess movements of the tongue from side to side.
- ❑ Ask the patient to press the tongue against the cheek and feel the strength of contraction and assess muscle bulk.
- ❑ Assess hypokinesis of tongue movements by asking the patient to say 'lah lah lah' as quickly as possible, and to make rapid in-and-out and side-to-side movements of the tongue.

Unilateral atrophy is usually easily recognised since the tongue becomes wrinkled and thinner. Sponta-

neous contraction (fasciculation) of small parts of the muscle may be apparent and is more easily seen when the tongue is protruded. Normally the tongue will protrude in the midline, but if there is unilateral XII lesion the tongue will deviate towards the side of the lesion. Slowness of tongue movement is seen in pseudobulbar palsy due to bilateral pyramidal lesions.

Interpretation

- Unilateral XII nerve lesions are usually seen with other cranial neuropathies, and the causes may be neoplastic (skull base tumour), vascular (medullary infarct, vetebral artery aneurysm) or traumatic.
- Bilateral lower motor neurone lesions may be seen as part of a wider clinical syndrome, e.g. motor neurone disease or syringobulbia.
- Myopathic disorders involving the tongue will generally be part of a more widespread syndrome (e.g. myasthenia gravis). Such lesions cause dysarthria, dysphagia and dysphonia.
- Unilateral upper motor neurone lesions may produce deviation of the protruded tongue which is not associated with fasciculation or wasting. This is most typically seen immediately after an acute cerebrovascular event; the asymmetry of tongue protrusion tends to resolve after several days.
- With bilateral upper motor neurone lesions, voluntary movements of the tongue are hypokinetic (slow) and the tongue tends to assume a more conical form. There tends to be dysarthria and dysphagia. Such dysfunction may occur in supranuclear or suprabulbar disorders, which may be vascular (e.g. bilateral insular infarction) or inflammatory (e.g. multiple sclerosis) in origin.
- Orofacial dyspraxias involve inability to move the tongue and parts of the face on command and are usually seen after parietal lobe lesions.
- Involuntary movements of the tongue (and usually parts of the facial musculature as well) may occur in a group of disorders called orofacial dyskinesias. These are most often drug induced (e.g. major tranquillisers, anti-parkinsonian drugs). They may be choreiform in type with Huntington's chorea or maybe tremulous in some cases (e.g. Parkinson's disease).

KEY POINTS

- The commonest cause of anosmia is obstruction of the nasal passages.

- The field for red colour vision is much smaller than that for monochrome.

- If a lesion occurs distal to the optic chiasma, the same side of each visual field will be affected in each eye and the defect is termed homonymous.

- The superior oblique muscle is supplied by the IV cranial nerve and is responsible for downward movement of the adducted eye.

- Conjugate ocular motility is dependent not only on the integrity of the cranial nerves but also on a central brain-stem tract, the medial longitudinal fasciculation (MLF).

- Parasympathetic fibres constrict and sympathetic fibres dilate the pupil.

- In many cases a VI cranial nerve palsy is a 'false localising' sign caused by raised intracranial pressure.

- Minor degrees of nystagmus are seen in normal patients at extremes of lateral gaze, particularly if maintained for more than 10 seconds.

- Pendular nystagmus is often due to long-standing poor vision.

- Unilateral loss of sensation in one or more branches of the trigeminal nerve is an important finding.

- A pathologically brisk jaw jerk occurs in patients with bilateral upper motor neurone lesions above the level of the pons.

- An upper motor neurone lesion affecting one corticobulbar (facial) tract results in relative sparing of the upper face because of bilateral innervation of those muscles.

- In clinical practice deafness is often best studied using audiometry.

- Many patients with vertigo and tinnitus have no detectable abnormality on clinical examination.

- IX cranial nerve dysfunction is usually seen with other signs of cranial nerve or brain-stem dysfunction.

- With lesions of the recurrent laryngeal branch of the vagus nerve, the voice will sound hoarse and the cough bovine.

- Inspect the trapezius muscle from behind.

- Orofacial dyskinesias are usually drug induced.

THE MOTOR SYSTEM

It is convenient to consider motor and sensory function separately, but precise movements require sensory and cerebellar input. The corticospinal motor pathways are outlined in Figure 7.22. This primary motor pathway is modulated by subcortical (basal ganglia), cerebellar and vestibular input. Patterns of motor dysfunction, therefore, may be determined by both focal and systematic neuropathology (Table 7.12). In the dyspraxias the organised sequence of complex motor activation is impaired although there is no deficit of spontaneous movement or pathways to individual muscles.

Inspection of muscles and limbs

The neurological examination incorporates:

- inspection of muscle groups (wasting, hypertrophy, and fasciculation)
- assessment of tone
- testing of power
- elicitation of deep tendon reflexes and plantar responses
- testing of coordination.

From these clinical parameters can be deduced whether the disease process is affecting the upper motor neurone, lower motor neurone, neuromuscular junction or the muscle.

The patient should be examined in underwear in order to observe the limbs and muscles clearly. Particular points to look for are:

- Is there muscle asymmetry?
- If so, is it due to atrophy or hypertrophy?
- If hypertrophy, is it physiological or pathological?
- Is there loss of muscle bulk?
- If so, is it focal or diffuse, proximal or distal, peripheral nerve or spinal segment in distribution?
- Does it involve scattered groups on both sides?
- Is there fasciculation?
- If so, is it confined to one limb or generalised?
- Is the posture or gait abnormal?

Table 7.12 Patterns of motor dysfunction

Paralysis or weakness
Impairment of coordination
Changes in tone and posture (dystonia)
Involuntary movements (dyskinesia)
Changes in the rate at which movements are performed (hypokinesis and bradykinesis)
Loss of learned movement patterns (dyspraxia)

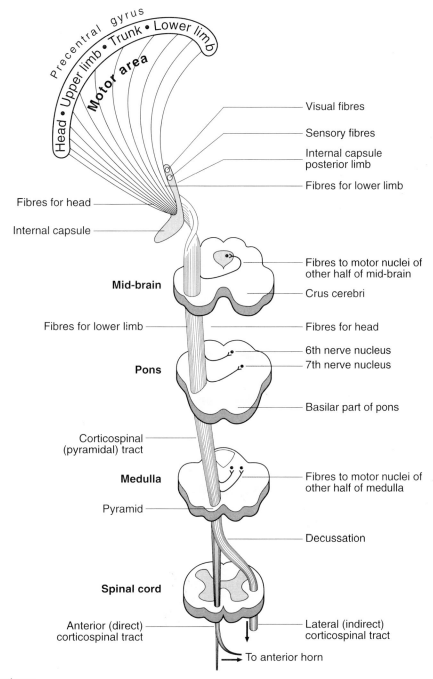

Fig. 7.22 The motor pathways.

- If so, what is the abnormality (see p. 203 and 281)?
- Are there involuntary movements (see p. 228)?
- If so, what is their nature?
- Is there incoordination of voluntary movement?

Interpretation

Muscle wasting can have a multiplicity of different causes (see Table 7.17 p. 231). Conversely, muscle hypertrophy may be occupational or a manifestation of certain rare forms of muscular dystrophy.

Fasciculations appear as subcutaneous twitches overlying muscle bellies when the muscles are at rest. They result from disease of lower motor neurones that innervate that particular muscle and are caused by brief contraction of single motor units. They may be coarse or fine in amplitude and are most commonly found in wasted muscles. They can occur in normal people after vigorous exercise. A similar usually benign phenomenon, myokymia, involves fasciculations of the orbicularis oculi. This condition is commonly caused by anxiety and tiredness.

Myoclonus is a sudden shock-like muscle contraction which involves one or more muscles of a whole limb. Myoclonic jerks may be focal or diffuse and may occur singly or repetitively. They may occur in normal people, particularly when falling asleep. Some patients with primary generalised epilepsy experience myoclonic jerks, especially after waking. Less common causes of myoclonic jerks are rare diseases such as subacute sclerosing panencephalitis, familial myoclonic epilepsies, anoxic cerebral damage and Creutzfeld–Jakob disease.

Choreiform movements are irregular, jerky, semi-purposeful and ill sustained. They tend to be multi-focal and are classically seen in Huntington's chorea.

Tics or habit spasms are much more stereotyped and localised than choreiform movements, and can be resisted at will by the patient.

Tremor is defined as rhythmic movement resulting from alternating contraction and relaxation of groups of muscles (see Table 7.13). Tremors produce oscillations about a joint or group of joints. The pattern of tremor most frequently seen is rapid and fine in amplitude and is an exaggeration of physiological tremor. It is more prominent in patients with hyperthyroidism and some patients who indulge excessively in alcohol, coffee or other drugs. A distal upper limb tremor is a cardinal feature of parkinsonism and characteristically involves a beating of the thumb towards the index finger. In its fully developed form, it is of 'pill rolling' type with the thumb moving across the tips of all fingers. Parkinsonian tremor is maximal at rest and reduced by voluntary movement. Tremor which is absent at rest, present on maintaining posture and exacerbated by movement is called intention tremor. It is due principally to disorders of the cerebellum or its connections. Much coarser and often more violent tremors usually involving the upper limb are induced by active movements (kinetic tremors) and abolished by rest in patients with multiple sclerosis, cerebrovascular disease involving the midbrain red nucleus (and thus termed 'rubral' type tremor) or subthalamic nucleus. The last classically causes hemiballismus, in which there are violent throwing movements of the limbs on one side.

Dystonic movements are slow and writhing and often lead to sustained abnormal contracture and limb posturing. These are often called torsion spasms and are most commonly seen in spasmodic torticollis, following infantile hemiplegia and in dystonia musculorum deformans. Athetosis describes slow writhing movements of distal parts, usually fingers and toes.

Palpation

Palpation of muscles is sometimes of value. Muscle bellies may feel:

- tender in inflammatory conditions (myositis);
- 'doughy' in Duchenne's dystrophy as a result of fatty infiltration of the pseudohypertrophied muscles;
- 'woody' in some forms of acute muscle necrosis (e.g. alcoholic rhabdomyolysis).

Tapping muscle bellies is a useful way of enhancing the production of fasciculations, or occasionally elicits sustained contraction (percussion myotonia) in myotonic disorders.

Tone

In clinical practice muscle tone may be defined as the resistance felt when a joint is moved passively through its range of movement. In normal people who are relaxed the manipulation of a joint evokes slight 'elastic' type of resistance from the adjacent muscles. The normal degree of this tension can be gauged only by repeated examination of healthy people. Abnormalities in tone must be interpreted in the light of other

Table 7.13 Types of tremor

Name	Frequency (Hz)	Examples	Rest	Posture	Movement
Action (or postural)	10	Hyperthyroidism Anxiety and fatigue	−	+	+
Intention	5	Cerebellar	−	+	++
Resting	5	Parkinsonism	++	±	±

clinical findings. Tone may be either normal, increased (hypertonia) or decreased (hypotonia).

Hypertonia may be manifest as either spasticity or rigidity. Spasticity is characterised by rapid build-up of resistance during the first few degrees of passive movement and then as the movement continues there is lessening of resistance. Spasticity in the upper limb is frequently more obvious in attempted extension, whereas in the lower limb it is more obvious with attempted flexion. Rigidity is a term used to describe sustained resistance to passive movement. The rigidity may be sustained throughout the range of movement or fluctuate in a jerky 'cogwheel' fashion.

Hypotonia may be very difficult to discern in a relaxed patient. In the upper limb hypotonia may be evident from the posture of the outstretched hands, which show flexion at the wrist and extension of the fingers (dinner fork deformity).

Clonus is a term applied to a rhythmic series of involuntary muscle contractions evoked by sudden stretch of the muscles.

Examination

Tone

❏ Ask the patient to relax and 'go floppy'.
❏ Passively flex and extend each joint in turn; do this slowly at first and then more rapidly to get a feel of muscle tension (Fig. 7.23A).
❏ In the upper limbs test muscle tone at the shoulder, elbow joint and wrist joint.
❏ In the lower limbs test tone by internally and externally rotating the resting leg (Fig. 7.23B) and by briskly raising the patient's knee off the bed and observing whether the ankle is also raised off the bed .

Knee clonus

❏ Sharply push the patella towards the foot while the patient lies supine and relaxed with the knee extended.
❏ Following the initial jerk, exert sustained pressure with the thumb and index finger in a downwards direction on the patella.

Ankle clonus

❏ Support the flexed knee with one hand in the popliteal fossa so that the ankle rests gently on the bed.
❏ Using the other hand briskly dorsiflex the foot and sustain the pressure (Fig. 7.24).

If knee clonus is present, the patella will jerk up and down following a solitary jerk stimulus. If sustained

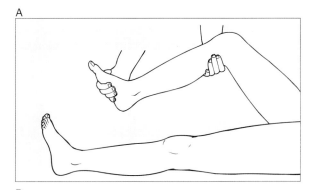
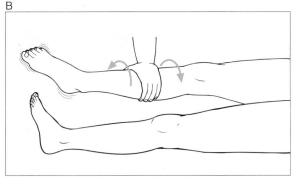

Fig. 7.23 Testing for tone. A. Check the full range of movement at the knee. **B.** Rock the relaxed leg to and fro.

ankle clonus is present there will be a rhythmical beating (alternating plantar and dorsiflexion) of the foot for as long as the pressure is maintained.

Interpretation

Although a few beats of clonus are present in some normal people, sustained clonus indicates damage to the upper motor neurones and is a 'hard' neurological sign.

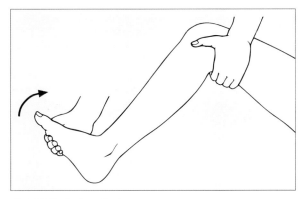

Fig. 7.24 Testing for ankle clonus.

Hypertonia is a common feature of upper motor neurone pathology. It is usually associated with increased deep tendon reflexes (see later), clonus, an extensor plantar reflex and typical patterns of weakness. It is a common finding in cerebrovascular disease, multiple sclerosis, traumatic spinal injury and degenerative spondylotic myelopathy.

Rigidity is most frequently encountered in patients with Parkinson's disease (who will often have the other manifestations of this disease such as bradykinesia, tremor, gait and postural abnormalities). Rigidity in parkinsonism often has a phasic component giving it a jerky feel (cogwheel rigidity).

Hypotonia is encountered in lower motor neurone and cerebellar disorders and in chorea. This is often associated with hyporeflexia, muscle wasting and paresis. Hypotonia is also seen transiently in the early phase following capsular cerebrovascular accidenty in which the plegic limb is atonic prior to becoming spastic and hyperreflexic. Cerebellar hypotonia is subtle and often difficult to detect but may be evident if knee reflexes are pendular (see below).

Power

When evaluating muscle power it is important to relate the strength of the muscles to the patient being tested. For example, a labourer may complain of weakness in an arm which to the examiner is extremely strong, while an elderly patient may have no symptoms despite being generally paretic.

There are two methods by which muscle power can be tested.

Examination

❏ *Isometric testing*; ask the patient to contract a group of muscles as powerfully as possible and then to maintain that position while the examiner tries to overpower the muscle group being tested.
❏ *Isotonic testing*; ask the patient to put the joint through a range of movement while attempting to halt movement progression.
❏ Examine individual muscle groups in both limbs alternately, or in some instances simultaneously, so that strength of the right and left can be directly compared.

Isometric testing is more sensitive in detecting subtle degrees of paresis.

One system of testing is shown Table 7.14. In some cases (e.g. pyramidal tract lesions) a pattern of weakness can be recognised (see Table 7.15).

Table 7.14 One method of testing the motor system

Test in a proximo-distal direction

In the upper limbs examine for:
 Abduction and adduction of the shoulder
 Flexion and extension of the shoulder
 Flexion and extension of the elbow
 Flexion and extension of the wrist
 Supination and pronation of the forearm
 Extension of the fingers at both the metacarpophalangeal and interphalangeal joints
 Finger and thumb flexion, extension, adduction and abduction

Test the abdominal muscles by asking the supine patient to flex the neck or sit forward.

In the lower limbs examine for:
 Hip flexion and extension, adduction and abduction
 Knee flexion and extension
 Foot dorsiflexion, plantar flexion, inversion and eversion, toe plantar flexion and dorsiflexion

Table 7.15 Patterns of muscle weakness due to pyramidal tract lesions

Affected	Relatively spared
Upper limbs	
Shoulder abduction	Shoulder adduction
Elbow extension	Elbow flexion
Finger extension	Finger flexion
Finger abduction	
Lower limbs	
Hip flexion	Hip extension
Knee flexion	Knee extension
Foot dorsiflexion	Foot plantar flexion

Muscle power is generally recorded using the grading recommended by the Medical Research Council (United Kingdom) (see Table 7.16).

In most clinical situations paresis occurs within the grade 4 range, and this can be subdivided into 4+ and 4– to give greater precision.

If a weakness is found in a particular muscle or limb, then a more detailed examination of muscles innervated by the same peripheral nerve or spinal segment should be undertaken (see Chapter 9).

Interpretation

In many patients the pattern of muscle weakness and the other clinical features will identify the category of the underlying disease (Table 7.17).

Deep tendon reflexes

A neurological reflex depends on an arc which consists of an afferent pathway, which is activated by a specific

Table 7.16 MRC scale for muscle power

0	No muscle contraction visible
1	Muscle contraction visible, but no movement of joint
2	Joint movement when effect of gravity eliminated
3	Movement sufficient to overcome effect of gravity
4	Movement overcomes gravity plus added resistance
5	Normal power

receptor, an efferent system, which activates a stereotyped response, and a simple or complex pathway that interconnects the afferent and efferent systems. Since the reflex response to an appropriate stimulus is involuntary, disturbances of reflexes afford objective signs of neural dysfunction. The deep tendon reflexes of the limbs provide essential information about the status of the central and peripheral nervous systems. They are phasic stretch reflexes which involve only two neurones (i.e. monosynaptic reflexes). They are evoked by sudden stretch of a muscle. This activates the muscle spindles, which produce an afferent volley that travels up 1A fibres, which enter the dorsal horn of the spinal cord and synapse on an α-motor neurone in the ventral horn of the cord. Excitation of the neurone leads to direct activation and contraction of the muscle. The important deep tendon reflexes are the biceps jerk (BJ), the supinator (SJ) jerk, the triceps (TJ) jerk and the knee (KJ) and ankle (AJ) jerks. It is important to strike the tendon since mechanical stimulation of a muscle belly may produce contraction of that muscle which is not dependent on the reflex arc. Since the deep tendon reflexes are monosynaptic they are subserved by a particular spinal cord segment. However suprasegmental influences modify activity of the reflex arc.

Elicitation of tendon reflexes

The five commonest reflexes and their segmental innervation are illustrated in Figures 7.25 to 7.30. The ankle jerk is usually elicited in the position shown in Figure 7.28. However, if it is difficult to obtain, the position shown in Figure 7.29 is particularly useful.

Other deep tendon reflexes which may be useful include the deltoid reflex (C5), the pectoral reflex (C7), the finger flexion jerk and the Hoffmann reflex (C7,C8,T1) and the hamstring jerk (L5,S1).

Examination

Tendon reflexes

❑ Place the patient in a comfortable relaxed position which allows the examiner to reach the limbs easily.

❑ Ensure that the muscle being tested is visible.

❑ Strike the tendon, not the muscle belly, with a sharp tap from a tendon hammer.

❑ Observe the muscle contraction.

❑ Test the symmetry of the reflex by comparing the amplitude of movement on one side with the other.

❑ In those patients in whom reflexes are difficult to elicit or appear to be absent, use the technique of reinforcement (the Jendrassik manoeuvre): for lower limb reflexes ask the patient to interlock the flexed fingers and to attempt to pull them apart at the time the tendon is being struck (Fig. 7.31). Ask the patient to tighten immediately before striking the tendon and to relax thereafter.

❑ When reinforcing upper limb reflexes, ask the patient to clench the teeth or squeeze the knees together whilst the tendon reflexes are being elicited.

Table 7.17 Causes of muscle weakness

Anatomical aetiology	Associated features		Common causes
Lower motor neurone	Muscle atrophy Fasciculation Reflexes absent or diminished Hypotonia	}	Peripheral neuropathies Radiculopathies Anterior horn cell damage (e.g. poliomyelitis) Motor neurone disease
Upper motor neurone	'Patterned' weakness Little or no muscle wasting Hyperreflexia Hypertonia Hypokinesia of movement	}	Cerebrovascular disease (e.g. hemiplegia) Spinal injury or disease (e.g. paraplegia) Multiple sclerosis
Myopathies	Muscle wasting (usually proximal) Hypotonia Tenderness (myositis)	}	Hereditary conditions (e.g. muscular dystrophy) Alcohol and other toxins
Psychological	Inconsistent weakness No associated features	}	Stress Anxiety Compensation claims

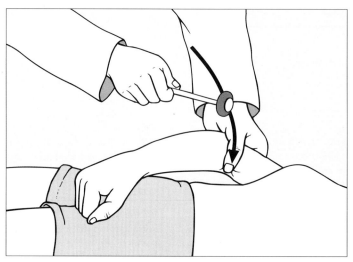

Fig. 7.25 Eliciting the biceps jerk, C5 (C6).

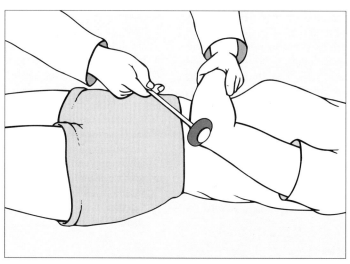

Fig. 7.26 Eliciting the triceps jerk, C6, C7.

The finger jerk

❏ Place the tips of the examiner's middle and index fingers across the palmar surface of the proximal phalanges of the patient's relaxed fingers.

❏ Tap the examiner's fingers lightly with a tendon hammer. The normal response is slight flexion of the patient's fingers. This becomes exaggerated if there is hyperreflexia.

The Hoffmann reflex

❏ Place the examining right index finger under the distal interphalangeal joint of the patient's middle finger.

❏ Briskly flick down the patient's fingertip with the examining right thumb tip, and allow it to spring back to the normal position while observing the patient's thumb for any movement. (Fig. 7.32).

Pectoral reflex

❏ Place the examiner's extended index and middle finger on the lateral border of the pectoralis muscle.

❏ Tap them with the tendon hammer.

Deltoid reflex

❏ Place the examiner's index finger across the tip of the shoulder (on the deltoid muscle belly).

❏ Tap the examiner's fingers with a tendon hammer.

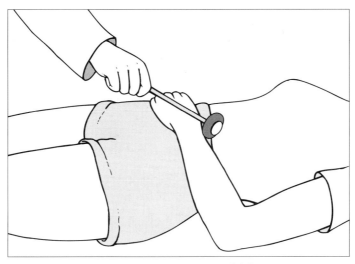

Fig. 7.27 Eliciting the supinator jerk (C5), C6.

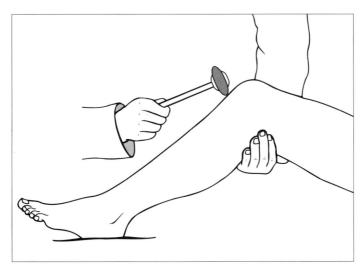

Fig. 7.28 Eliciting the knee jerk. (Note the legs must not be in contact with each other), L3, L4.

Interpretation

Normally during Hoffmann's test there is no response in the patient's adjoining thumb, however in states of hyperreflexia the thumb flexes in response to the manoeuvre.

In most patients a little response will be seen to either the pectoral or the deltoid jerk. However, in those with generalised hypertonicity and hyperreflexia a reflex contraction of the muscle will be seen and felt.

Deep tendon reflexes are classified as hyperactive (+++), normal (++), sluggish (+) or absent (–). If a reflex is present only with reinforcement it may be annotated as ±. It is only from examination of a large

number of patients that the clinician will get a feel for the normal spectrum.

Deciding whether deep tendon reflexes are pathologically brisk or a variant of normal can be very difficult. Ancillary clinical findings such as muscle tone, pattern of paresis, the presence of clonus and extensor plantar response will help clarify the significance of deep tendon hyperreflexia.

- Hyperreflexia is generally a sign of upper motor neurone pathology.
- Diminution or loss of ankle jerks may be present in some normal elderly people.
- In some patients who have myotonic pupils (see

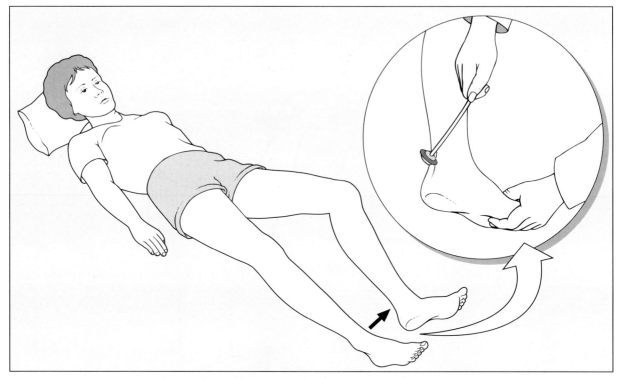

Fig. 7.29 Eliciting the ankle jerk of recumbent patient, S1.

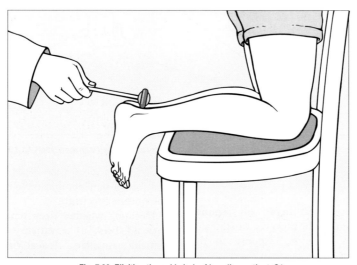

Fig. 7.30 Eliciting the ankle jerk of kneeling patient, S1.

p. 209) some of the deep tendon reflexes may be absent (Holmes–Adie syndrome).

- Isolated loss of a reflex may suggest a radiculopathy affecting that segment [e.g. loss of biceps jerk with C5–6 disc prolapse, loss of triceps jerk with C6–7 prolapse, loss of ankle jerk with lumbosacral (S1) disc prolapse].
- Symmetrical loss of reflexes may reflect generalised peripheral neuropathy.
- Lesions involving the anterior horn cell (poliomyelitis,

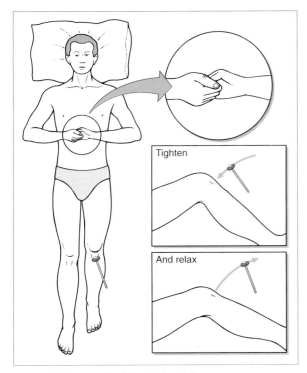

Fig. 7.31 Reinforcement in eliciting the knee jerk.

Tighten

And relax

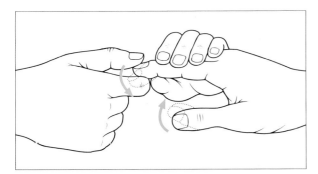

Fig. 7.32 Hoffman's sign.

motor neurone disease) will also lead to depressed or absent deep tendon reflexes.

A normal reflex contraction followed by delay in the relaxation time is a feature of hypothyroidism (Table 3.14 p. 78).

Diminished or absent tendon reflexes are in general caused by diseases of the lower motor neurone. Diseases of the neuromuscular junction and myopathies can produce hyporeflexia, but this tends to occur late in the disease process.

'Inversion' of deep tendon reflexes may be seen with combined spinal cord and root pathology (myelo-radiculopathy). This term refers to an absent or minimal response in the reflex arc being tested but with a much more obvious reflex response from muscles innervated from an adjoining spinal segment. This is most commonly seen when attempted elicitation of the biceps or supinator jerk evokes strong finger flexion. A similar but less common response may be seen when attempting to elicit the biceps jerk, the triceps reflex may be elicited. Such findings are common in cervical spondylotic myeloradiculopathy. Another finding in patients with spinal cord lesions is of crossed reflex induction. For example, elicitation of the knee jerk on one side may produce a reflex adduction response on the contralateral side.

Superficial reflexes

This group of reflexes includes the plantar response, the superficial abdominal reflex and cremasteric reflex. These are polysynaptic reflexes, which are evoked by cutaneous stimulation.

Plantar response (Fig. 7.33)

Following strong tactile stimulation of the lateral border of the sole of the foot, the normal plantar reflex is plantar flexion of the hallux with flexion and adduction of the other toes (S1,S2).

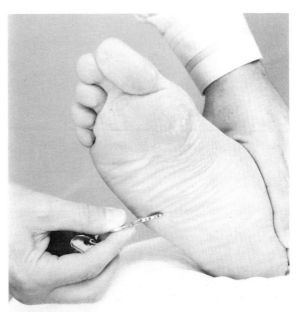

Fig. 7.33 Eliciting the plantar reflex.

An abnormal or extensor response occurs when the hallux dorsiflex and the other toes fan (abduct) and dorsiflex.

Superficial abdominal reflex

This involves reflex contraction of the anterior abdominal wall in response to light tactile stimulation. The segmental innervation of the reflex arc ranges from approximately T8 to T12.

The normal response is for the umbilicus to either elevate or depress and move laterally towards the quadrant of stimulation.

This reflex can be elicited easily in children and young adults but becomes much more sluggish in the elderly, the obese and after childbirth.

Cremasteric reflex

This involves brisk elevation of one testicle following ipsilateral stimulation of the inner thigh. This reflex is subserved by the genitofemoral nerve (L1,L2).

Examination

Plantar response
- ❏ Place the patient supine with the legs extended.
- ❏ Slowly rake a blunted point, such as an orange stick, the end of a car key or the examiner's thumbnail along the lateral border of the foot from heel towards the little toe.
- ❏ Stop as soon as the first movement of the big toe occurs.

Superficial abdominal reflex
- ❏ Position the relaxed patient supine.

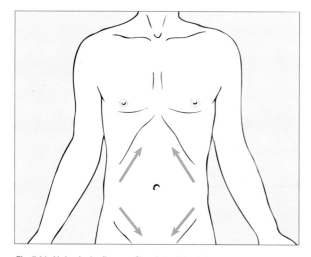

Fig. 7.34 Abdominal reflexes. Site of stimuli for their elicitation.

- ❏ Stroke the upper and lower quadrants of the abdominal wall on each side swiftly but lightly with an orange stick (Fig. 7.34).
- ❏ Observe any muscle contraction.

Cremasteric reflex
- ❏ Position the patient with the thigh externally rotated and abducted.
- ❏ Stroke the skin of the upper thigh using an orange stick.
- ❏ Observe the response of the ipsilateral testicle.

Interpretation

An extensor plantar response is an unequivocal sign of upper motor neurone lesion. It will often be associated with hyperreflexia, hypertonicity and clonus. In many people elicitation and interpretation of the reflex can be difficult because of either poor response or excessive ticklishness. In some instances, it is necessary to record the response as equivocal.

The superficial abdominal reflex is lost in upper and lower motor neurone lesions. However, because it is difficult to elicit in many patients it is at best only a useful ancillary sign.

The cremasteric reflex may be lost with either upper motor neurone disease or damage to the L1,2 spinal segment. However even in some normal patients, particularly the elderly, it may be difficult to elicit. In clinical practice many test this reflex only when assessing patients with spinal injury or other evidence of myelopathy.

Coordination: cerebellar function

The cerebellum plays an important role in the co-ordination of voluntary, automatic and reflex movement. The clinical subdivision of the cerebellum into the midline vermis and the lateral cerebellar hemispheres is useful.

- The *nucleus of the vermis* has multiple interconnections with the vestibular nuclei and is important in the maintenance of body posture and equilibrium.
- The *cerebellar cortex* and subcortical nuclei are important in smoothing and synchronising the timing of muscle contraction and relaxation when the limbs are moved.

The cerebellum also receives information from the spinal cord (spinocerebellar tracts), motor cortex (via the pontocerebellar fibres) and brain stem (red nucleus, reticular nuclei and the inferior olivary nuclear complex).

Clinical testing

Clinical tests of cerebellar function use movements of varying complexity to demonstrate the precision of motor function of both limb and postural musculature. The commonly used tests include *The finger-nose test.* This involves observing the speed, smoothness and accuracy of the movement and whether any tremor occurs. *Rapid alternating movement* of supination and pronation of the forearm. It is common for the test to be performed more quickly on the dominant side.

Other tests include the *heel–shin test* and the *heel–toe test of gait*. Additional tests that provide complementary information about the cerebellar function involve checking for nystagmus (p. 214), hypotonia (p. 230) and the presence of pendular reflexes (p. 231). Patients with cerebellar disorders also tend to have dysarthritic speech (p. 204).

Examination

The finger–nose test

- ❏ Ask the patient to hold one arm outstretched and then with the tip of the index finger to alternately touch the tip of the nose and then the examiner's fingertip as accurately as possible (Fig. 7.35).
- ❏ Make the test more discerning by moving the target fingertip so that the patient has to readjust 'aim'.
- ❏ Perform the test with the patient's eyes open and test each arm in turn.
- ❏ To test for ataxia due to proprioceptive deficit (sensory ataxia) now ask the patient to bring the outstretched fingertip to touch the tip of the nose with the eyes closed.

Rapid alternating movement

- ❏ Ask the patient to place one palm upwards and then alternately hit the upfacing palm with the palmar and then dorsal aspects of the fingertips of the other hand (Fig. 7.36).

The heel-shin test

- ❏ Ask the patient to raise one leg at the hip and then place the heel of the flexed leg on the contralateral knee and to then run the heel down the surface of the tibial shaft towards the ankle and then back again (Fig. 7.37A and B).
- ❏ To render the test more complex ask the patient first to raise the leg and touch the examiner's finger held in a suitable position with the big toe before placing the heel on the knee.

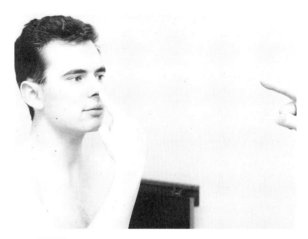

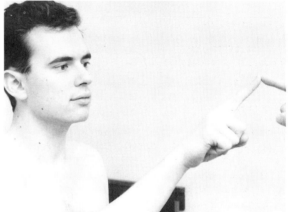

Fig. 7.35 The finger–nose test. Ask the patient to touch **A.** the tip of the nose and **B.** the examiner's finger.

The heel-toe test of gait

- ❏ Perform this test with the patient either barefoot or wearing flat shoes.
- ❏ Ask the patient to walk along a straight line so that the heel of one foot comes directly in contact with the toes of the other foot. The rear foot is then advanced so that its heel is then placed in front of the contralateral toe.
- ❏ Observe the gait in general, and in particular note any tendency to stagger and the side to which the patient preferentially falls.

Interpretation

Lesions of the cerebellar vermis. These cause truncal and gait ataxia.

- In severe lesions the patient may have difficulty maintaining balance when sitting, and unassisted walking may be impossible.

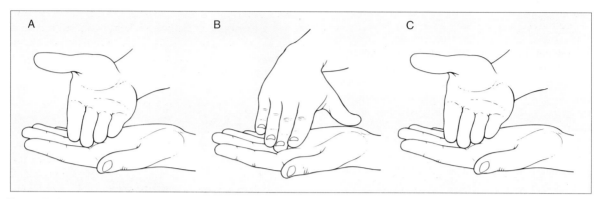

Fig. 7.36 Testing rapid alternating movement.

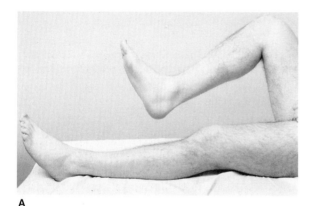

A

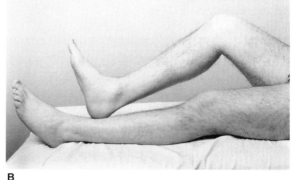

B

Fig. 7.37 The heel–shin test.

- The gait may be wide based (i.e. the legs are held further apart than normal), and there may be unsteadiness of both gait and standing posture.
- The patient may fall when attempting to do a heel–toe test.

Such phenomena are most commonly seen in patients with alcoholic cerebellar degeneration and neoplasms of the vermis. If the patient is examined only in bed such signs will be missed.

Disease of the cerebellar hemisphere.   There may be:

- abnormalities in the finger–nose test, impaired rapid alternating movement and heel–shin test
- horizontal phasic nystagmus towards the side of the lesion
- an intention tremor when performing the finger–nose test with past pointing or *dysmetria* (i.e. the patient under- or overshoots the examiner's finger)
- generalised incoordination and clumsiness of the movement (*dyssynergia*)
- slowness and incoordination when performing rapid

alternating movement (*dysdiadochokinesis*).

Cerebellar signs in adults are often due to cerebro-vascular disease or multiple sclerosis involving the cerebellum or its brain-stem connections. Specific syndromes due to occlusion of certain branches of the vertebrobasilar system are recognised by specific constellations of symptoms. Spontaneous intracerebellar haemorrhage, usually of hypertensive origin, is also a relatively common cause of acute-onset cerebellar signs in adults. Although cerebellar neoplasms are common in children, the predominant signs often tend to be those of intracranial hypertension with signs of cerebellar dysfunction occurring later. Metabolic intoxications (alcohol, phenytoin, carbamazepine) also frequently cause generalised cerebellar dysfunction. Generalised and progressive failure of cerebellar functions is seen in degenerative disorders with a genetic basis (the spinocerebellar degenerations) and as a non-metastatic effect of some malignancies, especially lung cancer.

KEY POINTS

- Patients should be examined in underwear.

- Abnormalities of tone need to be interpreted in the light of other clinical findings.

- Although a few beats of clonus are present in some normal people, sustained clonus indicates upper motor neurone damage and is a hard clinical sign.

- The pattern of weakness and associated clinical features will guide the examiner as to which category of disease underlies the paresis.

- Disturbances in deep tendon reflexes afford objective signs of neural dysfunction.

- It is important to strike the tendon, not the muscle, when eliciting a tendon reflex.

- Deciding whether or not a deep tendon reflex is pathologically brisk can be difficult.

- Diminished or absent tendon reflexes are usually caused by diseases of lower motor neurones.

- An extensor plantar response is an unequivocal sign of a pyramidal tract lesion.

- Rapid alternating movements in the upper limbs are normally performed more quickly on the dominant side.

- Lesions of the cerebellar vermis causing truncal and gait ataxia may be missed if the patient is examined only in bed.

THE SENSORY SYSTEM

Each of the modalities of light touch, pain, temperature, proprioception (joint position sense) and vibration have specific receptor systems and afferent pathways. Sensations of touch, pressure and position sense are carried in the peripheral nerves in relatively large fast-conducting fibres, while pain and temperature modalities are served principally by smaller, slower conducting fibres. The cells of origin of peripheral sensory fibres lie in the dorsal root ganglia. The central processes of those ganglion cells subserving pain, temperature and some light touch synapse in the laminae of the dorsal horn of the spinal cord then decussate (cross over the midline) into tracts in the contralateral spinal cord (anterior and lateral spinothalamic tracts). These fibres ascend to either the ventral posterior thalamic nuclei (25%) or the reticular nuclei of the brain stem and thalamus. The fibres carrying proprioception, discriminative, light touch and vibration sense ascend in the dorsal columns (cuneate and gracile fasciculi) to the spinal cord. They ascend to synapse in the gracile and cuneate nuclei of the caudal medulla.

Hypoaesthesia (decreased sensation)

This may be an awareness that the sensations of temperature, pain or light touch are diminished when compared with normal limbs. A patient may inadvertently burn the fingers if pain and temperature modalities are disturbed (as, for example, in cervical syringomyelia).

Altered sensations

These may be spontaneous (*paraesthesiae*) or elicited by touch or other stimuli (*dysaesthesiae*). They may be pins and needles, tightness or constriction or feelings of warmth or coldness.

Pain

Pain is an extremely common symptom. In some diseases, such as trigeminal neuralgia (V nerve distribution), glossopharyngeal neuralgia (IX nerve distribution), post-herpetic neuralgia and discogenic radiculopathies, the description of distribution of pain and its type may be diagnostic. In most cases, however, symptoms of pain do not conform to standard dermatomal or peripheral nerve distribution (Figs 7.39 and 7.40), and often pain may be perceived inappropriately (e.g. touch felt as pain); this phenomenon is termed hyperpathia or allodynia.

Numbness

Caution should be exercised when a patient describes a limb as 'numb' since this means weakness or heaviness to some people rather than loss of feeling.

The sensory modalities

From the clinical viewpoint, the important sensory modalities are joint position sense (proprioception), light touch, pinprick, vibration, temperature and two-point discrimination. Other aspects and sensory function are important but will be covered under the section on the cortical examination (see Table 7.18).

The aims of sensory testing are:

- to determine if any modalities are impaired;

Cerebral hemisphere

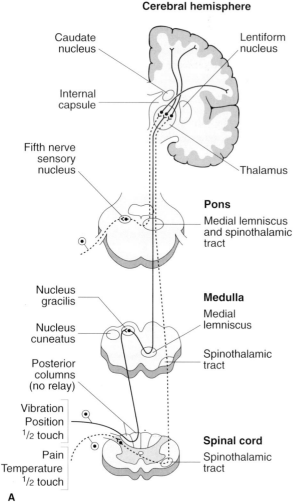

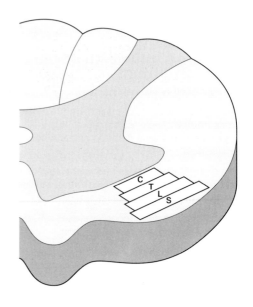

B

A

Fig. 7.38 A. The main sensory pathways. B. Spinothalamic tract. To show layering of the spinothalamic tract in the cervical region: C. represents fibres from cervical segments which lie centrally; fibres from thoracic lumbar and sacral segments (labelled T, L and S respectively) lie progressively more laterally.

• to determine the site of any lesion from the topographic pattern of dysfunction (dermatomal distribution, peripheral nerve distribution).

When performing these tests it is important to avoid inflicting unnecessary discomfort upon the patient and to explain what is being performed.

Examination

Touch

❏ Touch (do not stroke) the skin with a small piece of cotton wool; tissue paper and light digital touch are alternative stimuli.

❏ Avoid regularly timed stimuli so that the patient does not anticipate the test.

❏ Ask the patient to close the eyes and to respond verbally to each touch.

❏ Examine the spinal segments sequentially [e.g. in the upper limb start on the outer border of the arm (C5), then proceed downwards to the lateral border of the forearm (C6) then the thumb (C6), index finger, etc.].

❏ Compare sensation on each limb for symmetry.

❏ Outline the borders of any abnormal area of sensation by testing from the hypoaesthetic area towards normal.

Table 7.18 Tests of sensation

Modality	Pathway
Light touch Proprioception Vibration Two-point discrimination	Large fast-conducting axons Dorsal columns Medial lemniscus
Pinprick (superficial pain) Deep pain Temperature	Smaller slower conducting axons Spinothalamic tracts
Stereognosis Graphaesthesia Two-point discrimination	Parietal cortex (only valid if peripheral sensory function intact)

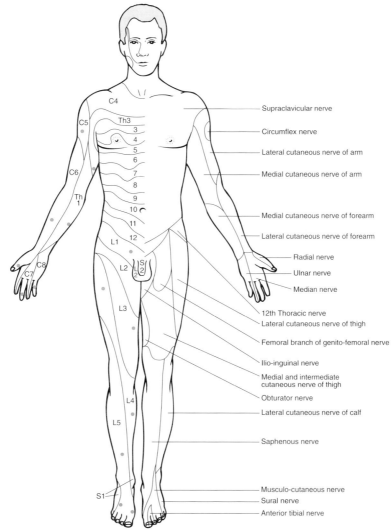

Fig. 7.39 Segmental and peripheral nerve innervation and points for testing anterior cutaneous sensation of limbs.   By applying stimuli at the points marked both the dermatomal and main peripheral nerve distribution are tested simultaneously.

❏ If the patient complains of dysaesthesia (an uncomfortable or abnormal feeling) map from the normal to the abnormal area.

Pain

❏ Because of the risk of transmitted hepatitis and HIV, use a new dressmaking pin or a dedicated disposable pin. Avoid using a hypodermic needle, which is too sharp.

❏ Establish a baseline for sharpness (e.g. sternal area) before examining the limb.

❏ Test pinprick sensation down each limb and over the trunk.

❏ Ask the patient to report if the quality of sensation changes, either becoming blunter (hypoaesthesia) or feeling sharper or more painful (hyperaesthesia).

❏ Test each dermatome in turn, but also bear in mind peripheral nerve distributions.

❏ Map out the boundaries of any abnormal area as described for light touch.

Deep pain

❏ Squeeze muscle bellies (e.g. calf, biceps or triceps) or apply firm compression over the patient's fingernail and toenail beds.

❏ Ask the patient to report as soon as the sensation becomes painful.

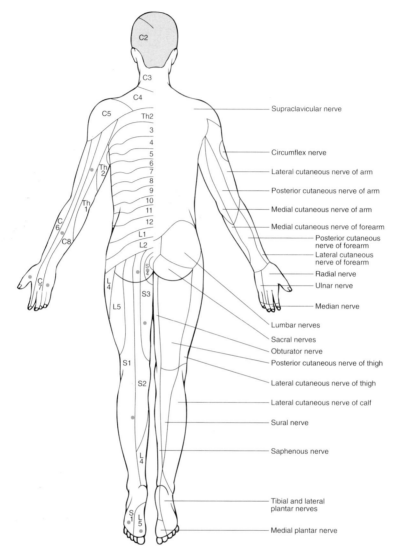

Fig. 7.40 Segmental and peripheral nerve innervation and points for testing posterior cutaneous sensation of limbs. By applying stimuli at the points marked both the dermatomal and main peripheral nerve distribution are tested simultaneously.

Temperature

❏ Touch the patient with a cold object (e.g. a tuning fork) and ask the patient about the quality of the temperature sensation. This can be performed on face, forearms, hands, trunk and legs.

❏ For improved discrimination fill two plastic containers (e.g. serum bottles) one with warm and the other with cool water. Ask the patient to close the eyes and to distinguish between warm and cool while applying the containers to the skin in a random sequence.

Joint position sense (JPS)

❏ Test this sensation initially at the most distal part of the limb. In the upper limb first test at the distal interphalangeal joint of the index finger.

❏ Show the patient the intended movements of the joint and name them (e.g. 'that's up' and 'that's down').

❏ Ask the patient to close the eyes.

❏ Grasp the proximal phalanx of the index finger with one hand and the medial and lateral borders of the distal phalanx with the other thumb and finger.

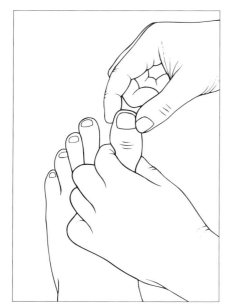

Fig. 7.41 Testing for position sense in the big toe.

❑ Move the patient's distal phalanx up and down.
❑ Ask the patient to identify the direction of movement during a random sequence of small movements (e.g. up, down, down, up).
❑ Then test the contralateral limb.
❑ If there is any abnormality of JPS at the distal interphalangeal joint, test at the proximal interphalangeal joint and, if necessary, at the metacarpophalangeal joint, progressing to the wrist and elbow if JPS remains impaired.
❑ In the lower limb start at the interphalangeal joint of the hallux, holding the proximal phalanx in the other hand (Fig. 7.41).
❑ Take care to ensure that the examiner's fingers do not rub against the patient's other toes.
❑ If there is impairment proceed to examine the metatarsophalangeal joint and, if necessary, the ankle and knee.
❑ Throughout the examination of JPS try to prevent the patient from guessing.

Vibration sense
❑ Examine the patient with his or her eyes closed.
❑ First hold the vibrating tuning fork (128 Hz) over the sternum so that the patient identifies the sensation.
❑ In the lower limbs test the big toe (Fig. 7.42A). If necessary, next move proximally in turn at the ankle (Fig. 7.42B), tibial shaft and tuberosity and the anterior iliac crest.

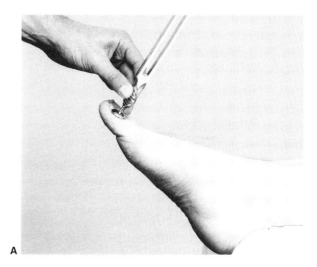

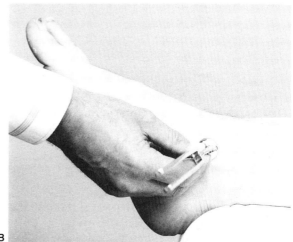

Fig. 7.42 Testing vibration sensation at A. the big toe and B. the ankle.

❑ In the upper limbs test the interphalangeal joint of the forefinger; if impaired, proceed to the metacarpophalangeal joint and then more proximal bony prominences.
❑ If in doubt, ask the patient to identify as soon as the tuning fork stops vibrating when 'blocked' by the examining fingers.

Two-point discrimination
❑ Use a two-point discriminator if one is available, or an opened-out paper clip.
❑ Perform the test with the patient's eyes closed.
❑ Hold the patient's index finger and apply either one or two of the test object points to the finger pulp.
❑ Ask the patient to determine if one or two stimuli were applied.

❏ Then determine the minimum distance at which two points are discriminated.

❏ Perform the test on the pulp of both index fingers and thumbs.

❏ Repeat the test several times during the course of the clinical examination to determine variation in two-point discriminatory distance.

Interpretation

Any impairment of JPS or vibration is first detected distally. Joint position is most commonly impaired in patients with large-fibre peripheral neuropathies and spinal cord disorders (myelopathies) affecting the dorsal columns. Disturbances of JPS may occur without paresis. In such patients the following findings may be noted:

• impaired fine-finger function and alterations of gait as a result of loss of feedback concerning muscle activity and joint position

• sensory ataxia when the finger–nose test is carried out with the eyes closed

• positive Romberg's test

• walking in the dark their gait becomes unsteady or they may fall when performing movements that require complex postural adjustments

• with the hands outstretched and eyes closed, the fingers may make small slow movements (pseudoathetosis).

Impaired vibration sense over bony prominences occurs with age and is often lost at the ankles over the age of 70. However, loss of vibration sense is seen in patients at an earlier stage than impairment of JPS. For example, it is an early feature in diabetic peripheral neuropathy.

In the normal person two separate stimuli can be discriminated when they are applied as close together as 3–5 mm on the pulps of the index finger. The test is rarely performed on the soles of the feet, where the distinguishing distance is anything up to 10 times greater. It is one of the few objective parameters of sensory function. Its documentation prior to surgery or any therapeutic endeavour is a useful way of gauging clinical response to treatment. Two-point discrimination in the fingers is impaired in many peripheral neuropathies, particularly those involving large sensory fibres, and in cervical myeloradiculopathies. In these conditions its loss is associated with other abnormal clinical findings suggestive of dorsal column dysfunction (light touch, JPS, vibration). Parietal lobe lesions may cause marked loss of two-point discrimination in the absence of other modality changes.

It may be difficult to decide whether there is significant sensory loss. Some patients may be particularly vague in their perception of the sensory stimulus, while others may be particularly obsessive and comment on minor variations in the intensity of the stimulus applied. Organic alterations of sensation are usually consistent and reproducible in their nature, degree and extent. Patients who have considerable alteration of superficial sensation will volunteer sensory symptoms. The finding of extensive or apparently severe sensory loss in the absence of such symptoms should cause the examiner to assess the signs sceptically.

Disorders of touch, pain and temperature perception (hypoaesthesia, dysaesthesia and hyperaesthesia), JPS and two-point discrimination are common in peripheral neuropathies and nerve injuries, discogenic radiculopathies and spinal injuries.

Lesions of individual peripheral nerves or sensory nerve roots commonly give rise to subjective feeling of numbness and diminution of all sensory modalities in their areas of distribution (Figs 7.38 and 7.39). Less commonly partial lesions of the peripheral nerve give rise to pain of a burning, unpleasant quality, as in causalgia, a condition occurring infrequently after injury to either the median or sciatic nerve. In polyneuropathies the numbness or paraesthesia and objective sensory features affect the distal parts of the limbs and often involve the legs before the arms. Superficial sensory loss in a polyneuropathy is found over the distal parts of the extremities and extends up the limbs to a level which may be relatively uniform around their whole circumference as a 'stocking and glove' type sensory disturbance.

With spinal cord lesions there may be a disassociated sensory loss (i.e. not all modalities are affected equally). Most commonly pain and temperature sensations are lost while touch, vibration and JPS are intact. This pattern results from lesions which damage the lateral spinothalamic pathways but not the dorsal columns. Disassociated sensory loss is classically found in patients with cervical syringomyelia but may arise from other intramedullary and brain-stem pathology. Other characteristic patterns of sensory (and motor) loss occur in the anterior spinal artery syndrome (preservation of dorsal column function, with loss of motor function and spinothalamic modalities) and in the Brown–Séquard syndrome (ipsilateral loss of motor function, vibration and JPS with contralateral loss of spinothalamic sensations). Lesions of the conus medullaris and cauda equina (central disc prolapse, neurofibroma, ependymoma, primary and metastatic neoplasia) cause sensory loss from the feet, up the back of the legs, to the buttocks, perineum and genitalia.

With intracranial lesions, which are frequently vascular in origin, other patterns of sensory abnormalities may be found:

- Unilateral lesions of the lower brain stem may cause impairment of pain and temperature on the ipsilateral side of the face (as a result of V nerve involvement) and on the contralateral side of the body below the neck (sometimes called alternating analgesia). Spinothalamic tract lesions above the mid-pontine level may damage both the spinothalamic tract and the medial lemniscus, which lie close together. This This will cause sensory impairment of all modalities on the contralateral face and body.
- Lesions of the thalamus may give rise to spontaneous, intense, burning pain on the contralateral side associated with diminution of touch over the same area. The pain threshold is usually raised. The pain is poorly localised and has a particularly unpleasant quality.
- Damage to the sensory cortex may not impair perception of pain, temperature and touch but causes alterations in the qualitative, affective and discriminatory aspects of sensory appreciation and is usually accompanied by loss of two-point discrimination or astereognosis (see below).

Cortical function

Tests that examine sensory cortical function depend on the integrity of the peripheral sensory pathways. If these are pathologically impaired, testing of cortical sensory function is pointless. This section deals with those aspects of cortical function which have not been discussed and which have moderately well localised anatomical substrates. When damaged these give rise to discrete patterns of clinical abnormality. The range of abnormalities can be detected by testing:

- speech and other language functions (e.g. reading, writing, verbal comprehension)
- calculating ability, body awareness, right and left orientation and integrative perception of sensory information (stereognosis).

If language functions are impaired many of these tests cannot be performed.

Point localisation tests (body awareness, finger gnosis, right/left orientation). These assess the ability of the patient to localise accurately parts of the body.

Stereognosis. Assesses the ability of the patient to identify common objects by touch alone.

Graphaesthesia. Tests the ability of the patient to recognise numbers or letters traced onto the skin with a blunt object.

Sensory extinction (inattention). Assesses perception of simultaneous stimuli applied to corresponding sites on both sides of the body requires an intact peripheral sensory system. The normal patient is aware when both sides are touched. However, if there is sensory extinction (also called sensory neglect or sensory inattention), the patient will perceive that only the unaffected side has been touched. Sensory inattention which is caused by lesions of the parietal lobe contralateral to the neglected side is often found with visual inattention (p. 210).

Calculating skills. The patient's ability to perform simple arithmetic is assessed by asking appropriate subtraction sums.

Examination

Point localisation

☐ Ask the patient with the eyes closed to localise tactile stimuli applied to various parts of the body, e.g. hands, fingers, different parts of the face.
☐ In addition, ask the patient to discriminate the right side from left, and to name individual fingers.

Stereognosis

☐ Ensure that the patient's eyes are fully closed.
☐ Place various identifiable objects in the palm of the patient's hands (e.g. pen top, coin, key, matchstick, piece of cotton wool).
☐ Ask the patient to identify the object using only sensory input from the hand and fingers.

Graphaesthesia

☐ Perform the test with the patient's eyes closed.
☐ Support the dorsum of the patient's hand and using a suitable object, such as the blunt end of a pencil, draw digits or letters on the patient's palm.
☐ Ask the patient to identify each symbol in turn.
☐ Repeat the test in the lower limb over the shin, if appropriate.

Sensory inattention

☐ Perform the test with the patient's eyes closed and arms outstretched.
☐ Confirm that the patient can feel a stimulus on either side when tested separately.
☐ Touch both hands simultaneously and ask the patient to report if the stimulus was applied to the left, right or both sides.

Calculating skills

☐ Ask the patient to perform subtraction sums. Alternatively, ask how much change would be expected from, say £10 if goods were bought costing a specific price.

Interpretation

- The inability to localise tactile discrimination in the various parts of the body occurs with lesions in the posterior inferior parietal cortex. *Finger agnosia* is a particular type of this deficit.
- The inability to recognise objects by touch alone (*astereognosis*) suggests an abnormality of the angular and supramarginal gyra in the parietal lobe.
- An inability to recognise symbols written on the palm of the hand (*dysgraphaesthesia*) also suggests an abnormality of the parietal sensory association cortex. Sensory inattention arises from lesions in a similar location.
- An inability to perform simple calculations (*dyscalculia*) suggests a lesion in the inferior parieto-occipital region.
- The association of right/left disorientation, finger agnosia, dyslexia and dyscalculia is termed Gerstmann's syndrome and is seen with lesions of the dominant angular gyral region.

Primitive reflexes

Primitive reflexes refer to a group of reflexes that are present in neonates and children (p. 347) but are lost with development and maturation of the central nervous system. Many of these reflexes return with generalised structural or functional diseases of the adult central nervous system (or with ageing), and indeed some remain present in a proportion of normal people. The commonly performed reflexes are the pout and snout reflex (rooty reflex), the grasp reflex and the palmomental reflex. As isolated signs they have minimal localising value, but in patients with neurological dysfunction their presence suggests a diffuse neuropathological process.

Arm drift

A very useful but non-specific sign in clinical neurology is termed 'drift'. A positive sign suggests some underlying abnormality in nervous function and is an indication for performing a more detailed neurological examination.

Examination

- ☐ Ask the patient to close the eyes and outstretch the limbs, placing palms uppermost and the fingers extended and adducted, and then to maintain this position.
- ☐ Observe the limbs for drift (i.e. a slow movement, usually downwards) from the initial position. This may be a subtle change in finger position (e.g. a slow flexion) or a more gross drift downwards or pronation of the whole arm.

KEY POINTS

- Caution should be exercised when a patient describes a limb as 'numb' since this means weakness or heaviness rather than loss of feeling to some people.

- When performing sensory tests it is important to explain what is being performed and to avoid unnecessary discomfort.

- Organic alterations of sensation are consistent and reproducible in nature, degree and extent.

- Parietal lobe lesions may cause marked loss of two-point discrimination in the absence of other sensory changes.

- Sensory cortical function cannot be evaluated if peripheral sensory pathways are impaired.

- Primitive reflexes have minimal localising value but suggest a diffuse neuropathological process affecting the cerebral hemispheres.

- A positive arm drift suggests some underlying abnormality of the nervous system and is an indication for performing a detailed examination.

EXAMINATION OF THE UNCONSCIOUS PATIENT

By definition patients are in coma if they do not open their eyes, utter sounds or obey commands in response to verbal or other stimuli. Wherever possible an account of events preceding coma should be obtained directly from friends or relatives and supplemented by any further information, e.g. from ambulance personnel. The history of medical conditions such as diabetes mellitus, renal, cardiac or hepatic dysfunction, drug abuse or a convulsive disorder is pertinent. The causes of coma in young patients are usually different from those in the elderly.

Examination should commence with assessment of the cardiac and respiratory status. Blood pressure, pulse rate and rhythm and respiratory rate, rhythm and volume may provide clues to the aetiology of the coma.

Table 7.19 The Glasgow coma scale

Motor response (score range 1–6)	
Obeys commands	6
Localises to pain	5
Flexion withdrawal to pain	4
Abnormal flexion	3
Extension	2
No response	1
Eye opening (score range 1–4)	
Spontaneous eye opening	4
Eye opening to voice	3
Eye opening to pain	2
No eye opening	1
Verbal response (score range 1–5)	
Normal speech, orientated	5
Normal speech, disorientated	4
Abnormal speech	3
Incomprehensible sounds	2
No verbal response	1

When assessing the patient's GCS the *best* scores from verbal, eye and motor assessments are used and added. The GCS will therefore range from 3 to 15. This scale gives an indication of the patient's conscious state and is not a substitute for neurological examination. For example, a patient may have had nondominant hemispheric stroke causing a dense hemiplegia yet still have a normal GCS.

Profound abnormalities in these parameters require emergency corrective or supportive therapy. Secondary insults from either hypoxia or systemic hypotension may cause catastrophic brain dysfunction. The degree of coma can be assessed by the Glasgow coma scale (GCS) (see Table 7.19). Only once the airway and cardiac output are satisfactory should further physical and neurological examination commence. Signs of trauma, acute or chronic medical disease, drug intake (needle marks or breath smelling of alcohol) or acute infection (pyrexia, neck stiffness (p. 207)) should be sought. If the patient has no obvious signs of injury a rapid estimation of blood glucose should be performed. If there is evidence of head injury, particular care should be taken since the cervical spine may also be injured. When assessing the GCS in an unconscious patient the response to pain is best tested by digital pressure on the supraorbital ridge. If pressure is applied to a limb, there may be no response because of spinal cord or peripheral nerve damage. In recording the various aspects of the GCS, the best response obtained is scored if there is asymmetry.

The size of the pupils and the response to the light reflex are particularly pertinent aspects of the neurological examination in coma. The temptation to dilate the pupils with mydriatics in order to obtain a better view of the fundus should be resisted at all costs.

Bilaterally fixed dilated pupils can occur with bilateral nerve III paresis (owing to massive brain swelling and tentorial herniation or midbrain damage) and following ingestion of anticholinergic drugs (e.g. magic mushrooms, tricyclic antidepressants). A unilateral fixed dilated pupil suggests an ipsilateral intracranial mass lesion (e.g. spontaneous intracerebral haemorrhage, traumatic haematoma) causing a III nerve palsy.

Pin-point pupils occur following pontine vascular lesions and after narcotic overdose, while in metabolic coma the pupils are normally reactive to light.

Unconscious patients are unable to fixate and will therefore have 'roving' eye movements. Not infrequently the ocular axes will not be conjugate.

In patients with severe raised intracranial pressure and signs of cerebral herniation the blood pressure will be high and the pulse slow (Cushing's response).

Assessment of asymmetry on the motor aspects of the GCS will give supportive evidence concerning unilateral intracranial pathology (e.g. with a right fixed dilated pupil, if the motor response is worse on the left side than the right, this further supports a diagnosis of an acute intracranial mass lesion).

Assessment of the corneal, oculocephalic, oculovestibular and gag reflexes will provide additional information about the integrity of brain-stem function.

Examination of the head should include a search for lacerations (? underlying depressed skull fracture), bruising over the mastoid process (Battle's sign indicative of a middle fossa fracture) and CSF or bloody discharge from the ears or nose. An anterior cranial fossa or nasal fracture may be associated with bilateral periorbital haematomas (racoon eyes). Palpation of the orbital margins may reveal a zygomatic or malar fracture. The severity of facial injuries can be gauged by checking the stability of the alveolar process of the mandible (grasp the upper jaw with a gloved hand and see if the alveolar process is stable).

Examination of limb tone and reflexes will provide information about the presence of spinal cord injury. Rectal examination may reveal poor anal tone in cauda equina damage. With cervical spinal cord injury there is usually associated hypotension (due to loss of sympathetic vascular tone) and bradycardia due to unopposed vagal activity to the heart.

KEY POINT

- It is essential that the airway is protected and both ventilation and cardiac output are satisfactory before further detailed physical and neurological examination is undertaken.

BRAIN DEATH TESTING

The diagnosis of brain death can be made following a clinical examination. This is now routine practice in intensive care units where people receive mechanical ventilatory support as part of the intensive management of many diverse conditions. Prior to performing brain death testing it is essential that the cause of irreversible brain damage and death is determined (e.g. intracerebral haemorrhage, encephalitis), and that hypothermia, drug intoxications, metabolic defects and neuromuscular blockade do not account for the absence of brain-stem activity at the time the tests are conducted. In patients who have previously been paralysed, restoration of normal neuromuscular function can be tested electrically or by elicitation of the deep tendon jerks. After these criteria are satisfied the following parameters are examined:

- pupil reflex to light (p. 209)
- corneal reflex (p. 216)
- oculovestibular reflex using iced-water irrigation of the external ear canal (p. 222)
- gag reflex (p. 223)
- cough reflex
- spontaneous respiration
- response to painful stimuli, within the cranial nerve territories.

In a brain-dead person all these reflexes are absent.

Spinal reflex activity in response to a peripheral stimulus (e.g. pressing the toenail bed) is usually absent but may be preserved in the brain-dead. The absence of spontaneous respiratory activity can only be confirmed if the $Pa\text{CO}_2$ is $>6.6\,\text{kPa}$ or $>50\,\text{mmHg}$. Normally the 'brain death tests' are performed by two experienced clinicians either together or separately. They are then repeated, after an interval, prior to the declaration of brain death. EEG testing is not necessary for a diagnosis of brain death, but is sometimes performed in the interval between the two sets of clinical tests. In brain death the EEG usually shows a flat isoelectric trace.

THE DIAGNOSTIC PROCESS

The completion of the neurological examination is followed by the correlation and interpretation of the information in order to reach a diagnosis. The diagnostic formulation should comprise:

- an assessment of the nature of the patient's dysfunction
- the definition of the distribution of lesions
- an assessment of the most likely pathological diagnosis.

In other words, what is disturbed, where and why?

DISTURBANCE OF FUNCTION

The combination of signs attributable to lesions of different parts and paths of the nervous system needs to be understood and memorised (Table 7.20).

These combinations of signs are those of fully developed dysfunction. Every abnormality is not to be expected in every case and the clinician must be prepared to deduce that a part of the nervous system has been damaged when incomplete patterns of signs have been demonstrated.

DISTRIBUTION OF LESIONS

The clinical recognition of neural dysfunction is followed by the identification of the site or sites of their involvement. All the observed signs may be due to a single localised lesion affecting adjacent structures or may be the consequence of more widespread damage.

Single lesions

The demonstration of cortical dysfunction will often enable the location of a lesion to be deduced fairly precisely.

Cerebral cortex. Impairment of specialised functions results in dementia, dysphasia, apraxia, astereognosis and other forms of agnosia. Cortical motor neurones are spread over a wide area and lesions typically affect function in only part of the opposite side of the body. Thus, unless the lesion is very large, paresis confined to one limb (monoplegia) or to one side of the face is more likely than a hemiplegia.

In contrast, a profound hemiplegia involving face, arm and leg, associated with loss of sensation of all modalities on the paralysed side, suggests a lesion affecting the *internal capsule*, where the upper motor neurone and sensory pathways are packed closely together.

Brain stem. Lesions are characterised by ipsilateral impairment of one or more cranial nerves with concurrent contralateral dysfunction in one or more long tracts. The cranial nerve dysfunction will depend on the part of the brain stem affected. A midbrain lesion is suggested by a III nerve palsy; pontine damage by VI and VII nerve signs accompanied by contralateral upper motor neurone signs. Occasionally

Table 7.20 Signs attributable to lesions in different parts and paths of the nervous system

Upper motor neurone (pyramidal tract) lesions
Weakness or paralysis of movement
Increase in tone of 'clasp-knife' type
Increased amplitude of tendon reflexes
Diminution of abdominal reflexes
An extensor plantar response

Lower motor neurone lesions
Weakness or paralysis of muscles
Wasting of muscles
There may be fasciculation in the involved muscles
Reduction in tone
Diminution or loss of tendon reflexes

Cerebellar lesions
Ataxia of gait
Intention tremor of limbs
Jerking nystagmus
Dysarthria of staccato or scanning type
Dysmetria and past-pointing
Impaired alternating movements
Hypotonia and pendular tendon reflexes
Smooth movements may be broken up into their constituent parts, producing
  jerking, marionette-like movements

Generalised neuropathies
Diminution of superficial sensation affecting the distal
  aspect of limbs with 'stocking' and 'glove' distributions
Wasting and weakness of distal limb musculature
Early loss of tendon reflexes

Sensory tracts
Dorsal columns:
Ataxia of gait and limb movements aggravated by eye closure (positive
  Romberg's test)
Impaired position sense
Diminished appreciation of vibration

Lateral spinothalamic tracts:
Impairment of pain and temperature sensation

Muscles
Wasting and weakness, usually proximal
Reduction in reflexes when muscle wasting is marked

Cerebral cortex dysfunction
Dysphasia
Dyscalculia
Right and left disorientation
Astereognosis sensory inattention
Apraxia
Amnesia and cognitive disorders
Visual field homonynous defects
Hemiparesis, monoparesis

other tracts such as the spinothalamic or sympathetic pathways are interrupted. Examples of lesions involving the midbrain, pons and medulla are given in Figures 7.43 and 7.44 (see also Fig. 7.14).

Spinal cord. Damage is localised by correlating motor, sensory and reflex changes.

Upper motor neurone signs arising from cord lesions are often, but not always, bilateral. Their presence helps to locate the site of lesion only very roughly. If they are present in the arms the lesion must be above the fifth cervical segment; if the abdominal reflexes are pathologically absent, a segment above the eighth thoracic must be implicated. Pyramidal tract signs in the legs indicate a lesion above the conus medullaris.

The site of spinal damage is localised much more precisely if the lesion also involves the anterior horn cells or motor roots, thereby causing lower motor neurone signs, with weakness and wasting in a segmental distribution. Sensory signs may help to delineate the position of cord lesions. Impairment of sensation over a segmental dermatome will indicate the level of a lesion. Interruption of sensory tracts may give rise to an upper level of sensory loss which corresponds to the site of the spinal lesion but which is often at a more caudal level. Spinal cord lesions which disrupt reflex arcs with loss of tendon reflexes indicate the segments which have been damaged.

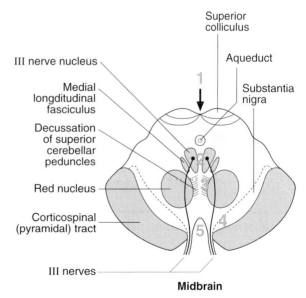

Fig. 7.43 Lesions of midbrain. Lesions at **1.**, e.g. pressure from a pineal tumour, cause weakness of upward gaze which may first be manifest as nystagmus in a vertical plane. Lesions at **2.** produce bilateral, partial lesions of the III nerve and anterior internuclear ophthalmoplegia (p. 214, damage to medial longitudinal fasciculus). Lesions at **3.** cause ipsilateral III nerve palsy and contralateral cerebellar signs (damage to decussating cerebellar peduncles) and/or tremors and athetoid movements (damage to red nucleus). Lesions at **4.** cause ipsilateral III nerve signs and contralateral pyramidal involvement. Lesions at **5.** cause bilateral pyramidal signs. Lesions which affect the midbrain immediately below this level also implicate the IV nerve.

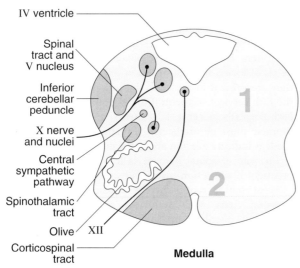

Fig. 7.44 Lesions of the medulla. Lesions affecting the lateral medulla **1.**, (e.g. thrombosis of the posterior inferior cerebellar artery), cause ataxia and intention tremor on the ipsilateral side; jerking nystagmus on turning the eyes to the side of the lesion (damage to the spinocerebellar tract in the inferior cerebellar peduncle); analgesia on the ipsilateral side of the face and contralateral limbs (affection of spinal tract of V nerve and the lateral spinothalamic tract); Horner's syndrome (involvement of the central sympathetic pathway); dysphonia, dysphagia and weakness of soft palate and paralysis of the vocal cords on the side of the lesion (damage to the X nerve). Lesions affecting the paramedian area **2.**, (e.g. infarction), cause a crossed paralysis – wasting and fasciculation of ipsilateral side of tongue (damage to XII nerve) and contralateral pyramidal signs.

Often the segmental level and the cross-sectional areas of a spinal cord lesion may be gauged (Fig. 7.45).

Below a hemisection of the cord on the ipsilateral side there will be found (1) upper motor neurone signs, (2) impaired joint position and vibration senses and sometimes (3) signs of vasomotor disturbance. On the contralateral side there will be reduced sensation to pain and temperature. This composite picture is called the *Brown–Séquard syndrome*.

Multiple lesions

Discrete lesions. An analysis of a patient's signs may show that they cannot be explained by a single lesion. Two or more discrete lesions may be required, as in multiple sclerosis, in which optic nerve and spinal dysfunction may be found concurrently.

Selective damage. Some neuropathological lesions afflict specific tracts in different parts of the nervous system. A polyneuropathy may be widespread, symmetrical or asymmetrical depending on aetiology. Involvement of motor or sensory fibres may predominate. Damage may be confined to upper and lower motor neurones, as in motor neurone disease, or to dorsal root ganglion cells, as in some forms of carcinomatous neuropathy. Spinal tracts may be selectively damaged, singly or in combination, as when dorsal and lateral columns are disrupted by vitamin B12 deficiency (subacute combined degeneration).

Diffuse damage. Diffuse damage may be demonstrated when disorders affect wide areas of grey and white matter and traverse structural and functional boundaries. Thus alcohol abuse may cause generalised cortical

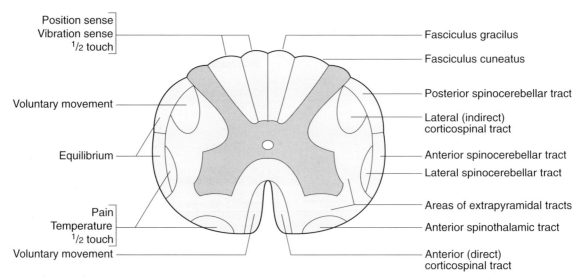

Fig. 7.45 Transverse section of the spinal cord.

neuronal loss, cerebellar degeneration, selective damage to the limbic circuitry and midbrain (as in Wernicke's encephalopathy) and peripheral neuropathy. All of these disturbances may not present concurrently, but combinations of several lesions are commonly found in the same patient. Repetitive head injuries may also cause randomised, diffuse cerebral atrophy resulting in the dementia of the 'punch-drunk' state.

PATHOLOGICAL DIAGNOSIS

Specific clues to aetiology may be contained in the history. The story of an antecedent head injury in an elderly patient with a progressive intracranial lesion may suggest a chronic subdural haematoma. A family history of epilepsy, muscle disease or ataxia may clarify the nature of a patient's illness.

The general medical examination may suggest that the neural lesion is due to a process which involves other systems. Evidence of peripheral vascular disease or a cardiac arrhythmia might imply that a cerebral lesion was vascular in nature. Anaemia and a smooth tongue could implicate vitamin B12 deficiency as the cause of a myelopathy. Features of hepatic cirrhosis may suggest an alcohol-related problem or Wilson's disease.

The nature and distribution of the neurological signs suggest some conditions and help to exclude others. Signs of focal brain dysfunction together with papilloedema suggest a space-occupying lesion, such as a tumour. Patients with multiple but transient neurological abnormalities, particularly drowsiness and nystagmus, may be suffering from alcohol intoxication or drug overdoseage.

With this approach, it is often possible to make a firm diagnosis on clinical grounds alone. On other occasions the probable causes should be considered and a rational scheme of investigation designed.

FURTHER INVESTIGATIONS

The general investigation of a patient with a neurological complaint is often important. Examples include assessing renal and hepatic function, checking for electrolyte abnormalities, testing for HIV status, checking for vitamin B_{12} deficiency and taking chest radiographs.

Some neurological investigations cause discomfort and may be hazardous. It is wise to start with those clinically appropriate investigations which are least disturbing and only proceed to invasive tests if these

become essential. Sometimes, however, the clinical urgency is such that the definitive investigation needs to be performed immediately.

Specific neurological investigations

The cerebrospinal fluid

The indications for lumbar puncture are limited. Examination of cerebrospinal fluid (CSF) is essential when acute or chronic infection of the brain or meninges is suspected. Lumbar puncture should usually be performed in patients in whom the diagnostic possibilities include multiple sclerosis, sarcoidosis, neurosyphilis and the Guillain–Barré syndrome. In suspected subarachnoid haemorrhage, computed tomography is the investigation of choice, but lumbar puncture may confirm the diagnosis if this is negative or unavailable.

A lumbar puncture should not be performed without preliminary brain imaging, such as CT scanning, if the patient is in coma or if there is suspicion of raised intracranial pressure, irrespective of whether or not papilloedema is present. The danger is of sudden death from 'coning' of the brain through either the tentorial hiatus or the foramen magnum. The CSF pressure can be measured by a simple manometer, and is usually 50–150 mm of CSF. The CSF is normally clear and colourless. It becomes turbid if it contains many cells. If blood-stained, the fluid should be collected in three successive tubes to distinguish between a traumatic puncture and a subarachnoid haemorrhage. In the former, the degree of blood staining becomes less; in the latter, it stays the same. Blood-stained fluid should be centrifuged to see whether the supernatant fluid has a yellow tinge (xanthochromia) which develops when blood has been present for at least 12 hours. The CSF may sometimes be yellowish in deeply jaundiced patients or when its protein content is much increased.

Laboratory examination of the CSF should include a cell count and an estimation of the protein and glucose content. In appropriate circumstances microbiological studies, bacterial or viral, and serological examination for syphilis and viral titres should be performed.

Cell count. Normal CSF contains fewer than five lymphocytes per mm^3. In bacterial meningitis the cell count may be markedly raised with a predominance of polymorphs. Lymphocytosis is found in tuberculous meningitis and viral meningitis, though in the initial stages of these conditions there may be an increase in polymorphs. A slight to moderate rise in the lymphocyte count may be found in viral encephalitis, active neurosyphilis, multiple sclerosis and sarcoidosis.

Protein. The total protein content in normal CSF lies between 0.2 and 0.5 g/l. A moderate elevation of protein may be found in many intracranial diseases and some systemic conditions, including hypothyroidism and diabetes. Very high protein contents are found in the Guillain-Barré syndrome and when compression of the spinal cord blocks the CSF flow.

Although the total protein is usually within normal limits, the IgG fraction is significantly raised in approximately two-thirds of patients with multiple sclerosis. Another feature of multiple sclerosis is the presence of oligoclonal bands in the gammaglobulin region. Similar bands may be seen in other disorders, e.g. neurosyphilis and systemic lupus erythematosus (SLE).

Glucose. The CSF glucose is normally between 2.2 and 4.5 mmol/l and is approximately 1.7 mmol/l below the blood level. A marked reduction in CSF glucose occurs in bacterial meningitis; in severe cases glucose may be absent. A moderate reduction may be found in tuberculous and carcinomatous meningitis and neurosarcoidosis.

Serology. Tests for syphilis are still performed routinely. They include the Venereal Disease Research Laboratories (VDRL) flocculation test. The *treponema pallidum* haemagglutination test (TPHA) and the fluorescent *treponema* antibody test (FTA) are more specific and more sensitive, but may remain positive for life even after effective treatment. An enzyme-linked immunosorbent assay (ELISA) for antitreponomal IgG is easier to perform but it is not more specific. A similar ELISA for antitreponomal IgM can be used to detect recent or active infection.

Anti-nuclear factor (ANF) and DNA-binding antibodies, may be positive in connective tissue disorders (e.g. SLE) involving the nervous system. Antibodies against phospholipids (e.g. cardiolipin) may be elevated in some younger patients with cerebral infarction. Serum antibodies directed against skeletal muscle acetylcholine receptors are present in more than 80% of patients with myasthenia gravis, and may be valuable in early stages of diagnosis.

Microbiological investigation. Whenever infection is suspected the CSF should be centrifuged and the sediment examined microscopically after Gram staining, and, if tuberculous meningitis is a possibility, after Ziehl–Neelsen staining. Occasionally fungi and cryptococci are found in the CSF, and the latter are best demonstrated by staining with Indian ink.

Cultures should be prepared from the CSF in cases of suspected infection and antibiotic sensitivities determined. If the initial examination is negative, but the clinical suspicion remains high, lumbar puncture should be repeated.

Certain viruses may be cultured from the CSF, but the diagnosis of viral infection usually depends on detecting rising antibody titres in serum or CSF. In some special circumstances (e.g. herpes simplex encephalitis) viral DNA can be detected by the polymerase chain reaction.

Miscellaneous tests. In certain situations, more specialised examinations of the CSF may be carried out. For example, in carcinomatous meningitis and cerebral lymphoma, examination of fresh CSF after cytocentrifugation may reveal malignant cells.

Intracranial disease

Numerous investigations are available. The choice is influenced by many factors including the nature and site of the neurological problem.

Skull radiography. A plain radiograph of the skull may be of value in identifying expanding tumours in the pituitary fossa, abnormal calcification, skull vault metastases fractures, or altered bone configuration, as in Paget's disease. It is not a useful screening test in patients with headache or seizures.

The electroencephalogram (EEG). This records the electrical potentials of the brain. Intracranial disease may cause normal electrical rhythms to be suppressed or, more commonly, there may be abnormal wave forms. Such abnormalities may be generalised or localised. Usually EEG abnormalities are more marked in acute cerebral hemisphere lesions. The EEG is less valuable in chronic lesions, extracerebral lesions (such as meningiomas) and in posterior fossa lesions. The EEG may be of diagnostic value in epilepsy. Generalised or localised paroxysmal spikes or sharp wave forms may be detected between fits and may be induced by hyperventilation, photic flicker stimulation, sleep or drugs. Twenty-four-hour ambulant EEG recordings from selected patients may prove helpful, but a normal EEG does not exclude the diagnosis of epilepsy. Examples of normal and abnormal EEG records are shown in Figure 7.46A and B.

Evoked potential recording. The development of signal averaging has permitted the measurement of small cerebral and spinal potential changes evoked by visual, auditory (AEP) and peripheral nerve stimuli (SSEP). Visually evoked potentials (VEPs) are the most useful. Stimulation is usually with a reversing chequerboard pattern projected on to a screen or displayed on a television set. The dominant response from a normal eye is a positive wave with a peak at about 100 ms (Fig. 7.47). Lesions of the retina, optic nerve, chiasma, tract, radiation or occipital cortex may all disrupt or

A   B

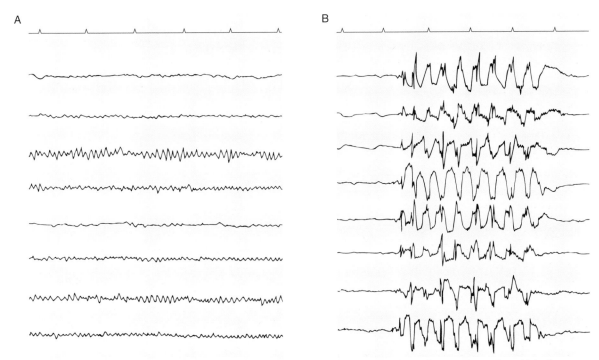

Fig. 7.46 EEG.   A. Portion of an eight-channel EEG record taken from a normal adolescent. Four channels running anterior to posterior over the parietal regions are displayed from each side. Top four traces − right side; lower four − left side. Uppermost trace is a 1-second time marker. Note the posteriorly dominant 10/s waves − the alpha rhythm. **B.** Abnormal EEG from a patient suffering generalised tonic–clonic seizures. This interictal record shows a paroxysm of generalised spike and slow-wave activity lasting about 3 seconds, during which the patient showed no clinical abnormality.

delay the response, but demyelinating lesions of the optic nerve often cause marked delay with relatively good preservation of the wave form. The test may be of diagnostic value in patients with possible multiple sclerosis with clinically normal vision.

Radionuclide cerebral scanning. An injected radioisotope

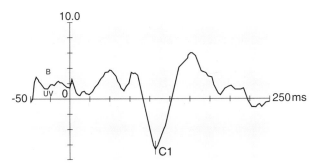

Fig. 7.47 Normal visual evoked responses elicited by reversing chequerboard pattern stimulus to the right eye. The trace shown is mid-occipital. One hundred individual responses are computer averaged to produce these traces. The major positive (downward) deflection occurs about 110 ms after the stimulus (marked C1) and is called the P100 response.

(such as technetium) is taken up differentially by diseased intracranial tissue. In its original form this technique is inferior to CT scanning; but tomographic modifications (see below: PET, SPET) have research uses for functional brain imaging.

Computed tomography (CT scan). This technique detects and displays the differing X-ray densities of cranial and brain structures. White and grey matter and the fluid-filled spaces can be visualised in tomographic 'slices' at various levels through the brain and spine (Fig. 7.48). The technique is atraumatic, takes a matter of minutes and involves very little radiation. Its sensitivity can be increased by the intravenous injection of a water-soluble contrast agent containing iodine. With 'contrast enhancement' CT scanning will reveal the vast majority of cerebral tumours, infarcts, haemorrhages, abscesses, arteriovenous malformations and also cerebral atrophy and hydrocephalus. However, small lesions, particularly those of low density, such as infarcts and some gliomas, may be missed. It is also of limited value for disease involving the craniocervical junction and posterior fossa structures. CT scanning cannot reliably distinguish between infarction and haemorrhage if performed 2 weeks after the acute event.

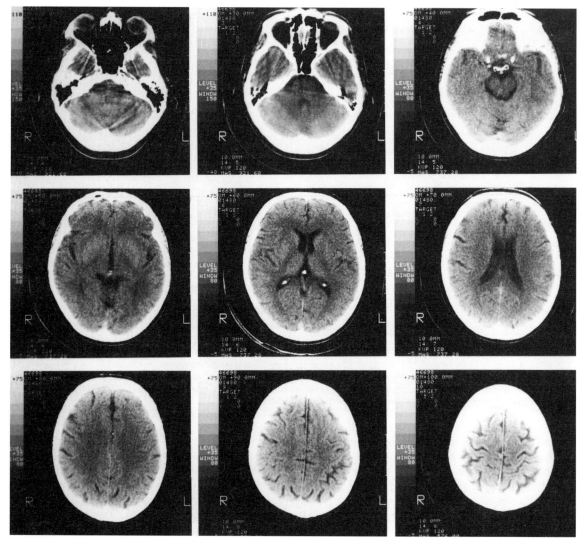

Fig. 7.48 Normal CT scan.

Magnetic resonance imaging (MRI). This utilises the magnetic properties of hydrogen nuclei. Since grey matter contains much more water (and hence hydrogen nuclei) than white matter, the technique vividly differentiates grey and white matter. MRI produces multiplanar images similar to those of conventional CT scanning (Fig. 7.49). It is a sensitive method of imaging which is of particular value in looking for:

- areas of demyelination
- lesions of the posterior fossa
- lesions of the foramen magnum and spinal cord (e.g. syringomyelia) (Figs 7.50 A and B)

Emission computed tomography. The two most common

emission computed axial tomographic techniques are single photon emission tomography (SPET) and position emission tomography (PET). Both involve recording the radiation emitted from the brain following the intravenous injection of radionuclides. They are sensitive but spatial resolution is low. Areas of altered brain function (e.g. epileptic foci or changes in cerebral blood flow, oxygen uptake, glucose metabolism, monoamine storage) can be detected in the absence of structural defects. PET requires a cyclotron, and its use is therefore restricted to major research centres. PET may be of valve in diagnosing Parkinson's disease.

Ultrasound scanning. Doppler ultrasound scanning can be used to image the cervical carotid arteries for the

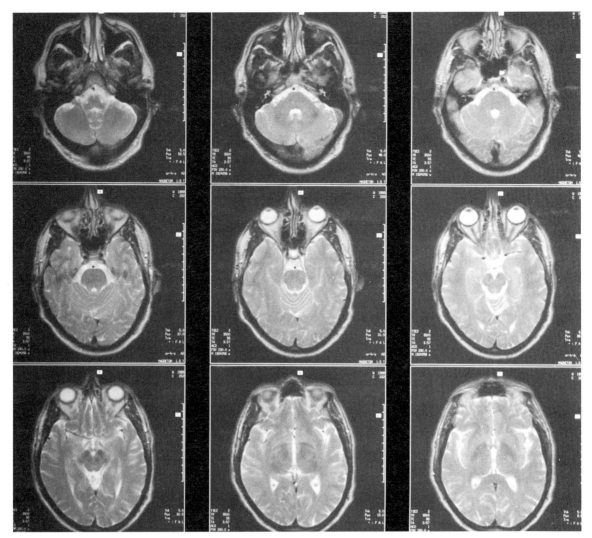

Fig. 7.49 Axial MRI scans of normal brain.

presence, and estimated severity, of atheroma sufficient to cause a stenotic lesion. This is a valuable
'screening' procedure in the investigation of patients
presenting with TIAs and minor strokes. Blood flow
velocity in intracranial vessels can now also be
measured transcranially.

In infants the fontanelle can be used as an acoustic
window to image some intracranial structures.
Neonatal cerebral haemorrhages and hydrocephalus
can be demonstrated.

Cerebral angiography. Angiography is the definitive
technique for defining a lesion of a cerebral blood
vessel such as an aneurysm or stenosis. It is also of
value in demonstrating the precise vascular anatomy of

a cerebral tumour when embolization is contemplated.
The investigation is uncomfortable and potentially
hazardous.

Digital subtraction angiography involves the injection
of either arterial or venous contrast. Venous injection
reduces the risks but often produces images of the
extracranial arteries that are of indifferent quality, with
less satisfactory views of intracranial vessels. Small
arterial injections produce much better image quality
with the technique. High-resolution magnetic resonance
angiography provides a non-invasive technique of
obtaining good images of the cerebral arteries and
venous circulations.

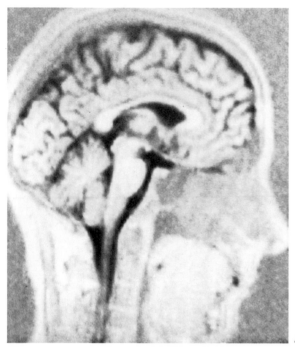
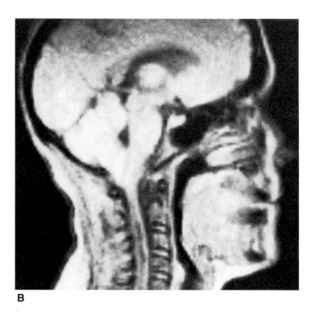

Fig. 7.50 Sagittal MRI scans: A showing medial aspect of cerebral hemisphere brain stem, cerebellum and cervical spinal cord. In **B** there is herniation of the cerebellar tonsils and a syrinx cavity in the cervical cord in a normal subject

Spinal cord

Myelography. Myelography, or radiculography, remains a widely used investigation of localised damage to the spinal cord or to outline abnormalities of the nerve roots. It requires the introduction of a radio-opaque dye into the subarachnoid space by lumbar puncture.

CT scanning. CT scanning also has a place in the imaging of the spine with or without the addition of contrast. It is especially useful in sorting out problems in patients who have had previous disc surgery in whom it may be important to distinguish between fibrosis and a recurrent disc lesion. Bony stenosis of the spinal canal can also be readily demonstrated.

MRI. MRI provides the ability to produce longitudinal (sagittal) as well as axial sections of the entire spinal cord and, when available, is the optimal method of studying the spinal cord, nerve rootlets and disc spaces.

Peripheral nerves

Electromyography. This is useful in the investigation of disorders of muscles and peripheral nerves. Needle electrode studies of muscles during voluntary contraction helps identify denervation and differentiates it from myopathic disorders. Many peripheral nerves can be stimulated electrically and conduction velocities in motor and sensory fibres measured separately. These studies help gauge the type and severity in polyneuropathies, and may define the site of localised nerve compression, as in the carpal tunnel syndrome.

Autonomic nervous system

Tests of the autonomic nervous system, dependent on measuring cardiovascular responses to standing, Valsalva manoeuvre, deep breathing and sustained hand grip, can be performed in selected patients. Abnormalities are seen particularly in polyneuropathy due to diabetes mellitus, alcoholism and amyloidosis.

The examination of the eye

This chapter describes the clinical examination of the eye except those aspects dealt with elsewhere.

THE HISTORY

An accurate history is essential. As vision is the most important sense in man, fear of blindness makes patients especially anxious about eye problems. This should be recalled when approaching the patient.

Symptoms fall into three main categories:

- abnormal appearance
- pain
- disturbance of vision.

Abnormal appearance

Abnormal appearance may be a presenting symptom, or may be noted as a sign during examination. It is important to establish whether the abnormality is congenital or acquired, its speed of onset and whether there are any associated features. Table 8.1 gives a few examples of conditions which may present with an abnormal appearance of the head or face and eyes.

Pain

The character of pain in eye disease falls into four main categories:

- foreign body sensation
- deep severe pain
- eye strain
- headache unrelated to the eye but with visual symptoms.

Foreign body sensation. This ranges from a feeling of mild discomfort and grittiness to severe burning with

Table 8.1 Abnormal appearance of head, face and eyes

Site	Appearance	Associated features	Cause
Head	Abnormal posture	Squint and diplopia on straightening head	Vertical muscle palsy
Face	Asymmetry Fullness of supraorbital ridge	Cranial nerve palsies	Sphenoidal ridge meningioma
Eyes	Proptosis	Lid lag Lid retraction	Dysthyroid eye disease
Lids	Xanthelasma	Corneal arcus	Hypercholesterolaemia

photophobia (light sensitivity) and discharge. It is characteristic of corneal epithelial damage. There may, for example, be a history of rheumatoid disease (Sjögren's dry eye syndrome), cold sores (herpes simplex corneal ulcers) or of using ultraviolet light (welder's flash burns).

Deep severe pain. Severe eye pain is distressing and often associated with nausea and vomiting. It is vaguely localised to the eye and brow. It is characteristic of intraocular inflammatory disease (uveitis, scleritis and endophthalmitis) and of high intraocular pressure (acute glaucoma). Similar pain occurs in herpes zoster ophthalmicus (shingles affecting the first division of the V nerve) and intracranial aneurysms pressing on the V nerve.

Eye strain. This symptom is generally vague. The eyes feel tired and aching, often with frontal headache. The most usual cause is tension headache or fatigue. Occasionally it is caused by uncorrected optical errors or problems with binocular vision and requires an optician's advice.

Headache. Pain in the head is often associated with visual symptoms. A migraine attack classically begins with the flashing or zig-zag lights of a visual aura but may also be associated with a hemianopia. Visual obscurations (temporary visual loss when bending) occur with headache in chronic raised intracranial pressure.

Disturbance of vision

When taking the history it is important to establish time sequences, associated features and whether the disturbance is unilateral or bilateral. Apparent sudden loss of vision may have only been noticed suddenly when the normal eye was covered. The main disturbances of vision are:

- blurred vision
- loss of vision
- double vision
- photopsia and haloes
- floaters.

Blurred vision. Blurring is usually due to an ocular problem. When the media (cornea, lens, aqueous or vitreous) are hazy, vision blurs and there is often dazzle in bright light. Cataracts cause such symptoms. The blur caused by refractive errors is cured by spectacles.

Loss of vision. Sudden visual loss suggests a vascular aetiology. The nature of the loss may help localise the lesion. Loss of vision in one eye indicates that the problem is anterior to the chiasm; hemianopic field defects in both eyes that it is post chiasmal. Patients often state that they cannot see out of the right eye when they cannot see the right side of the visual field (right hemianopia), and likewise those with a left hemianopia may equate this with loss of vision in the left eye. Scotomas or blind spots are often observed accurately by the patient, who will describe the defect in the field of vision.

Double vision. Patients may describe double vision when they mean blurred vision. True double vision becomes single when one eye is covered. Sudden onset of double vision usually indicates a neurological problem.

Photopsia and haloes. Seeing flashes and zig-zags of light is called photopsia. It occurs when the retina is stimulated by the vitreous tugging on it. Very similar sensations are noted in both eyes in migraine. Haloes are due to prismatic effects, usually water drops in the cornea or lens in corneal oedema or cataract.

Floaters. Seeing occasional small 'floaters' is physiological, but patients may be alarmed when they are first noticed. A sudden rush of many floaters or large black 'tadpoles' suggest a vitreous haemorrhage.

KEY POINTS

- Migraine is commonly associated with visual symptoms, including hemianopia.
- Sudden loss of vision is usually vascular; sudden onset of diplopia is frequently neurological in origin.
- Patients may mistake hemianopia for loss of vision in one eye.

THE EXAMINATION

Eye examination can be divided into five main parts:

- inspection
- pupil reactions
- ocular movements
- ophthalmoscopy
- visual function tests.

INSPECTION

Eyelids

The lids normally cover the upper and lower margins of the iris. The palpebral fissures should be symmetri-

cal. The palpebral aperture is narrowed in blepharospasm (spasm of the eyelids) and photophobia (light sensitivity), which are often associated with painful eye conditions. Photophobia also occurs in migraine and is associated with meningeal irritation.

Ptosis (upper lid drooping) can be due to congenital or acquired levator palpebrae paresis (third nerve palsy), or to sympathetic paresis (Horner's syndrome, Fig. 3.16A p. 59).

Lid retraction, with widening of the palpable aperture, is obvious when sclera is visible above and below the iris (Fig. 8.1). It occurs in hyperthyroidism, usually with a lag of the upper lid on looking down (lid-lag) and when the eye is pushed forward (proptosed) by retrobulbar tumours, inflammation or in dysthyroid eye disease. Bilateral proptosis is also called exophthalmos. The periorbital tissues are loose and the lids swell easily. Periorbital oedema occurs commonly in congestive heart failure, glomerulonephritis, hypersensitivity reactions and thyroid disease. There may be associated conjunctival oedema (chemosis).

The lids may turn in (*entropion*) (Fig. 8.2), causing corneal damage, or out (*ectropion*), causing watering. Both malpositions occur in the lax tissues of the elderly but can also result from conjunctival or skin scarring respectively.

Common lumps on the lids include styes (microabscesses of lash follicles), tarsal cysts (pea-like swellings of the tarsal glands) and rodent ulcers (basal cell carcinoma).

Conjunctiva

Conjunctival inflammation (conjunctivitis) is common and causes a red eye with the injection maximal towards the fornix (the fold between globe and lid). It

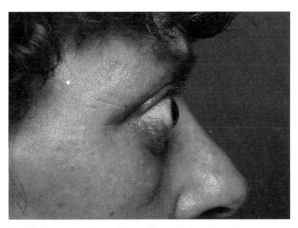

Fig. 8.1 Proptosis and lower lid retraction in dysthyroid eye disease.

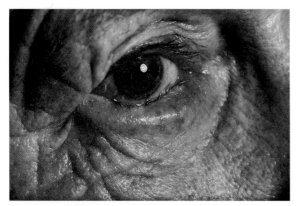

Fig. 8.2 Senile entropion of the lower lid.

is often accompanied by photophobia and excessive lacrimation. Infective causes are associated with a sticky yellow discharge which glues the lashes together. Lymph follicles may be seen as sago-like lumps on the tarsal conjunctiva and are particularly characteristic of acute trachomatous conjunctivitis. Allergic inflammation is characterised by itch, a white discharge and conjunctival oedema (*chemosis*). Other causes of chemosis include alcoholism, chronic respiratory failure and superior vena cava obstruction (p. 41).

Subconjunctival haemorrhage (Fig. 8.3) causes an alarming bright-red splash of blood which usually occurs spontaneously but may appear in whooping cough or labour or as a result of local trauma or bleeding disorders. *Pingueculae* are triangular yellow deposits beneath the conjunctiva between the canthus and the edge of the cornea. They develop with advancing years and are of no clinical significance. *Pterygium* is a patch of progressive fibrosis in the same area which may encroach upon the cornea, particularly in tropical countries. Foreign bodies stuck under the upper lid

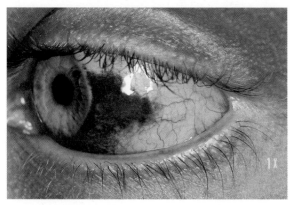

Fig. 8.3 Subconjunctival haemorrhage.

cause severe irritation and photophobia. They are easily removed on everting the lid.

Sclera

Normal sclera is white, often with small brown spots of pigmentation marking perforating blood vessels in the elderly. The sclera are yellow in jaundice (Fig. 3.2A p. 42–3). In osteogenesis imperfecta and severe iron deficiency anaemia the sclera are thin and appear blue (Fig. 3.1A p. 40). Inflammation (scleritis) causes a dusky red colour, severe eye pain and tenderness. It is often a feature of connective tissue disease. The condition scleromalacia may also be found in rheumatoid arthritis and may rarely progress to perforation (scleromalacia perforans).

Cornea

Normal cornea is transparent with blood vessels only at the limbus, the junction between cornea and conjunctiva. General loss of transparency and lustre occurs in corneal oedema and extensive epithelial damage. Acute glaucoma characteristically causes corneal oedema. Extensive damage to the corneal epithelium occurs in advanced exophthalmos, chemical corneal injuries, vitamin A deficiency and severe dry eye syndrome, which may be associated with connective tissue disease (Sjögren's syndrome), or occur as part of the sicca syndrome.

More localised corneal haze is often caused by trauma with foreign bodies or ulcers due to infection, the herpes simplex virus being a common cause. Damage to the epithelium may be difficult to see but can be detected by instilling yellow fluoroscein drops, which stain the affected area.

The blood vessels around the limbus dilate in response to corneal disease or injury (an appearance known as ciliary flush). They may also invade the cornea when they are visible as a little leash growing from the limbus with surrounding haze.

Corneal arcus (Fig. 3.1A p. 40) is a white ring near the outer margin of the cornea. In elderly subjects it is common and of no significance. In younger patients it may indicate hypercholesterolaemia.

A *Kayser–Fleischer ring* is a yellow or brown deposit of copper at the periphery of the cornea found in Wilson's disease (hepatolenticular degeneration). *Corneal calcification* at the medial and lateral aspects of the corneo-scleral junction is a useful sign suggesting long-standing hypercalcaemia.

Loss of corneal sensation is associated with V nerve lesions (p. 214–7). An insensitive cornea (Fig. 8.4) is

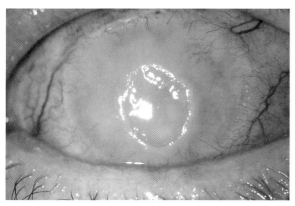

Fig. 8.4 Loss of transparency, ulceration and vascularisation in an insensitive cornea.

very vulnerable to trauma and infection and may need to be protected with a shield or by a tarsorrhaphy (artificial closure of the lids).

Iris

Heterochromia (different colours of the irides) may indicate intraocular disease. In inflammation (*iritis*) the iris looks muddy with a small pupil and there is ciliary flush. Iritis may be a manifestation of systemic disease.

Lens

The normal lens is not visible on inspection. Advanced cataracts can be seen as a milky whiteness in the pupil.

Intraocular pressure

This is low in dehydration and high in glaucoma.

Examination

❏ Stand back a little to overview the head, face and eyes, inspecting them from the front, side and above.
❏ Note abnormal head postures, asymmetry, prominent or squinting eyes, bony abnormalities – anything which looks out of the ordinary.
❏ Inspect the eyes closely using a pen torch.
❏ Evert both lids to examine the palpebral conjunctiva and the fornix.
❏ Pull down the lower lid while the patient looks up.
❏ To evert the upper lid ask the patient to look down, grasp the lashes, press gently on the upper border of the tarsal plate with a cotton tip and swing the lashes up (Fig. 8.5).
❏ Make a rough estimation of intraocular pressure by fluctuating the eye gently with the index finger (Fig. 8.6). Accurate measurements are made with a tonometer.
❏ Use slit lamp microscopy for detailed inspection of the eye.

PUPIL REACTIONS

Normal pupils are round, regular and nearly equal in size. They are miotic (constricted) in infancy, old age, bright light, sleep and convergence. They are mydriatic

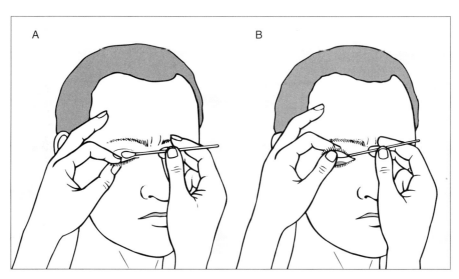

Fig. 8.5 Everting the upper lid.

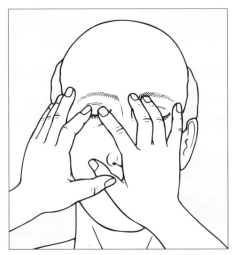

Fig. 8.6 Testing intraocular tension.

(dilated) in excitement and in the dark. When light is directed at one pupil, it constricts (direct light reflex), as does the other pupil (consensual light reflex). When the eyes converge both pupils constrict (accommodative reflex). Normal pupils are often described as PERLA in case notes (pupils equal and reactive to light and accommodation). Table 8.2 lists some

Table 8.2 Pupil abnormalities

Cause	Appearance	Reaction
Retinal/optic nerve disease	Abnormal > normal side	'Afferent pupil defect' Poor direct light reaction Normal consensual reaction and accommodation on affected side. Consensual reaction on normal side reduced
Neurosyphilis producing a pretectal lesion	Small, irregular, unequal	'Argyll Robertson' No reaction to light Normal reaction to accommodation
III nerve palsy Parasympathetic blocking drops	Abnormal > normal side	'Efferent pupil defect' No reaction to light or accommodation Other pupil reacts consensually
Ciliary ganglion lesion	Abnormal > normal side	'Holmes–Adie' No reaction to light. Slow sustained reaction to accommodation
Sympathetic lesion	Abnormal < normal side	'Horner's' Reacts to light/accommodation Does not dilate with cocaine drops
Inflammation of iris	Abnormal < normal side Festooned	No reaction to light/accommodation Other pupil reacts consensually
Iris ischaemia in acute glaucoma	Abnormal > normal side	No reaction to light/accommodation Other pupil may not react consensually

examples of pupil abnormalities. A detailed description of the pupillary reflexes and their examination is given in Chapter 7.

OCULAR MOVEMENTS

The eyes are normally parallel in all positions of gaze except convergence. When they are not, a squint is present. Squints may be associated with paresis of one of the extraocular muscles (paralytic or inconcomitant squint) or with defective binocular vision (non-paralytic or concomitant squints).

Acquired paralytic squints cause diplopia, the images being maximally separated and squint greatest in the direction of action of the paretic muscle. Congenital and long-standing paralytic squints often result in abnormal head postures with the head turned or tilted to minimise the diplopia.

Concomitant squints are the same in all positions of gaze. They usually become manifest in childhood (Fig. 8.7) when they are not associated with diplopia, as this symptom is suppressed centrally in young children. Central suppression causes amblyopia (lazy eye).

Eye movements should be examined by:

- Testing movements in all positions of gaze (p. 212–4). Both eyes should move symmetrically with no diplopia. If diplopia is present, the most peripheral double image is the one from the paretic eye (Fig. 8.8).
- The cover test. The cover/uncover test is particularly helpful in detecting small concomitant squints in children.

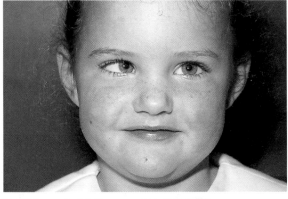

Fig. 8.7 Concomitant right convergent squint in a child.

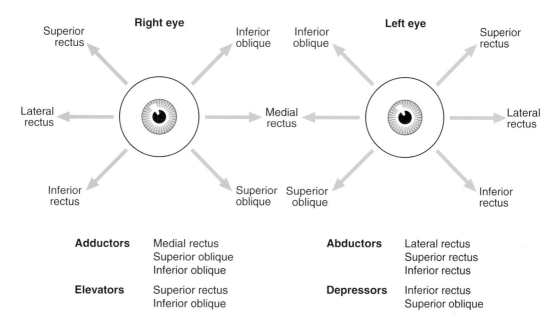

Adductors	Medial rectus	**Abductors**	Lateral rectus
	Superior oblique		Superior rectus
	Inferior oblique		Inferior rectus
Elevators	Superior rectus	**Depressors**	Inferior rectus
	Inferior oblique		Superior oblique

Fig. 8.8 Actions of extra-ocular muscles.   This diagram will help to work out which eye muscle is paretic. For example, a patient whose diplopia is maximum on looking down and to the right has either a weak right inferior rectus or a weak left superior oblique. Cover one of the patient's eyes and ask which image disappears – the most peripheral image comes from the affected eye.

Examination

❏ Ask the patient to look into the distance (using an interesting toy for a child).
❏ Cover one eye.
❏ Closely observe the uncovered eye for any movements. If it moves to take up fixation, that eye was squinting.
❏ Repeat the sequence for the other eye.

OPHTHALMOSCOPY

Ophthalmoscopy can be used to:

• detect opacities in the media
• estimate optical errors
• examine the fundus.

Technique

The direct ophthalmoscope is the most commonly used instrument. It provides a 15 × magnified upright image of the retina. A beam of light from the instrument is deflected by a mirror into the patient's eye, illuminating the retina, which the examiner observes through a hole in the mirror. Lenses can be rotated into place to compensate for short sight (myopia) (Fig. 8.9) or long sight (hypermetropia) (Fig. 8.10) in examiner and/or patient.

Learning to use the ophthalmoscope successfully takes a lot of practice. Rough handling, prolonged dazzling, poking the eye with the ophthalmoscope and garlicky breath do not help patient cooperation! The key points are summarised in Table 8.3 and the techniques illustrated in Figures 8.11 and 8.12.

Ophthalmoscopy is much easier through a dilated pupil. Dilation is essential in infants and children and for accurate examination of the periphery and macula and is advised when screening for diabetic retinopathy. The pupils should not be dilated when intracranial pathology requires pupillary monitoring. There is a very small risk of precipitating angle closure glaucoma by dilating eyes with shallow anterior chambers. Patients should be warned that after dilation vision will be slightly blurred and easily dazzled, that driving and reading may be affected and that medical advice is required should prolonged blur, haloes or eye pain occur. Tropicamide 0.5% drops are recommended as they work in 20 minutes and wear off in 8 hours. Do not constrict the pupil with pilocarpine drops after the

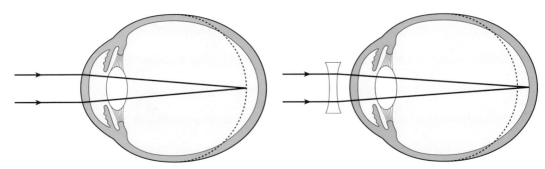

Fig. 8.9 The myopic (short-sighted) eye. **A.** The eye is too long and the retina is not in focus when no lens is used. **B.** The use of a concave (minus) lens brings the retina into focus.

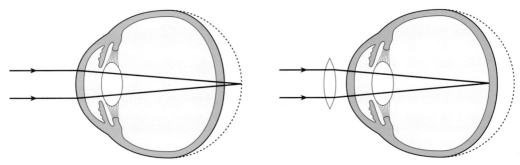

Fig. 8.10 The hypermetropic (long-sighted) eye. **A.** The eye is too short and the retina is not in focus when no lens is used. **B.** The use of a convex (plus) lens brings the retina into focus.

examination; they cause eyeache, blurring and do not protect against glaucoma. Remember to record pupil reactions before instilling drops and to note the drops used.

Examination

☐ Use a dark room and new ophthalmoscope batteries.

☐ Ask the patient to look at a distant object and blink and breathe normally.

☐ Stand or sit on the side to be examined an arm's length from the patient and with eyes level with the patient's.

☐ To look at the right eye, hold the ophthalmoscope with the lenses at zero in the right hand.

Table 8.3 Key points for successful ophthalmoscopy

- Dark room
- Bright ophthalmoscope light
- Correct position of patient
- Correct position of examiner
- Use correct eye and hand
- Dilating drops if possible
- Practice

☐ Use the right eye to examine the patient's right eye (and use the left eye while examining the patient's left eye).

☐ If the examiner has difficulty using the non-dominant eye, examine the patient from above to permit the patient to continue to fix on a distant object (Fig. 8.11B).

☐ Switch on the instrument and shine it at the pupil, angling it slightly towards the nose.

☐ If the eye closes, open it gently.

☐ Demonstrate the red reflex and note the nature of any opacities in the media, which will be outlined black against the glow.

☐ Keeping the beam pointing in the same slightly nasal direction and the red reflex in view, move close to the patient, stopping just clear of the lashes.

☐ Steady the instrument by resting the middle and ring fingers of the right hand against the patient's cheek.

☐ The optic nerve (disc) should now be in view because of the angle of approach. If, instead of the disc, retinal blood vessels are seen, the 'arrow' made at bifurcations points to the disc.

☐ If the image is out of focus, use the index finger of the right hand to rotate the lens wheel until the view is clear.

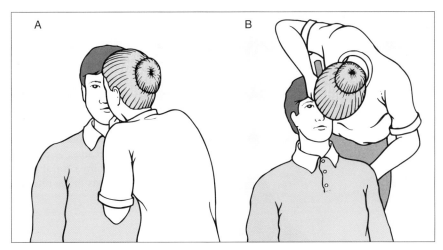

Fig. 8.11 Ophthalmoscopy: correct methods. **A.** The patient's gaze can be fixed on a distant point. **B.** Using the right (dominant) eye to inspect the patient's left eye from above by an examiner who has difficulty in using the left eye. The patient's gaze is not obstructed.

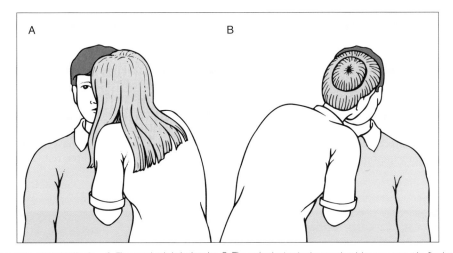

Fig. 8.12 Ophthalmoscopy: wrong methods. **A.** The examiner's hair obtrudes. **B.** The patient's view is obstructed and the gaze cannot be fixed on a distant point.

❏ Examine the fundus systematically.
❏ Note any abnormality as though the fundus were a clock with the disc at the centre. The disc diameter (1.5 mm) is used as the unit of measurement, e.g. 'haemorrhage at 6 o'clock two disc diameters from disc'.
❏ Examine the macula last; it is difficult to see through an undilated pupil. Use a narrow beam and ask the patient to look straight at the light.

Opacities in the media

The ocular media (cornea, aqueous lens and vitreous) are normally clear. Any opacities are noted when observing the red reflex. Dense opacities completely obscure the reflex – an example is advanced cataract. The depth of the opacity can be determined by moving the ophthalmoscope. Corneal opacities move in the opposite direction, lens opacities stay still and vitreous opacities move in the same direction.

Refractive errors

Providing the examiner does not have an uncorrected refractive error, the lenses required to focus on the patient's retina give an indication of any optical abnormality.

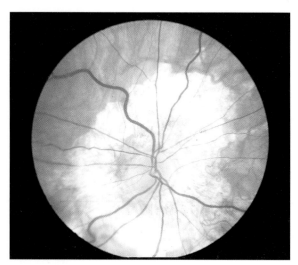

Fig. 8.13 Highly myopic disc.

Myopia. Minus (concave) lenses are required. In high myopia it may not be possible to focus on the retina unless patients wear their glasses. The optic disc often looks abnormal in high myopia, appearing very large and pale with surrounding chorioretinal atrophy (Fig. 8.13).

Hypermetropia. Plus (convex) lenses are required. The discs may look pink and slightly swollen (pseudopapill-oedema).

Astigmatism. When severe, the refractive error cannot be fully corrected with the ophthalmoscope. The disc may look distorted.

The normal fundus

Retina

The colour of the retina varies considerably according to skin pigmentation, from reddish black in those with black skin to pale pink in albinos (Fig. 8.14). Retinal pigment is often clumped, giving a tigroid appearance. Large choroidal vessels are visible if pigment is very sparse. The normal macula lies temporal to the disc within the vascular arcades, is darker than the rest of the retina and has a shiny central (foveal) reflex. There are normally no deposits in the retina.

Optic disc

The optic disc is pink with slight temporal pallor. The margin is well demarcated except nasally. Quite commonly there is a surrounding pigment rim or partial white crescent of exposed sclera. The optic cup is paler than the rest of the disc and varies in depth and size but the diameter should not exceed more than 50% of the disc.

Blood vessels. The bifurcation of the central artery and vein are visible at the disc. Physiological pulsation of the vein may be present; arterial pulsation is abnormal. The upper and lower branches of the artery divide into nasal and temporal arterioles (lacking internal elastic lamina) with corresponding venous tributaries. The arterioles have a smaller calibre than the veins and are a brighter red. Healthy vessel walls are invisible.

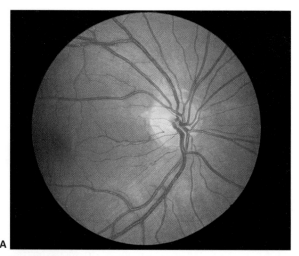

A

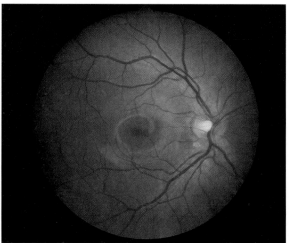

B

Fig. 8.14 Normal fundus.   A. Caucasian; **B.** Asian.

The abnormal fundus

Retinal atrophy

Old injuries and inflammation result in atrophic scars. The white sclera is exposed and there is often surrounding hyperpigmentation. White patches of atrophic retina also occur in congenital coloboma, high myopia and retinal degeneration.

Abnormal pigmentation

The commonest pigmentary abnormality is that associated with age-related macular degeneration in which retinal pigment epithelial changes cause hypopigmentation and pigment clumping at the macula. Central vision is poor.

Benign choroidal melanomas are flat dark lesions (Fig. 8.15). Malignant melanomas are raised, enlarge progressively and often metastasise.

Retinitis pigmentosa is associated with pigment deposits shaped like bone spicules.

Abnormal deposits

Hard exudates. These are well-defined, yellowish-white deposits in the retina, often arranged in rings. They are caused by lipoproteins leaking out of an abnormally permeable blood vessel, which may be visible in the centre of the ring. At the macula they tend to accumulate in a star shape because of the unique horizontal arrangement of the deep retinal layers around the fovea (Fig. 8.16). They are

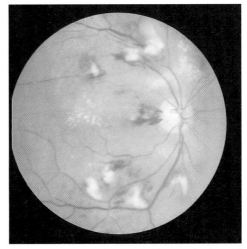

Fig. 8.16 Retinal soft exudates, flame haemorrhages and early macular star of hard exudate in hypertensive diabetic patient.

commonly seen in hypertension, diabetes and following retinal vascular occlusions.

Soft exudates. These look like deposits of cotton wool in the superficial retina. They occur around areas of infarcted retina and may be associated with other features of retinal ischaemia (venous dilation, haemorrhages and new blood vessels). They are due to swelling of the nerve fibre layer axons (Fig. 8.16).

Colloid bodies. These may be mistaken for hard exudates. They are small, round yellow deposits in the deepest retinal layer appearing most commonly in the elderly and around the macula (Fig. 8.17). Other abnormal deposits include foci of active chorioretinal

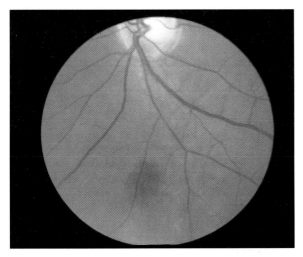

Fig. 8.15 Benign melanoma at 6 o'clock two disc diameters from the disc.

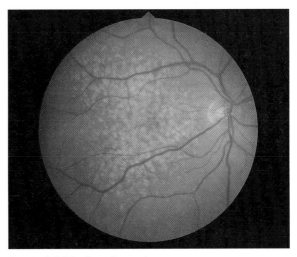

Fig. 8.17 Colloid bodies at the macula.

inflammation, metastatic infections (miliary tuberculosis) and carcinomas.

Congenital abnormalities of the optic nerve

Examples include myelinated nerve fibres and persistent hyaloid artery remnants. The appearance in refractive errors has already been mentioned.

Glaucoma

A larger and deeper than normal cup suggests glaucoma (Fig. 8.18). Such a finding is an indication for measuring intraocular pressure by tonometry.

Optic atrophy

An atrophic optic disc is pale. Subtle changes are hard to interpret – it is helpful to compare the two discs, as marked asymmetry in colour is significant. The terms primary, secondary and consecutive optic atrophy are confusing and are best avoided. Optic atrophy is usually associated with decreased vision and afferent pupillary defects. It is not a diagnosis but a sign. Causes include extensive retinal destruction, glaucoma (Fig. 8.18), toxins and cerebral tumours.

Papilloedema

Swelling of the disc is called papilloedema. The swollen disc is pink with congested veins and surrounding small haemorrhages, the margins are blurred and the cup is lost (Fig. 8.19). It can be due to inflammation of the optic nerve head (papillitis) or to increased intracranial pressure or cerebral oedema. In papillitis there is associated marked visual loss, an afferent pupil defect and the papilloedema is most likely to be

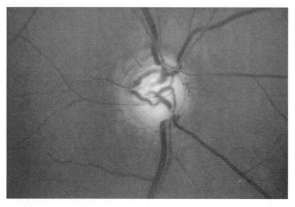

Fig. 8.18 Optic disc atrophy and cupping in glaucoma.

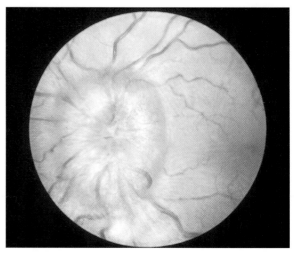

Fig. 8.19 Papilloedema.

unilateral. In increased intracranial pressure the vision is normal at first, papilloedema is most likely to be bilateral and there are other characteristic features such as headache and vomiting. In accelerated hypertension cerebral oedema and papilloedema are features.

Retinal vascular abnormalities

Haemorrhages. Superficial retinal haemorrhages are flame shaped because of tracking of blood along the horizontally arranged nerve fibres. They occur in hypertension (Fig. 8.16).

Deep haemorrhages are dark-red blots contained by the vertically arranged deep retinal layers. Microaneurysms look very similar. Both occur in the dots and blots of background diabetic retinopathy (Fig. 8.22).

Preretinal haemorrhages obscure the underlying retina. Initially round, they form a flat-topped fluid level and may burst into the vitreous (Fig. 8.20). They may occur following subarachnoid haemorrhage or follow bleeding from retinal new vessels.

In *vitreous haemorrhage* the fundus view is hazy or absent and the red reflex abnormal. The blood may be distributed diffusely through the vitreous gel or form clots which cause tadpole-like floaters.

Choroidal haemorrhages are very dark red and often large with wavy margins. They occur in trauma and age-related choroidal vascular disease.

Retinal artery occlusion. Obstruction of the central retinal artery results in sudden, and often total, loss of vision. The retina is pale and swollen and the macula stands out a bright cherry red. In branch artery occlusion the affected arteriole is attenuated and the

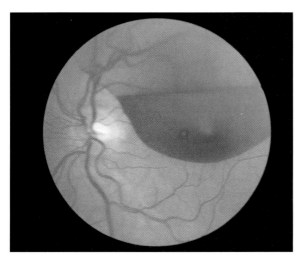

Fig. 8.20 Pre-retinal haemorrhage.

corresponding retinal segment pale. Emboli may be visible in the arterioles as shiny (cholesterol) or white (platelet) plaques. They cause transient loss of vision (amaurosis fugax) as well as arterial occlusions.

Retinal vein occlusion. In central vein occlusion a little vision is retained. The ophthalmoscopic picture is a dramatic 'stormy sunset' with large flame haemorrhages and cotton wool spots splashed over the fundus (Fig. 8.21). In branch vein occlusion the same picture is confined to the affected segment and marked nipping often marks the site of the occluded vein.

Ischaemic optic neuropathy. Occlusion of the blood supply to the optic nerve head results in pale papilloedema. There is irreversible loss of sight. Giant cell arteritis is a common cause of ischaemic optic neuropathy.

Hypertension. Chronic hypertension leads to diffuse or segmental narrowing of the arteriolar blood column as the vessel walls thicken. In extreme sclerosis the sheathing of the vessel walls is visible. The thick-walled arterioles compress the veins at crossings, causing venous nipping. Flame haemorrhages, hard exudates and papilloedema are features of accelerated hypertension. Hypertension seldom affects vision.

Diabetic retinopathy. Microangiopathy affects the retinal capillaries in diabetes, leading to widespread capillary non-perfusion. Early (background) disease is characterised by dot and blot haemorrhages and microaneurysms; as capillary non-perfusion increases, signs of retinal ischaemia appear. These are cotton wool spots, venous dilation and intraretinal new vessels. Neovascularisation sprouting from the optic nerve and surface of the retina characterises proliferative retinopathy (Fig. 8.22). Blindness often follows.

VISUAL FUNCTION TESTS

Visual acuity

Visual acuity (VA) is measured by testing the ability of the retinal cones to distinguish test objects, most commonly letters. It should be assessed at the beginning of an eye examination for several reasons. Firstly, it ensures that the test is not forgotten, a common omission of potential medicolegal significance. Moreover, as patients occasionally attribute visual loss to the

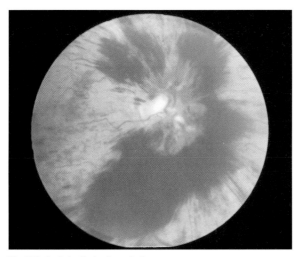

Fig. 8.21 Central retinal vein occlusion.

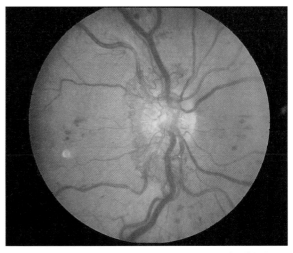

Fig. 8.22 Dots, blots and optic disc new vessels in proliferative diabetic retinopathy.

eye examination itself, it is best to measure and record it at the start. The bright light of the ophthalmoscope may dazzle the patient if it is used before testing vision.

Distance visual acuity should be measured using distance spectacles if worn, with a Snellen chart at 6 metres (Fig. 8.23). Distance VA is recorded as two numbers written one over the other. The first is the distance separating the test letter from the patient, generally 6 metres. The second records the smallest line of letters read. Each line is marked with a number – 60, 36, 24, 18, 12, 9 and 6. This represents the distance in metres at which a normally sighted person could read that line. Normal VA is 6/6, subnormal 6/9, etc. Vision of 6/12 is needed for driving and VA of less than 3/60 is legal blindness.

Examination

- ❏ Test each eye separately ensuring the other is totally occluded.
- ❏ If possible, use a line rather than single letters and use different letters for each eye as patients, especially children, memorise quickly.
- ❏ If the vision is abnormal, check it again using a pinhole which partially corrects optic errors, though children and the elderly often find this difficult to use.
- ❏ If VA is less than 6/60 repeat the test with the chart 3 metres away as 3/60, etc.
- ❏ If the vision is less than 3/60, ask the patient to count fingers held 1 metre from the face, to detect a moving hand or perceive light.
- ❏ Measure near vision in each eye using reading glasses and standard reading charts.
- ❏ If no charts are available, use a newspaper and record the smallest print seen.

Other methods of testing VA are available for children and people who cannot read.

Colour vision

Tests of colour vision assess the function of the retinal cones and optic nerve. Colour vision tends to fail early in a number of conditions. Abnormalities are found in:

- congenital red/green colour blindness, which is carried on the X chromosome and affects 7% of males
- age-related macular disease
- optic neuritis.

Ishihara plates are the most commonly used test. They consist of a series of plates in which coloured spots contain numerical shapes which the patient is asked to pick out. Errors are made when colour vision is defective.

Visual fields

Testing fields assesses the function of the peripheral and central retina, the optic pathways and the cortex. The normal field extends 160° horizontally and 130° vertically with a blind spot 15° from fixation in the temporal field.

Defects in fields are described as central or peripheral. A scotoma is a field defect surrounded by a seeing area. Lesions anterior to the chiasm cause binocular field defects only if both eyes or optic nerves are affected.

Central scotomas involve fixation and are characteristic of disease affecting the macula and the axons leading from it.

Centrocaecal scotomas lie between fixation and the physiological blind spot and occur in toxic optic neuro-

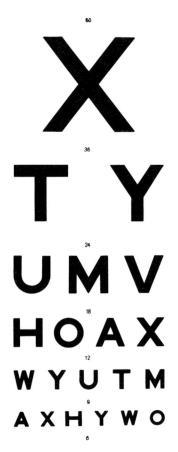

Fig. 8.23 Snellen test.

pathy. *Ring scotomas* forming a circular defect around fixation are typical of retinitis pigmentosa; *arcuate scotomas* of glaucoma. Both may progress to 'tunnel vision' with extensive loss of visual field almost to fixation.

Altitudinal hemianopia is loss of the upper or lower field in one eye, common in vascular disease of the optic nerve.

Posterior to the chiasm, lesions result in binocular field defects and are discussed in Chapter 7.

Examination of visual fields can be carried out at the bedside by confrontation (Fig. 7.5). The technique is described on page 210. An accurate and permanent record of visual fields can be made using a perimeter. Patients unable to cooperate with confrontation testing are not suitable for perimetry.

EXAMINATION OF INJURED EYES

It may be very difficult to inspect a painful or injured eye without an anaesthetic. Avoid forcing open an injured eye as pressure on an eye with an open wound may cause further damage. Local anaesthetic drops may relieve pain enough to allow the eye to open itself. In small children an examination under a general anaesthetic may be required.

EXAMINATION CHECKLIST

A normal eye examination can be carried out quickly using simple equipment and should conclude that:

- External inspection is normal.
- Vision in each eye is normal.
- Confrontation visual fields are full.
- Ocular movements are normal.
- Pupil reactions are normal.
- Optic discs are flat and of normal colour.
- Retinal vessels are normal.

KEY POINTS

- An insensitive cornea requires protection; it is very vulnerable to infection or trauma.
- Corneal damage is best detected by applying fluoroscein drops.
- Acquired paralytic squints cause diplopia.
- The cover/uncover test is valuable in detecting small concomitant squints.
- Ophthalmoscopy is easier to perform through a dilated pupil. This is particularly important when examining the periphery and the macula (as in diabetic retinopathy) and in infants and children.
- The pupils should not be dilated if pupillary reflexes require monitoring because of intracranial pathology.
- Retinal haemorrhages are flame shaped if superficial, blot shaped when deep.

REFERENCES

Elkington A, Khaw P 1988 ABC of eyes. British Medical Journal
Kanski J 1990 The eye in systemic disease. Butterworths, London

Trevor-Roper P 1986 Lecture notes on ophthalmology. Blackwell Scientific Publications, Oxford

P. J. Abernethy • N. Hurst

9

The locomotor system

THE HISTORY

General features of rheumatic disorders

The principal clinical features of rheumatic disease are joint pain, stiffness and swelling, bone pain and muscle weakness. Many rheumatic diseases are easily recognised by the anatomical pattern of involvement of joints and other connective tissues. Recognition of these patterns, when combined with observation of 'extra-articular' or systemic features, forms the basis for formulating a differential diagnosis. Other important diagnostic clues are obtained from the family history and social history, including the patient's occupation and personal habits. Since rheumatic symptoms are frequently the presenting complaint of many systemic disorders, a careful general medical history must also be taken (Table 9.1).

Patterns of joint involvement

It should be established which joints or groups of joints have been affected, the pattern of involvement of joints, i.e. whether monoarticular (single joint), oligo-articular (a few joints) or polyarticular (many joints) (Table 9.2). This in itself will provide some useful clinical clues, particularly when considered along with the mode of onset, i.e. acute, chronic, insidious, migratory, etc.

Rheumatic symptoms

Pain. This should be analysed as described in Chapter 2 (p. 29). In particular, the severity, type of onset (acute or chronic), time pattern and relationship to activities should be assessed. Sometimes the history alone, in the absence of clinical signs, allows a diagnosis to be made. For example, in some patients with carpal tunnel syndrome there may be no objective signs, but patients may describe intense discomfort and numbness in the fingers, often wakening them

Table 9.1 The history summarised

- Pattern of joint involvement
- Mode of onset
- Character of pain – relieving and exacerbating factors
- Stiffness – early morning and after immobility
- Extra-articular features
- Family history
- Social history
- General medical history
- Past medical history

Table 9.2 Some common anatomical patterns of rheumatic disease

Inflammatory disorders (synovitis)	
Polyarticular	
MCP, PIP and MTP joints*	RA[+], SLE[+], psoriasis
DIP joints	Psoriasis
Girdle joints	Polymyalgia rheumatica, RA
Oligoarticular	
Asymmetrical large joints or dactylitis (sausage digit)	Reactive arthritis, Reiter's syndrome, psoriasis or AS[+]
Monoarticular	
Acute	Gout, pseudogout, infection, psoriasis
Chronic	Psoriasis, RA, AS, chronic infection (e.g. TB)
Axial, sacroiliac and girdle joints	AS
Degenerative disorders (bony swelling ± synovitis)	
Polyarticular	
DIP or PIP joints and/or first CMC joint*	Nodal OA[+]
Monoarticular	
Chronic	OA
Axial joints	Lumbar or cervical spondylosis

* MCP, metacarpophalangeal; PIP, proximal interphalangeal; DIP, distal interphalangeal; MTP, metatarsophalangeal; CMC, carpometacarpal.
[+] RA, rheumatoid arthritis; SLE, systemic lupus erythematosus; OA, osteoarthritis; AS, ankylosing spondylitis.

from sleep in the early hours of the morning and relieved by shaking the hand or hanging it out of bed.

Stiffness of joints. This occurs with both inflammatory and degenerative lesions. In inflammatory joint disease, such as rheumatoid arthritis, there is characteristically a diurnal variation in stiffness and pain which is worse on rising in the morning, typically lasts at least 30 minutes, and may return at the end of the day. Such patients also describe marked 'immobility stiffness' or 'gelling' after periods of inactivity. Patients with degenerative joint disease may complain similarly of stiffness, but this tends to show much less or no diurnal exacerbation, and may persist even with use of the joint.

Swelling. This is an important feature of joint disease, and although usually identified during the physical examination should be sought from the history where the condition is episodic. Swelling, in the absence of trauma, is highly suggestive, but not pathognomonic of inflammation. Conversely, some inflammatory joint diseases may be associated with little or no swelling (e.g. viral arthritis, SLE).

Weakness. This may occur as a result of joint

disease, but where weakness is the presenting dominant symptom it is highly suggestive of a myopathy.

Typical questions which may be used to elicit the main characteristics of the patient's symptoms of pain and stiffness include the following:

- Is your pain or stiffness worse or better
  — in the morning or at the end of the day?
  — during sleep?
  — after sitting?
  — during or after walking?
- How long does it take to wear off or improve?
- How far can you walk?

The following examples provide a guide to the features of pain and stiffness encountered in specific conditions.

Inflammatory disease

Acute lesions. In acute lesions such as osteomyelitis, septic arthritis or gout, the pain is severe and throbbing, disturbs sleep and prevents use of the limb or affected joint. When a joint is involved all movement is inhibited by protective spasm and any attempt at movement causes severe pain. If the patient sleeps deeply, the spasm may relax and the patient wakes with a characteristic cry if some movement occurs causing recurrent painful muscle spasm. Infection of bone near a joint may also give rise to protective spasm, but in contrast to septic arthritis gentle examination should reveal a small range of joint movement.

Chronic lesions. The local and systemic features are less severe than in acute lesions and often exhibit diurnal variation. For example, rheumatoid arthritis often has an insidious onset, with pain and stiffness which is worse in the morning and eases with gentle activity. In a severe case, the symptoms may return towards the end of the day or persist throughout the day and disturb sleep at night. Similarly, in ankylosing spondylitis, back pain and stiffness may be quite severe on rising, last up to several hours and ease with physical activity.

Inflammatory muscle disease. The major symptom of inflammatory muscle disease, such as polymyositis, is progressive weakness. This predominantly affects proximal girdle and truncal muscles, and patients complain of difficulty getting up from a lying or sitting position, climbing stairs or brushing their hair. Bulbar muscles may become affected, causing nasal regurgitation or inhalation of liquids with dysphagia and dysphonia.

Degenerative lesions

Degenerative joint disease is often associated with a mild inflammatory reaction. Some immobility, stiffness and early morning exacerbation therefore may be present but is usually short-lived and much less marked than in inflammatory joint disease.

Osteoarthritis. The patient with peripheral or axial joint osteoarthritis will usually give a history of gradually increasing pain over months or years, with loss of movement of the joint. Early morning stiffness and pain usually settles after gentle use of the joint over about 15–30 minutes, but may return with use as the day progresses. With lower limb joint osteoarthritis daily activities such as dressing, walking and climbing steps will become progressively impaired. Rest pain and night pain may become a disturbing feature.

Prolapsed intervertebral disc. Acute back pain may occur without prior warning or there may be several years' history of minor backache associated with physical activity. Usually the acute episode occurs when bending or lifting, or the day after such activities, but sometimes it occurs for no discernible reason. The pain subsides with rest over a period of several weeks, and is often followed by further major or minor episodes. Over years this episodic pattern develops into that of osteoarthritis of the spine.

Spinal stenosis. Narrowing of the spinal canal or neural exit foramina is usually caused by degenerative changes in the intervertebral discs and facet joints and can result in back pain or radicular pain. The back pain is often diffuse, radiates to the buttocks and thighs and may be accompanied by tingling and numbness. These symptoms, which the patient may find difficult to describe, increase with standing or walking, and are relieved by sitting or lying down. Leaning forward or holding a supermarket trolley may also help to ease the pain and increase exercise tolerance.

Joint instability. Unstable joints become increasingly painful as the day progresses. As the supporting muscles tire, the related ligaments stretch and pain increases.

Tumours

With the exception of osteoid osteoma, benign bone tumours are painless unless they press on neighbouring structures. Pain is a variable feature of malignant tumours and when present is not related to activity, is not relieved by rest and may be worse at night. Pathological fractures may occur as a result of trivial trauma and cause sudden pain.

Psychogenic symptoms

The complaint of chronic polyarthralgia or myalgia, which is constant day and night and does not conform to any clear pattern, should raise the suspicion that this may be a somatic presentation of an underlying psychological or psychosocial problem. Closer questioning may result in the presenting symptom evaporating only to be replaced by multiple new symptoms. Other clues include the lack of associated organic symptoms such as stiffness or joint swelling and the presence of features such as tiredness, lack of energy, change in mood and sleep patterns or appetite. Conversely, however, the pain and disability of chronic joint disease may also result in lowered mood, sleep disturbance and tiredness.

Traumatic lesions

Sprained ligaments. Immediately after a sprain, the pain may be severe and constant. Subsequently, pain only occurs with movement which stretches the damaged structure and is relieved when the ligament is relaxed.

Chronic strain of ligaments. In weight-bearing ligaments, in the back or foot for example, the patient is most comfortable in the morning. As the day progresses the supporting muscles tire and an aching pain develops which is relieved by rest.

Traumatic arthritis. Following severe joint injury there may be immediate swelling due to haemarthrosis as a result of damage to bone or ligaments. Injury may also cause slower onset of swelling due to damage to avascular structures such as the menisci of the knee. However, trauma may also precipitate an underlying 'latent' disorder such as osteoarthritis, rheumatoid arthritis or gout, and when symptoms of inflammation following trauma persist longer than expected, this possibility must be considered.

Non-articular or systemic features

Non-articular features are often crucial to making a correct diagnosis of inflammatory joint disease and should be carefully sought in the history and examination. The pattern of joint involvement should suggest possible diagnoses which will prompt enquiry about particular non-articular features. For example, in a patient with an acute lower limb oligoarthritis suggestive of reactive arthritis such as Reiter's syndrome a careful history should be taken to identify recent enteric infection including a possible source. A sensitive enquiry into sexual contacts should also be made to identify possible exposure to sexually transmitted infection. Similarly, night sweats and 'flu-like' symptoms in a patient with acute monoarthritis suggests sepsis. Examples of non-articular features and their disease associations are shown in Table 9.3.

General medical background, family and social history

The medical background may be very important, and a careful enquiry into past illnesses, family history, social history and medication often brings out diagnostic clues.

A number of commonly used drugs can precipitate rheumatic disease. In hospital practice, for example, the commonest precipitant of gout is diuretic therapy. Certain antibiotics may cause hypersensitivity vasculitis, and hydralazine and procainamide cause drug-induced SLE.

Certain ethnic and racial groups are predisposed to particular conditions, for example SLE in Afro-Caribbeans and Asians, and gout in Polynesians with a Western lifestyle.

In some rheumatic diseases the family history may be crucial to making the diagnosis (Table 9.4). A common example is a family history of psoriasis in a patient presenting with undiagnosed chronic oligoarthritis.

A careful social history is essential. Factors in the patient's domestic or working environment may be the cause of the patient's symptoms (Table 9.5); con-

Table 9.3 Examples of non-articular features associated with rheumatic diseases

Disease	Non-articular features
Symmetrical polyarthritis	
RA	Subcutaneous nodules, Raynaud's phenomenon, sicca syndrome, pleurisy, episcleritis
SLE	Raynaud's phenomenon, serositis, alopecia, photosensitivity, rash, fever, episcleritis
Asymmetrical oligoarthritis	
Psoriatic arthritis	Psoriasis, nail dystrophy
Reactive arthritis (including Reiter's syndrome)	Urethritis, conjunctivitis, fever, penile ulcers, psoriasiform rash, iritis, mouth ulcers, diarrhoea, enthesitis (e.g. Achilles tendonitis, plantar fasciitis)
Ankylosing spondylitis	Iritis, enthesitis,
Sarcoidosis	Erythema nodosum and hilar adenopathy
Monoarthritis	
Gout	Tophi, obesity, renal impairment
Septic arthritis	Fever, malaise, source (usually skin), throat

Table 9.4 Conditions in which the family history may be diagnostically helpful

Diseases linked to the HLA-B27 tissue type – ankylosing spondylitis, iritis, reactive arthritis, weaker association with psoriasis, inflammatory bowel disease

Psoriasis – psoriatic genes may be expressed in either skin, joints or both in any order and at any time

Hypermobile joints – Marfan's syndrome, Ehlers–Danlos syndrome, benign familial hypermobility, floppy (prolapsing) mitral valve

Gout

Table 9.5 Some social factors associated with rheumatic disorders

	Condition
Carpet layers and miners	Prepatellar bursitis
Exposure to vinyl chloride monomer	Raynaud's phenomenon and acro-osteolysis
Smoking	Lung cancer and hypertrophic osteoarthropathy
Excess alcohol, obesity	Gout
Frequent sexual partners	Chlamydial infection and reactive arthritis, gonococcal arthritis
Intravenous drug abuse	Septic arthritis, rheumatic syndromes associated with HIV infection
Sport	Torn menisci or ligaments, stress fractures

versely the development of rheumatic disease also may have profound social and economic consequences, particularly for people in manual or unskilled jobs.

The assessment of any patient with significant rheumatic disorder should include assessment of activities of daily living, i.e. ability to dress, wash, use a lavatory, walk, climb steps, perform hand functions (turning taps, writing, etc.) and do daily chores such as shopping and housework. Simple self-assessed questionnaires are available for this purpose (e.g. The Stanford Health Assessment Questionnaire).

KEY POINTS

- Establishing the pattern of joint involvement from the history often provides information of diagnostic importance.

- In inflammatory joint disease there is often marked diurnal variation in pain and stiffness which tends to be worse on rising.

- Chronic and constant polyarthralgia or myalgia which does not conform to any organic pattern raises the possibility of an underlying psychological problem.

- Non-articular or systemic features and family history are often crucial in making a correct diagnosis.

- A careful social history is important in assessing the level of handicap.

PRINCIPLES OF A LOCOMOTOR EXAMINATION

General inspection

The examination begins on first meeting the patient, with observation of the patient's overall posture, gait,

ease of movement and demeanour. Features such as facial rash, stiff neck posture, abnormal gait, difficulty getting out of the waiting room chair or a despondent appearance may give immediate clues as to the nature of the problem.

Guided by the history a careful search for relevant non-articular features of joint disease should be made along with a thorough general medical examination since many common rheumatic diseases are accompanied or complicated by pathology in other systems.

Aims of examination

The physical examination is aimed at identifying the site of pathology, signs of inflammation, loss of function, and associated complications (Table 9.6).

This is achieved by inspecting the joints, palpating them, observing their movement and performing specific manoeuvres to test the integrity and function of supporting structures.

Table 9.6 Physical examination – the principles

Anatomy	Bony, articular, ligamentous, tendinous, muscular or neurological
Inflammation	Tenderness, erythema, warmth, effusion synovial swelling
Function	Range of movement and specific functions (e.g. walking, rising, power grip)
Complications	Deformity, instability, muscle wasting, calluses, extra-articular features

Basic techniques and signs

Initial inspection of joints will allow identification of erythema, obvious swelling, local muscle wasting and calluses. Although joint deformity is usually readily identified, in certain joints, such as the hip and shoulder, deformities may have to be 'unmasked' during formal examination. The terms valgus and varus are used to describe deviation of the limb distal to the joint away from (valgus, e.g. knock knee) or towards (varus, e.g. bow-leg) the midline.

Disorders of tendons, ligaments and their attachments (entheses) and bursae are associated with tenderness localised to the site of pathology.

During active (i.e. unassisted) movement, while one hand gently palpates the joint to detect crepitus or clicks, the examiner's other hand can if necessary be used to give gentle assistance to the patient in the direction of movement of the joint. Restriction is usually obvious using the patient's opposite limb as a 'normal control'.

The movements of some joints such as the subtalar joint of the hind foot are most easily examined passively. Other relatively immobile joints, including sternoclavicular, acromio-clavicular, manubriosternal, costochondral and sacroiliac joints, have to be examined by palpation or stressing manoeuvres to detect abnormality.

The neutral zero method of recording is recommended. All joints are considered to be in the neutral position when the body is in the classical anatomical position, with two exceptions, namely the hands are flat against the thighs in the sagittal and not the coronal plane; the feet are at right angles to the leg and not plantar flexed (Fig. 9.1).

In some joints, such as the elbow and knee, movement can normally occur in only one direction from neutral. Extension beyond neutral normally does not occur, and when it does is referred to as hyper-extension. Certain joints such as the shoulders and hips allow movements in all directions from the neutral position. Such movements are defined as flexion, extension, abduction, adduction and internal and external rotation. Combined they result in circumduction.

Measurement of the range of movement. A goniometer (Fig. 9.2) is particularly helpful to assess the rate of progression of a deformity or improvement with therapy. Although typical normal ranges of movement are quoted in the text, there are quite wide variations between individuals and with age. The joints where a goniometer is most commonly used are the knee, hip and elbow.

Both the active and passive movements are measured

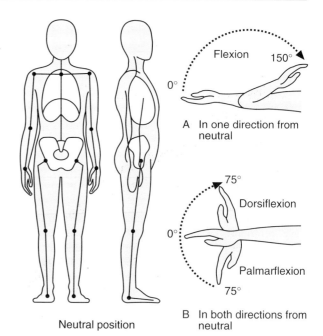

Fig. 9.1 Measuring movements of joints.

and separately recorded if they differ. When limitation of movement is present it is best described by the arc of movement present. For example, if a patient lacks 30° of extension of the elbow and can flex to 90° from that position, the range of movement is described as 30–90° of flexion.

Examination

Inspection
- ☐ Inspect the joint and surrounding tissue for abnormalities.

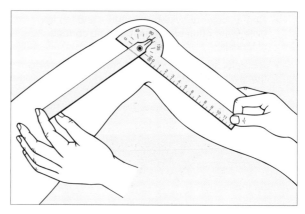

Fig. 9.2 Goniometer.

Palpation
☐ Palpate carefully for warmth, swelling and tenderness.

Movement
☐ Observe the range of active movement while gently palpating the joint for abnormal clicks or crepitus.
☐ If restricted, gently perform passive movement and check again for crepitus.
☐ Where appropriate perform passive stretching manoeuvres to detect joint instability or ligamentous injury.

Interpretation of signs

The aim of the examination is to determine the anatomical site and type of pathology involved. Pain, swelling and restriction or laxity may be due to pathology in the joint or an adjacent structure, and can often be diagnosed by a thorough examination.

Intra-articular structures. Articular disorders are characterised by joint line tenderness on palpation, pain and restriction of movement with possible swelling and crepitus. In acute lesions, the whole joint is tender to palpation (Fig. 9.3). Crepitus arising from soft tissues or cartilage is common in many joint disorders and is distinguishable from the grinding bone-on-bone crepitus following complete erosion of cartilage.

Bony swelling of a joint due to osteophytes feels hard on palpation, while synovitis is usually warm and causes a diffuse and somewhat rubbery swelling of the joint, usually with an associated fluctuant effusion. The diffuse swelling caused by joint synovitis should be readily distinguishable from the synovitis of bursae and tendon sheaths, which is well localised to the involved structure.

Joint restriction due to bone as in osteoarthritis has an 'inelastic' feel to the examiner at the end of range, but when due to soft-tissue contracture or damaged intra-articular tissue (e.g. cartilage) may feel slightly elastic.

Complete lack of movement accompanied by severe pain is due to acute inflammation or recent trauma, and these are differentiated by the history. Complete lack of movement without pain indicates spontaneous fusion (ankylosis) or surgical fusion (arthrodesis) of the joint.

Pain may be elicited from a structure such as a torn semilunar cartilage by palpation or by manoeuvres which compress it (Fig. 9.4). Locking of the joint may also occur (p. 307). Reducing pressure on the damaged structure reduces or relieves pain (Fig. 9.4). An effusion is usually present.

Capsule or ligament. A sprained or strained capsule or ligament is painful when stretched by active or passive movements. Such movements are restricted by protective muscle spasm. Movement which eases tension on the structure relieves the pain and is not limited (Fig. 9.5A). Tenderness is localised to the sprained area. An effusion may be present if the capsule is intact.

A completely ruptured ligament will give rise to instability and swelling over the ligament rather than within the joint, owing to escape of joint fluid. Passive stretching of the ligament is painful and demonstrates an excess degree of movement (Fig. 9.5B).

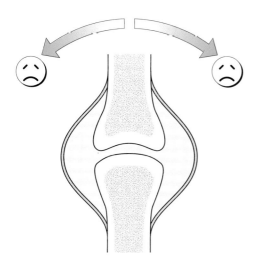

Fig. 9.3 Inflammation of a joint.

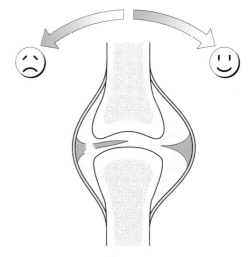

Fig. 9.4 Rupture of semilunar cartilage.

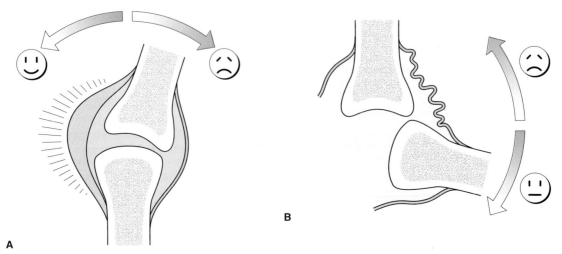

Fig. 9.5 A. Sprain of capsule or ligament. B. Rupture of capsule or ligament.

Tendons. When a tendon or tendon attachment (enthesis) is damaged or inflamed there is focal tenderness at the site of pathology. Pain arising in the tendinous attachment of a muscle close to a joint can be distinguished from that due to a strained ligament. Contraction of the suspected muscle without moving the joint (isometric contraction) will produce pain if the muscle or its tendon, rather than the joint ligament, is the cause (e.g. tennis elbow, p. 297).

Tenosynovitis results in swelling of the tendon sheath and limitation of active, but not passive, movement of the related joints sometimes accompanied by tenderness and crepitus in the line of the sheath.

Tendon rupture is associated with complete loss of active movement but a normal range of passive movement.

Muscles. A painful lesion in muscle causes pain during isometric contraction, and active movement is restricted. Passive movement which relaxes the muscles relieves pain and is not restricted. Both active and passive movements which stretch the muscle are restricted by pain (Fig. 9.6). Contracture of muscles caused by either disuse or certain neurological or muscle diseases may result in painless restriction of joint movement.

Derangement of muscles acting over two joints will result in the position of one joint affecting the range of movement in the neighbouring joint. For example, a fixed talipes equinus deformity could be due to a contracture of the ankle joint or to a tight Achilles tendon. To distinguish these the knee is flexed, effectively lengthening the Achilles tendon. The ankle can now be dorsiflexed if the joint is normal (Fig. 9.7).

When a muscle is paralysed or its tendon divided, active movements are abolished but passive movement in the opposite direction is excessive. Left untreated the uncontrolled action of the antagonists will produce joint deformity.

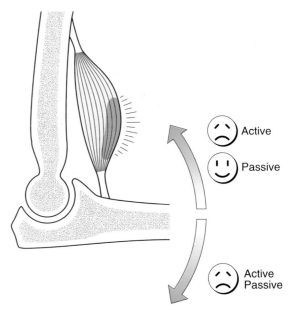

Fig. 9.6 Painful lesions in a muscle.

A

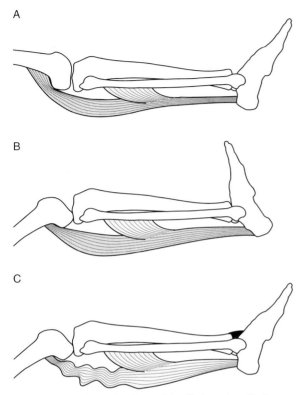

B

C

Fig. 9.7 Demonstrating that impairment of dorsiflexion at the ankle A. may be corrected by knee flexion if the cause is contraction of gastrocnemius muscle B. but will not correct if the pathology is in the ankle C.

KEY POINTS

- Articular disorders are characterised by joint line tenderness, pain and restriction of movement with or without swelling and crepitus.

- A lesion affecting capsule or ligament is painful when stretched by active or passive movements.

- Tendon rupture is associated with complete loss of active, but a normal range of passive, movement.

- A painful lesion in a muscle causes pain during active contraction, even without movement.

DETAILED REGIONAL EXAMINATION OF LIMBS AND SPINE

ANALYSIS OF GAIT

Normal gait consists of even, undulating co-ordinated movements of the spine, pelvis, hip, knee, ankle and foot. An abnormality at any level disturbs this coordination and results in a limp and, quite frequently, symptoms at other normal levels. Abnormal gaits may be divided into two types – *painless* or *painful (antalgic)*.

When the abnormal gait is painful the rhythm more than the contour of the gait is disturbed. The patient takes weight off the painful limb more quickly than usual, spending more time on the painless limb. The only sign may be shortening of the stride on the affected side. When the pain is severe, the limb, flexed at hip, knee and ankle, is placed delicately on the ground and the patient hops quickly onto the sound leg. The painful region, if it is within reach, is supported by one hand and the other arm is outstretched for counterbalance.

In a painless abnormal gait the contour rather than the rhythm is affected. The different causes are described below.

Osteogenic gait. With the patient clothed and wearing special footwear a shortened limb may cause little or no evidence of gait disturbance, but when stripped for examination the gait and its cause should be readily apparent.

Arthrogenic gait. If the hip is arthrodesed or ankylosed in only a few degrees of flexion and without significant abduction or adduction, the contour of the gait is little disturbed. With the more common deformity of severe fixed flexion of the hip, the buttock becomes prominent as the leg extends and the gait is awkward. With bilateral hip flexion contractures of this magnitude, the patient adopts a 'Charlie Chaplin' type of gait with both buttocks prominent. If the hip has an abduction deformity, the patient has to swing the resulting 'long' leg out and round with each step.

The effect of a stiff or painful knee is immediately obvious, particularly on stairs. The patient has to climb stairs one at a time, with the sound leg leading up and the stiff leg leading down (good leg up to heaven and bad leg down to hell).

A stiff ankle or foot causes little interference with normal gait unless accompanied by deformity. If the foot is plantar flexed in equinus the gait will resemble that of a foot drop, but this may be disguised if high heels are worn.

Myogenic gait. The effect of muscle weakness will depend on the site and degree. In muscular dystrophy or the myopathy of severe osteomalacia there is a characteristic waddling gait due to weak gluteal muscles.

Neurogenic gait. See page 203.

Psychogenic gait. If the gait is bizarre or seems greatly exaggerated in comparison with other, more objective, physical findings, psychological causes should be considered.

EXAMINATION OF THE SPINE

The key to accurate diagnosis of spinal complaints lies in taking a careful history, with attention to eliciting symptoms which help to distinguish mechanical, or non-inflammatory, from inflammatory spinal disease. Spinal disease may occur in the absence of local symptoms and present with pain or neurological symptoms or signs in the limbs. Knee or hip synovitis in a young person may also be the first clue to the presence of associated, but previously unsuspected, spinal disease such as ankylosing spondylitis.

Although the examination can be divided into examination of the movements of individual cervical, thoracic and lumbar segments, many spinal diseases are not confined to one segment and cause generalised alterations in spinal posture or function.

Spinal posture

The posture of the spine should be viewed as a whole. At all times the normal spine should present as a straight line viewed from behind. Normal posture varies with age (Fig. 9.8), but in the juvenile and young adult there is a lumbar lordosis, slight thoracic kyphosis and cervical lordosis. In pregnancy or obesity the lumbar lordosis is exaggerated. With advancing age the lumbar curve is slowly lost, the kyphotic posture exaggerated and the hips may become flexed. Eventually in advanced age the general kyphosis of the fetus may be reproduced in the wheelchair. Thus variations in the spinal curves are to be expected through life and only become abnormal when exaggerated or angular rather than curved.

Certain spinal diseases produce characteristic alterations in posture (Table 9.7).

Scoliosis. Scoliosis, or lateral curvature of the spine, is always abnormal. In the cervical spine this is termed torticollis or wry neck. In the thoracolumbar region the scoliosis may be due to faulty posture and is correctable, or due to protective spasm in the presence of a painful lesion or to some underlying structural abnormality. These can be distinguished by getting the patient to bend forward keeping the legs straight. A postural scoliosis will be corrected, but a curve due to a painful condition will be associated with limitation of flexion. Scoliosis due to an underlying painless structural lesion (e.g. paralysis following polio) will persist even on flexion and a hump will be revealed on the convex side of the curve (razor back deformity) because the lateral curvature of the spine is accompanied by rotation of the vertebra at the apex of the curve. The consequent distortion and narrowing of the rib cage may interfere with respiratory and cardiac function and shorten life expectancy.

Ankylosing spondylitis. This is often associated with abnormal spinal posture. In advanced cases the lumbar spine loses the normal lordosis and becomes straight, the thoracic spine becomes increasingly kyphotic with a stiff immobile rib cage, and there is often a compensatory exaggerated cervical lordosis.

Spinal osteoporosis. The most obvious feature is

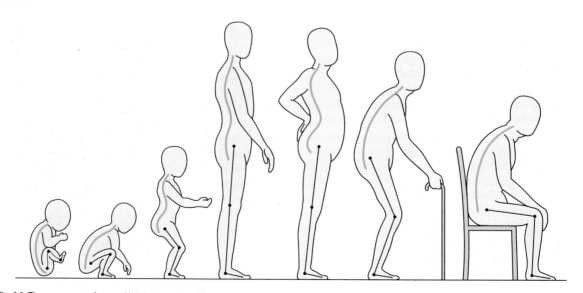

Fig. 9.8 The seven ages of man. Variation in posture with age.

Table 9.7 Causes of abnormal spinal posture

Increased thoracic kyphosis	Ageing, osteoporosis, ankylosing spondylitis
Loss of lumbar lordosis	Ageing, ankylosing spondylitis
Lumbar scoliosis (painful)	Disc protrusion
Lumbar scoliosis (painless)	Leg length inequality, hip deformity
Thoracolumbar scoliosis (painless)	Congenital, paralytic conditions (e.g. polio), idiopathic

exaggeration of the thoracic kyphosis giving the appearance of the 'dowager's hump' as a result of multiple wedge fractures of thoracic vertebral bodies.

Cervical spine

The cervical spine is the most mobile section of the vertebral column. The neck is seldom in the same position for any length of time. Degenerative changes are therefore common but are not necessarily accompanied by symptoms. Mobility is also a factor in the liability of the cervical spine to injury.

Anatomical features

In the cervical spine (Fig. 9.9) the transverse processes project laterally from the body of the vertebrae, protecting the more easily crushed cancellous bone of the body in the event of injury. The facet joints lie more horizontally than at other levels of the spine. Thus forced flexion of the neck is more likely to result in an anterior dislocation rather than a crush fracture. The other synovial articulations between the vertebrae are small saddle-shaped 'neurocentral' joints (joints of Luschka), which join the posterolateral borders of the bodies of each vertebrae.

The neural canal is almost filled by the cervical enlargement of the spinal cord, and the emerging cervical roots pass through the exit foramina bounded by the facet joints posteriorly and the intervertebral discs and neurocentral joints anteriorly. The nerve roots, particularly in the lower cervical spine, may be compressed or irritated either by lateral disc prolapse or by osteophytes arising from facet or neurocentral joints. A central disc prolapse may produce pressure on the cord itself. Nodding of the head occurs at the atlanto-occipital joint; rotational neck movements take place mainly at the atlanto-axial joint and flexion, extension and lateral flexion mainly at mid-cervical level.

Special points in the history

Neck pathology may cause local or referred pain in either the shoulder, arm, chest wall, and head. Disease of the upper cervical spine at the atlantoaxial joints, as in rheumatoid arthritis, usually gives rise to pain, sometimes with dysaesthesiae or other neuropathic

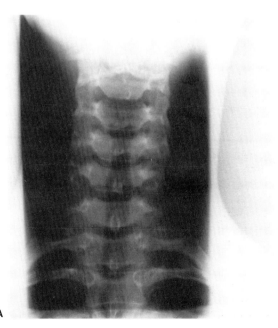

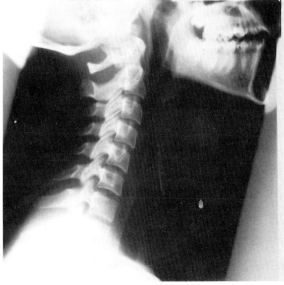

A   B

Fig. 9.9 Cervical spine – anterior (A) and lateral (B) views.

symptoms, radiating up into the occiput in the distribution of the C2 nerve root. Disease of the middle and lower cervical spine tends to cause pain radiating into the upper border of the trapezius, the interscapular region or into the arms. It may be accompanied by dysaesthesiae in the distribution of the affected nerve roots. Irritation of C6 and C7 nerve roots may give rise to widely referred pain around the chest wall. In any patient complaining of upper limb, shoulder or upper trunk pain, neck pathology should be considered as a potential cause. In many patients, poor neck posture is either the main cause of pain or, where there is underlying pathology, a significant exacerbating factor.

Examination of the cervical spine

Because of the close relationship of the bones, joints, blood vessels, spinal cord and nerve roots, a lesion of the cervical region may produce both local and referred symptoms. Examination of the neck must therefore include a neurological examination of the upper and lower limbs for lower and upper motor neurone signs (see Table 7.20 p. 249).

Inspection. Deformity is easily detected. Where an acute painful lesion is present the gait is characteristic. The patient walks with care to avoid jarring the neck, moving the whole body to look to the side. Patients may even support their chin with their hand. Torticollis (wry neck) is the most common deformity. If this has been present for several years asymmetry of the face will have developed. In rheumatoid arthritis, a flexion deformity may develop as a result of mid-cervical erosive damage and subluxation, and a 'cock robin' posture (i.e. lateral flexion deformity of the upper cervical spine) may arise as a consequence of erosive damage to the lateral masses of the atlas. In established ankylosing spondylitis, the neck is often hyperextended to compensate for increased thoracic kyphosis.

Palpation. Tender spots in the muscles are often associated with nerve root irritation or neck pathology. These may be over the cervical spine or at some distance in the upper border of trapezius. If a cervical disc lesion is present the foraminal compression test (Fig. 9.10) will elicit the characteristic pain.

Movement. Causes of neck restriction include degenerative disease, traumatic cervical syndrome or inflammatory arthritis. Loss of lateral flexion is a useful and sensitive sign of neck pathology. Nodding tests movement at the atlanto-occipital joint.

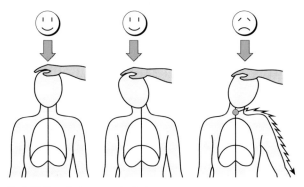

Fig. 9.10 Foraminal compression test.

Examination

Inspection
❏ Inspect the neck for deformity.

Palpation
❏ Palpate the bony contour and note any tender spots in paraspinal muscles.

Movement
❏ Ask the patient to look right and left (80° of rotation each way), and to tilt the head right and left (45° lateral flexion each way) and to flex (75°) and extend (60°) the neck. Note any asymmetry of movement and loss of the normal contour of the spine.
❏ Gently perform passive movements if there is impairment of active range. Note whether the end point of movement feels elastic or inelastic.
❏ Perform upper and lower limb reflexes and note any sensory or motor abnormalities.

Thoracic spine

This segment of the spinal column is the least mobile and maintains a kyphosis throughout life. Performing chest expansion to assess movement of the costovertebral joints is an essential part of examining the thoracic spine. In the absence of underlying pulmonary disease the chest expansion should be at least 5 cm. Developmental lesions of the thoracic spine such as epiphysitis are relatively common and may cause exaggeration of the kyphosis, as can acquired diseases such as osteoporosis or ankylosing spondylitis. Restriction of chest expansion is an important feature of ankylosing spondylitis. Infection of the spine may result in a sharp angular deformity or 'gibbus'. Deformity due to faulty posture will correct on forward flexion, while that due to structural abnormality will not.

Anatomical features

Movement in the thoracic spine is mainly rotational, but there is a very small amount of flexion, extension and lateral flexion.

Special points in the history

Tender costal cartilages are found in a number of rheumatic conditions (e.g. ankylosing spondylitis, SLE), or can occur without apparent cause (Tietze's syndrome). The importance of this feature lies in distinguishing it from visceral causes of chest pain, by identifying the tender areas on palpation of the chest wall. Pain in the thoracic spine is less common than in either the cervical or lumbar spine. Disc lesions are infrequent but can occur and may be accompanied by girdle pain radiating round the chest mimicking cardiac or pleural disease. Chest pain arising from the joints at the thoracolumbar junction also occurs in ankylosing spondylitis and is sometimes confused with pleuritic, renal or cardiac pain. Pyogenic or tuberculous infection of the spine should also be considered, especially in patients from poorer socioeconomic groups or who are immunosuppressed. In middle and old age vertebral collapse from osteoporosis or malignancy is a common cause of pain. When thoracic pain is poorly localised and there is no satisfactory explanation, intrathoracic causes (e.g. aortic aneurysm) should be considered.

Examination

Inspection
- With the patient standing, inspect the posture from the front, back and side and note any deformity.

Palpation
- Examine the bony contour and define areas of tenderness.
- Where local tenderness is not detected, repeat the gentle percussion with the fist or tendon hammer.

Movement
- Observe rotation of the thoracolumbar spine from behind with the patient seated on the couch, thereby splinting the pelvis.
- Note the effect of forward flexion on any deformity present.
- Measure chest expansion.

Lumbar spine

Lumbar spinal symptoms are very common and may be due to trauma, degenerative disc disease, osteoarthritis of the facet joints, osteoporosis or inflammatory disease such as ankylosing spondylitis. Referred pain due to intra-abdominal causes should also be considered.

In many patients backache is related to poor posture or related ligamentous stresses, and often no specific pathology can be identified. In such individuals contributory factors such as inequality of leg length or psychosocial problems should be identified and addressed.

Anatomical features

The principal movements are flexion, extension, lateral flexion and rotation. On forward flexion the upper segments move first, followed by the lower segments to produce a smooth lumbar curve. Similarly, on lateral flexion a smooth curve should develop and the patient's fingertips should reach the top of the knees. In the adult the spinal cord ends to the level of the second lumbar vertebra (L2). Injury above this level may cause serious damage at the cord, which is permanent, and to the nerve roots, which may be temporary. Below the level of L2 only nerve roots can be damaged.

Congenital anomalies are very common in the lumbar or sacral segments but are rarely symptomatic. Such anomalies include vestigial ribs on the upper lumbar vertebrae, partial or complete fusion of the fifth lumbar vertebrae with the sacrum (sacralisation) or, conversely, segmentation of the first sacral vertebra (lumbarisation).

The intervertebral disc contains a tough outer ring of fibrous tissue, the annulus, and a central nucleus surrounded by jelly-like material with a high water content (Fig. 9.11). Degenerative change in the lower lumbar discs begins in the third decade. The annulus may tear, causing pain and, if extrusion of the nucleus occurs, nerve root compression may result. Initially there is no radiological change, but with time gradual narrowing of the intervertebral space becomes apparent. The corresponding facet joints also develop osteoarthrosis. Such changes are present in the majority of individuals by the fifth decade but are frequently an asymptomatic radiological finding.

Special points in the history

- Acute disc protrusion usually causes sudden onset of back pain, with or without nerve root symptoms, and is usually associated with bending or lifting. Sudden movements, such as coughing or straining at

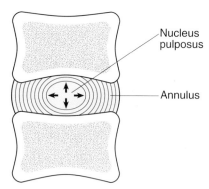

Fig. 9.11 Intervertebral disc.

Nucleus pulposus

Annulus

stool, will exacerbate the pain. The acute episode may be superimposed on a background of preceding mild episodic backache, due to disc degeneration, to which the patient has become accustomed.

- Osteoarthrosis and degenerative disc disease in the lumbar spine cause typical symptoms of intermittent discomfort or pain in the lower back, short-lived morning or immobility stiffness and gradual loss of mobility of the lumbar spine over years or decades. The pain and stiffness are relieved by gentle activity but recur with excessive activity.
- Chronic ligamentous strain and spinal instability cause pain on standing and towards the end of the day, with freedom from pain at the beginning of the day.
- Ankylosing spondylitis usually presents in young adults with a history of low backache and stiffness worse in the morning or after inactivity and eased by activity. Morning stiffness is usually more marked than in osteoarthrosis, lasting at least 30–60 minutes. There are often other clues to the diagnosis such as a family history (p. 277).
- Spinal stenosis, i.e. the narrowing of the spinal canal or neural exit foramina, is usually caused by degenerative changes in the intervertebral discs and facet joints and can result in back pain or radicular pain. The back pain is often diffuse, radiating to the buttocks and legs, and is accompanied by tingling and numbness. These symptoms, which may be difficult to describe, increase with standing or walking, and are relieved by sitting or lying down. Forward flexion by stooping or holding a supermarket trolley or bicycling may also help to ease the pain and increase exercise tolerance.

- Pyogenic or tuberculous infection of the lumbar spine or sacroiliac joint may track into the sheath of the psoas muscle, presenting as a painful flexed hip or as a swelling in the groin. Active flexion or attempted passive extension of the hip will exacerbate the pain, while passive flexion is relatively painless. This contrasts with infection of the hip joint, when all movements are painful, and with a lesion causing femoral nerve root (L2,3) irritation (p. 289), when active or passive hip flexion relieves the pain by reducing tension on the nerve root.
- Unremitting spinal pain of recent onset may also suggest infection or, in older patients, malignant disease. When the history is of many years' duration, however, a serious organic cause is unlikely.

Examination of the lumbar spine

The commonest cause of scoliosis is disc protrusion. The direction of convexity of the scoliosis depends on the relationship of the disc prolapse to the adjacent root, not on the side of the midline to which the disc is protruding. If the prolapse is lateral to the root, the patient leans towards the opposite side, relieving the pressure on the root. If the prolapse is medial to the root, the patient leans towards the same side as the lesion (Fig. 9.12).

Accentuation, absence of, or reversal of the normal lordosis is also abnormal. For example in ankylosing spondylitis the lordosis may be lost or reversed.

Muscle tenderness indicates local spasm, while bone tenderness may signify a more serious problem such as infection or neoplasm.

The changes in the lumbar curve which occur during flexion will be interrupted if there is a stiff segment or if there is irritation of a nerve root. For example, in early ankylosing spondylitis the lower segments may remain immobile during flexion. Even with a completely rigid lumbar spine, patients may still be able to touch their toes providing that they have mobile hips. A quantitative assessment of flexion may be obtained using Schober's test. This method provides a measure of the distraction of the lumbar spinous processes and is useful in the assessment of progression in ankylosing spondylitis (Fig. 9.13).

Examination

Inspection

❏ With the patient standing, observe the posture from behind, checking that the spine is straight, and from the side, checking that there is a normal lordosis.

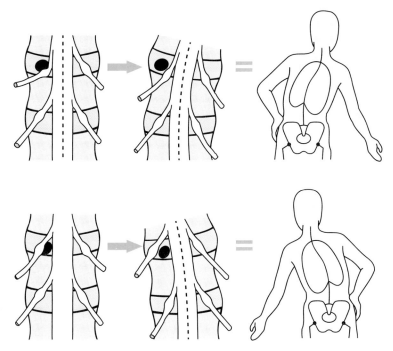

Fig. 9.12 Deviation of spine in prolapsed intervertebral disc.

Palpation
- ❏ Note the presence of tenderness over the spinous processes or in the paraspinal muscles.
- ❏ Perform light percussion with the fist to elicit bone tenderness.

Movement
- ❏ Ask the patient to extend backwards, then to bend forward keeping legs straight, and then to each side trying to touch the side of the knees, while observing the contour formed by the spine.

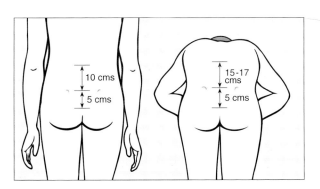

Fig. 9.13 Schober's test. Measuring forward flexion of spine.

Schober's test (Fig. 9.13)
- ❏ Make a mark on the skin at the level of the lumbosacral junction at the dimples of Venus, and two other marks 5 cm below and 10 cm above the first.
- ❏ Place a tape measure over the lower spine with the end (0 cm) at the lower mark and ask the patient to bend forwards.
- ❏ Record the movement of the upper skin mark up the tape measure.

On forward flexion the upper mark will normally move upwards by at least 5 cm.

Tests for nerve root compression

Sciatic roots. Prolapse of intervertebral discs occurs most commonly at the L4/5 or L5/S1 level, producing compression of the L5 and S1 nerve roots respectively. Tension is put on these roots by flexing the hip with the knee straight – so-called *straight leg raising*. Normally about 90° of hip flexion should be possible but this varies considerably (70–120°). When the root is stretched over a prolapsed disc, straight leg raising will be restricted, and pain will usually be felt in the lumbar region, not just in the leg (Fig. 9.14).

The 'Bowstring sign' is another useful test and may be used to confirm nerve root irritation and to exclude malingering.

If there is still doubt as to whether there is genuinely sciatic nerve root irritation, two other manoeuvres may be tried, namely the 'flip' test and the 'sitting' test.

Examination

Straight leg raising
❑ Examine the patient lying supine (Fig. 9.14A).
❑ With the knee flexed, check that passive hip flexion is normal.
❑ With the knee extended, raise the leg on the unaffected side by lifting the heel with one hand while preventing knee flexion with the other hand. Note the range of movement.
❑ Repeat this on the affected side, asking the patient to report as soon as it is painful and where the pain or paraesthesiae is felt (Fig. 9.14B).
❑ When this limit is reached, gently dorsiflex the ankle, thereby applying further tension on the nerve root (Bragaard test) (Fig. 9.14C).

Bowstring sign
❑ Perform straight leg raising and at the limit, flex the knee, reducing tension on the sciatic roots and hamstrings.
❑ Now further flex the hip to 90° (Fig. 9.14D).
❑ Gently extend the knee until pain is once again reproduced (Lasègue's sign) (Fig. 9.14E).
❑ Apply firm pressure with the thumb first over the hamstring nearest the examiner, then in the middle of the popliteal fossa and finally over the other hamstring tendon. Ask the patient which manoeuvre exacerbated the pain (Fig. 9.14F). The test is positive if the second manoeuvre is painful and if the resultant pain radiates from the knee to the back.

Sitting test
❑ Ask the patient to sit up from the lying position, ostensibly to inspect the back. Only in the absence of sciatic nerve irritation will the patient be able to sit up straight with legs flat on the bed.

Flip test
❑ Ask the patient to sit with hips and knees flexed to 90° on the edge of the couch and test the knee reflexes. Then extend the knee, ostensibly to examine the ankle jerk. When there is genuine root irritation the patient will 'flip' backwards to relieve the tension. The malingerer, distracted by attention

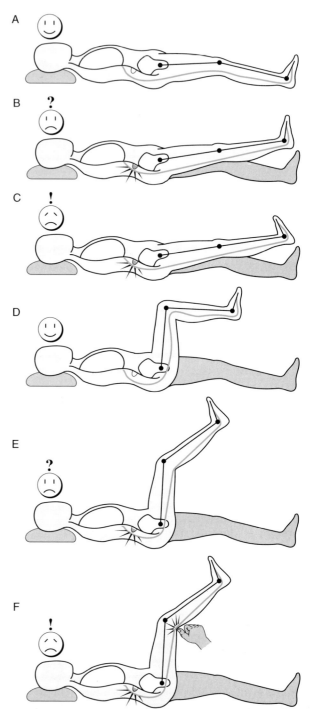

Fig. 9.14 Stretch tests – sciatic nerve roots. A. Neutral; nerve roots slack. **B.** Straight leg raising limited by tension of root over prolapsed disc. **C.** Tension increased by dorsiflexion of foot (Bragaard test). **D.** Root tension relieved by flexion at the knee. **E.** Knee extended, root tightens over prolapsed disc causing pain radiating to the back (Lasegue test). **F.** Pressure over centre of popliteal fossa bears on posterior tibial nerve which is 'bow stinging' across the fossa causing pain locally and radiation into back.

to the ankle jerk test, may permit full extension of the knee, which is the equivalent of full 90° straight leg raising (Fig. 9.15).

The accompanying neurological signs of L5 and S1 nerve root irritation include weakness of dorsiflexion of the great toe (extensor hallucis longus, L5), weakness of ankle dorsiflexion and inability to walk on heel (L5), loss of ankle reflex and inability to walk on tiptoe (S1), and numbness, paraesthesiae or hyperalgesia in the first interdigital cleft and lateral aspect of calf (L5), lateral border of foot and sole (S1) (Fig. 7.39 p. 241).

Femoral roots. Disc prolapse at higher levels may involve the L2, L3 or L4 roots of the femoral nerve. The femoral nerve passes into the thigh anterior to the pubic ramus, and hip flexion or straight leg raising will relieve any tension on these roots. They are stretched by extending the hip with the knee flexed.

Examination

Femoral stretch test
- Ask the patient to lie prone, or on the unaffected side if there is a painful flexion deformity of hip.
- Flex the knee slowly asking the patient to report onset of pain.
- If this fails to produce pain gently extend the hip with the knee still flexed.

If the test is positive pain radiates into the back and thigh (Fig. 9.16). Knee flexion alone may be sufficient to exacerbate pain and cause the patient to flex the hip to reduce tension on the nerve root.

When limitation of hip extension is due to a hip lesion, knee flexion should have no effect on the pain.

The accompanying neurological signs of femoral nerve root irritation may include altered sensation over the anteromedial thigh and reduced knee jerk (L3/4).

Sacroiliac and other paraspinal or central joints

Examination of the sacroiliac joints is an essential part of the spinal examination, although the available clinical tests are not wholly reliable. Pain arising from these joints may radiate into the buttocks and posterior thighs, but unlike sciatica rarely goes below the knee. Local palpation is often unhelpful and may give rise to false-positive and false-negative results. Stressing the pelvis may produce buttock pain if these joints are inflamed.

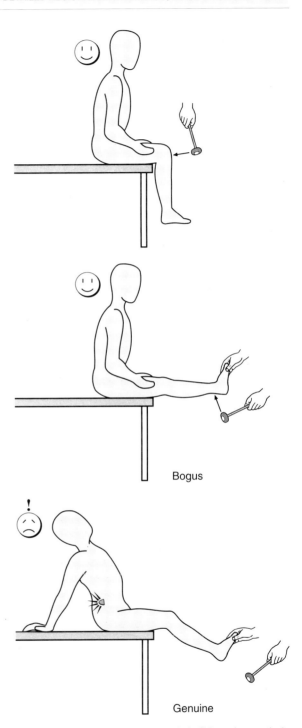

Bogus

Genuine

Fig. 9.15 Stretch test – sciatic nerve roots. In the 'flip' test when attention is diverted to the tendon reflexes the genuine patient will not permit full extension of the leg.

The sternoclavicular and manubriosternal joints may be involved, for example, in ankylosing spondylitis, psoriasis or polymyalgia rheumatica, while the acromio-clavicular joints may be affected by osteoarthritis.

Examination

Sacroiliacs
❑ Ask the patient to lie prone on a firm surface and apply firm pressure with the heel of the hand over the sacrum.
❑ Alternatively, lie the patient on the side on a firm surface and press down on the pelvic brim.

Other joints
❑ Inspect and palpate the sternoclavicular, acromioclavicular and manubriosternal joints for swelling or tenderness.

KEY POINTS

• Scoliosis of the spine is always abnormal.

• Spinal disease may occur in the absence of local symptoms and present with neurological features or pain in the limbs.

• Neck pathology may cause local or referred pain in either the shoulder, arm, chest wall, head or face.

• Chest expansion is an essential part of assessing the thoracic spine.

• Lumbar spinal symptoms are very common and frequently no underlying cause can be found.

• Even with a rigid spine, patients with mobile hips may be able to touch their toes.

EXAMINATION OF THE UPPER LIMBS

Many everyday activities involving the upper limb depend on normal function at all levels, i.e. hand, wrist, elbow and shoulder. For example, eating requires not only a functional hand but also the ability to flex the elbow and internally rotate and flex the shoulder. Similarly, cleaning the perineum after defecation is extremely difficult unless the wrist can be supinated, the elbow flexed and shoulder internally rotated. A proper assessment of the upper limb must include examination of the integrity and function of all of the joints and never of one joint in isolation.

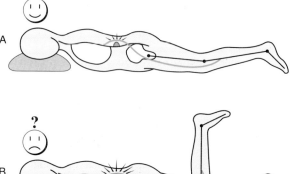

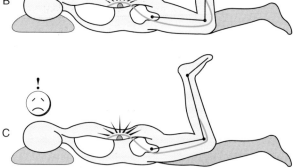

Fig. 9.16 Stretch test – femoral nerve. **A.** Patient prone and free from pain because femoral roots are slack. **B.** When femoral roots are tightened by flexion of the knee, pain may be felt in the back. **C.** If still no pain, femoral roots are further stretched by extension of the hip.

The hand, wrist and forearm

Although the hand and wrist may be affected by regional or local conditions, they are also frequently involved in polyarthritis.

Anatomy

Skin and deep fascia. In the palm both structures are thickened and are bound together at the skin creases. On the dorsum the skin and fascia are thin and elastic. Because of these differences any swelling of the joints, tendon sheaths or other tissues tends to be much more evident over the dorsum.

Muscles. The flexor and extensor muscles of the forearm are the power-house of the hand and wrist. However, without the help of intrinsic muscles of the hand neither a proper grip nor fine movements are possible. If the intrinsics are paralysed, for example by neuropathy, the forearm muscles acting alone may cause clawing of the fingers, rendering the hand almost useless.

Joints. The interphalangeal joints allow only flexion and extension. The metacarpophalangeal joints allow flexion and extension, and a little abduction and adduction when they are extended. The wrist allows flexion and extension, radial and ulnar deviation and circumduction.

Rotation of the forearm depends on the superior and inferior radioulnar joints and on the concavity of the volar aspects of the shafts of the radius and ulna. In pronation, these two concavities fit into one another. Pronation is limited if the curve is distorted, such as after a fracture.

Nerve supply. The radial, ulnar and median nerves are all essential for normal hand function. Variation in nerve supply is common, particularly as a result of overlap between the median and ulnar nerves.

The *radial nerve* supplies the wrist and finger extensors and an area of skin on the dorsum of the first interosseous space. Damage to the nerve is most common in the spiral groove of the humerus and results in wrist drop and weak grip because the flexors no longer have an antagonist to steady the wrist.

The *ulnar nerve* supplies sensation to the ulnar border of the hand. Its motor fibres supply the adductor of the thumb, the interossei and lumbricals except those to the index and sometimes the middle finger. When the nerve is damaged close to the wrist, the unopposed action of the long flexors and extensors produce a claw hand deformity (Fig. 9.17). The ring and little fingers are clawed and the wasting of the muscles between the metacarpals is most obvious between the thumb and index finger.

The *median nerve* supplies the main bulk of the flexor muscles in the forearm, the short flexor, abductor and opponens of the thumb and the lumbricals to the index and middle fingers. The common site of damage is at the wrist. If untreated, this results in wasting of the thenar eminence, with the thumb developing a simian posture. The sensory disturbance may be very disabling since the sensation over the volar aspect of index and middle fingers is essential to almost all aspects of hand dexterity and fine function.

Special points in the history

Symptoms of arthralgia and stiffness in the hand are frequently the earliest indication of polyarthritis. The pattern of joint involvement often provides an essential clue to the differential diagnosis (Table 9.2). Paraesthesiae and nocturnal discomfort in the hand may be due to the carpal tunnel syndrome. While often idiopathic, this may be the first manifestation of rheumatoid arthritis or other systemic diseases such as hypothyroidism or acromegaly.

Examination

Examination of the hand consists of inspection, palpation and assessment of function. Since a full examination of function is lengthy, it is essential to tailor the examination to the clinical history and nature of the problem. For example, in a patient with lacerations of the digits a thorough assessment of the integrity of tendons, nerves and circulation is essential. In contrast, in a patient presenting with stiffness and swelling of small joints the examination will be directed towards establishing the pattern of joint and tendon synovitis and testing the principal hand functions such as power grip and fine pinch.

Inspection. Changes in nails, skin or soft tissues (Table 9.8), muscles, joints or hand posture may provide immediate clues to the nature of the problem. The presence and distribution of synovitis, which is apparent as fusiform swelling around joints or as swelling of tendon sheaths, should be noted (Table 9.2). Postural abnormalities may arise from damage to the joints and their supporting soft tissues (e.g. ulnar deviation of the fingers in rheumatoid arthritis) or from tendon rupture or a combination of these (p. 279).

Palpation. Palpation of the hands will elicit tenderness and help to assess the cause of swelling of joints, tendon sheaths or other tissues. Osteophytes in the hand are apparent as small hard bony outgrowths over the dorsum of the DIP or PIP joints, while synovitis causes tender, rubbery fusiform swelling of the joints. Other abnormalities are listed (Table 9.8). Thickening and loss of laxity of the skin of the fingers (sclerodactyly) is a feature of progressive systemic sclerosis and some patients with SLE and occurs in long-standing diabetes mellitus (diabetic cheirarthropathy).

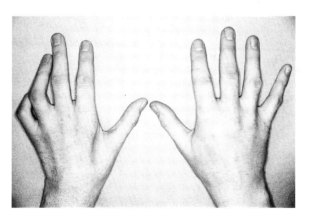

Fig. 9.17 Left claw hand deformity. Note the wasting of the dorsal interosseous muscle, the extension of the MP joints and flexions at the PIP joints of the ring and little fingers.

Table 9.8 Examples of visible 'non-articular' abnormalities of the hands associated with rheumatic diseases

Abnormality	Appearance and consistency	Typical site	Associated rheumatic disease
Heberden's nodes	Small bony nodules	Dorsum of DIP joints	OA
Bouchard's nodes	Small bony nodules	Dorsum of PIP joints	OA
Rheumatoid nodules	Fleshy and firm	Extensor surface and flexor tendons	RA
Tophi	White subcutaneous	Juxta-articular	Gout
Calcific deposits	White subcutaneous	Finger pulp	SCL, DM
Dilated capillaries	(Use magnifying glass)	Nail folds	SCL, DM, SLE

OA, osteoarthritis; RA, rheumatoid arthritis; SCL, scleroderma; DM, dermatomyositis; SLE, systemic lupus erythematosus.

There may also be swelling associated with tendon sheaths. Synovitis of the flexor tendon sheaths causes a firm diffuse swelling of the volar surface of the digit and the palm. In a normal finger the tissues over the volar surface of the proximal phalanx are lax and can be readily pinched into a fold; however, if synovitis is present the tissues become firm and tense with the consistency of a cooked sausage (Savill pinch test). Localised swelling or palpable thickening of a tendon may cause 'triggering' of the fingers or thumb. The patient is able to flex the digit normally, but on attempting to extend the finger, it sticks and then either suddenly straightens or has to be passively straightened. The nodule is usually palpable at the level of the distal palmar crease, or the base of the thumb.

Extensor tenosynovitis presents as a swelling which may extend above and below the extensor retinaculum to produce an hourglass deformity. If the synovium is adherent to the tendon, the synovial swelling may sometimes move with the tendon on flexion and extension of the fingers. Synovitis of the wrist joint causes less obvious swelling with loss of the normal contour. This is usually more apparent on the dorsum and sides than on the flexor aspect.

The distal radioulnar joint is frequently involved in rheumatoid arthritis. The supporting ligaments become weakened and dorsal subluxation of the ulnar head occurs. Rotation of the wrist becomes painful and the distal ulna is painful when pressed down like a piano key (piano key sign).

Movement. The value of the hand as a tool is largely dependent on opposition. The abductor brevis and opponens combine to produce opposition. The position of the thumbnail helps to distinguish opposition (median nerve) from adduction (ulnar nerve). On adduction the nail is seen in side view, while in opposition it is rotated and the plane of the nail lies in the plane of the palm (Fig. 9.18). The principal functions of the hand are pinch, which requires opposition of the thumb to the fingertips, and power grip which requires flexion of the fingers. This depends on the integrity not only of the joints and finger flexors but also of the intrinsic muscles.

Examination

Inspection
- ❏ Inspect the hands and wrists carefully.

Palpation
- ❏ Palpate the joints of the hands and wrists and periarticular soft tissues to elicit tenderness and identify the nature of any swelling.
- ❏ Palpate the flexor tendon sheaths (Savill pinch test) to detect synovial swelling.
- ❏ Feel for local swellings of tendons, especially at the mouth of flexor sheaths, while asking the patient to flex and extend the digits.

Movement
- ❏ Ask the patient to grip one or two of the examiner's fingers and to perform fine pinch (as if threading a needle).
- ❏ Ask the patient to put the hands in the position of prayer and then lower the hands keeping the palms together. This demonstrates the range of wrist dorsiflexion.
- ❏ Ask the patient to place the backs of the hands together and to raise the arms. This demonstrates the range of wrist flexion.

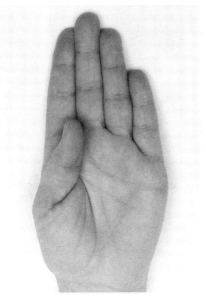

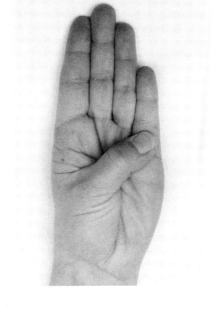

| A | B |

Fig. 9.18 A. Adduction and B. opposition of the thumb.

Specific muscles and tendons

❑ Undertake detailed testing of individual muscles and tendons only if indicated.

❑ *Flexor digitorum profundus (FDP)* (flexes the DIP joint). Ask the patient to flex the DIP joint while holding the finger in extension at the PIP joint (Fig. 9.19A).

❑ *Flexor digitorum sublimis (FDS)* (flexes the PIP joints). Ask the patient to flex the PIP joint while the other fingers are held in full extension to eliminate the action of FDP (Fig. 9.19B).

❑ *Lumbricals* (flex the MCP joints and extends the PIP joints). Ask the patient to extend the IP joints with the MCP joints held in flexion to exclude the

action of the long extensors (Fig. 9.20A).

❑ *Palmar interossei* (adduct the fingers and assist the lumbricals). Ask the patient to grip a card between the fingers (Fig. 9.20B), while the examiner attempts to pull it away.

❑ *Dorsal interossei* (abduct the fingers and assist the lumbricals). Ask the patient to spread the fingers and press the side of the index fingers against each other (Fig. 9.20C). Weakness will be obvious on the abnormal side.

❑ *Thenar muscles supplied by median nerve* (abduction and opposition of the thumb). Ask the patient to abduct the thumb vertically off the palm from the position shown in Fig. 9.18A and to hold it against

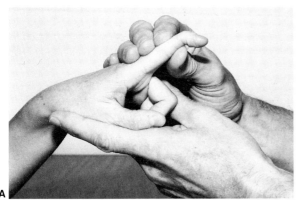

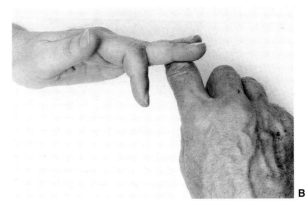

| A | B |

Fig. 9.19 A. Flexor digitorum produndus. B. Flexor digitorum sublimis.

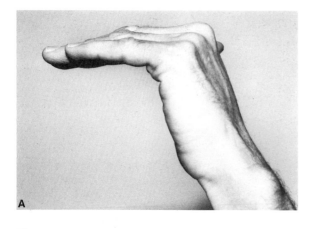

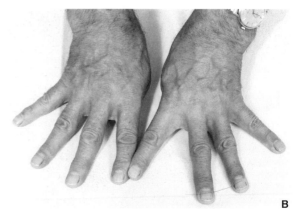

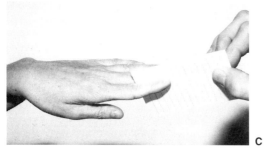

Fig. 9.20 A. Lumbricals. B. Palmar interossei. C. Left dorsal interossei.

resistance. Test opposition by asking the patient to touch the terminal phalanx of the little finger with the thumb and to maintain this against resistance.

❑ *Thenar muscle supplied by ulnar nerve* (adduction of the thumb). Ask the patient to hold a card between the radial side of the fingers and the extended thumb. If the adductor is weak, the thumb cannot be held straight and flexes at the MCP and IP joints (Froment's sign) (Fig. 9.21A).

❑ *Extensor pollicis longus* principally elevates the thumb (hitch-hiker's thumb). Ask the patient to place the palm on a flat surface and to lift the thumb like a hitch-hiker. The patient will only be able to do this if the tendon is intact (Fig. 9.21B).

Common hand deformities and syndromes

Rupture of extensor tendons may occur at various sites and cause a deformity such as mallet finger or boutonnière deformity, or weakness of extension of thumb or fingers.

Mallet finger (Fig. 9.22). This is due to separation of the extensor slip from the distal phalanx.

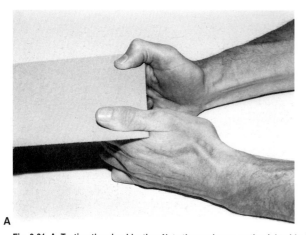

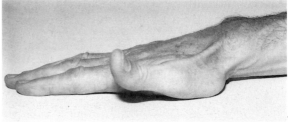

Fig. 9.21 A. Testing thumb adduction. Note the weakness on the right side. B. Intact extensor policis longus elevating the thumb off a flat surface.

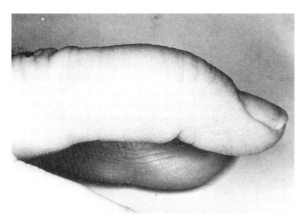

Fig. 9.22 Mallet finger.

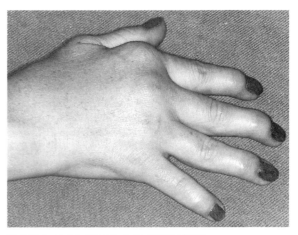

Fig. 9.24 Swan neck deformity in rheumatoid arthritis.

Boutonnière deformity (Fig. 9.23). This occurs as a result of rupture of the extensor slip to the middle phalanx. The lateral extensor bands may then slip to the side of the proximal interphalangeal joint, causing flexion at this joint and extension at the distal interphalangeal joint.

Rupture of extensor pollicis longus. Rupture of EPL at the wrist may occur after a Colles fracture or in rheumatoid arthritis and causes loss of thumb extension. This tendon normally elevates the thumb when seen from the side (hitch-hiker's thumb) (Fig. 9.21B).

Rupture of extensor tendons to the little and ring fingers. This causes these two fingers to droop at the level of the wrist. This is a common problem in rheumatoid arthritis because of the effect of local synovitis or mechanical attrition associated with a subluxed distal ulna.

Swan neck deformity (Fig. 9.24). This is relatively common in rheumatoid arthritis. The intrinsic muscles waste and become contracted causing flexion of the metacarpophalangeal joints, extension of the proximal interphalangeal joints and flexion of the distal interphalangeal joints. With further destruction of soft tissues the metacarpophalangeal joints may undergo volar subluxation.

Ulnar deviation of the fingers (Fig. 9.25). This is common in, but not unique to, rheumatoid arthritis and occurs because of disruption of the normal slings and supports which maintain the direction of pull of extensor tendons. The tendons are allowed to slip between the metacarpal heads, resulting in an abnormal pull on the fingers in an ulnar direction. Intrinsic muscle contracture may also contribute to this deformity as the ulnar interossei are stronger than those on the radial side.

Carpal tunnel syndrome. This occurs as a result of compression of the median nerve in the carpal tunnel (p. 291). The principal symptoms are of progressive

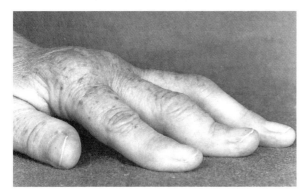

Fig. 9.23 Boutonnière deformity.

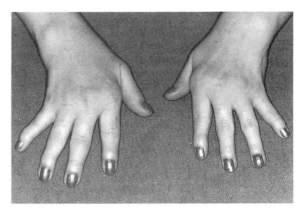

Fig. 9.25 Ulnar deviation of the fingers in rheumatoid arthritis.

paraesthesiae and numbness in the fingers which often correlate poorly with the distribution of the median nerve. In the early stages the symptoms are usually worse during the night and tend to regress in the morning. If neglected, sensory loss becomes more severe and wasting of the thenar eminence and weakness of thumb abduction and opposition occur. Tinel's or Phalen's sign may be useful in diagnosis but neither test is wholly reliable. To elicit Phalen's sign the wrist is flexed passively for a minute or two. This should reproduce or exacerbate the symptoms if carpal tunnel syndrome is present. Tinel's test involves percussing over the carpal tunnel for about half a minute. If positive, the test reproduces or exacerbates the patient's symptoms. A better 'test' is to provide a night resting splint, which often alleviates the patient's nocturnal symptoms.

De Quervain's tenosynovitis. This painful condition affects the tendons of abductor pollicis longus and extensor pollicis brevis as they pass through their retinacular compartment and traverse the radial styloid. The patient complains of local tenderness and pain on thumb movement. The main signs are of local tenderness and sometimes swelling just proximal to the radial styloid. The pain is reproduced by passively moving the wrist into ulnar deviation while the patient holds the thumb clenched into the palm (Finkelstein's test) (Fig. 9.26).

The elbow

Fracture of the elbow at the supracondylar level may damage the brachial artery causing Volkmann's

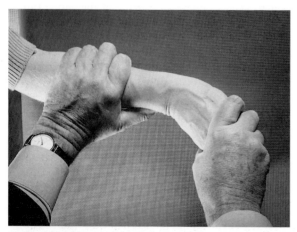

Fig. 9.26 Finkelstein's test. The patient's right thumb and fingers are grasped by the examiner and the wrist brought into ulnar deviation. In the presence of de Quervain's teno synovitis, acute pain is produced by this manoeuvre.

ischaemic contracture of the forearm flexor muscles. Trauma may also cause ulnar nerve damage.

The elbow is also commonly involved in inflammatory arthritides. In rheumatoid arthritis the elbow joint may become eroded and quickly develops a fixed flexion deformity; rheumatoid nodules and bursae may develop over the olecranon. Olecranon bursae may also occur in gout.

Soft-tissue conditions such as lateral epicondylitis (tennis elbow) and medial epicondylitis (golfer's elbow) are relatively common and are not confined to keen sports people.

Anatomy

The joint is composed of two parts, that between the humerus, and the radius and ulna, and the superior radioulnar joint. The former allows flexion through a range of 150° and the latter rotation of the forearm through 180°.

Special points in the history

Although intra-articular pathology is usually localised to the elbow by the patient, periarticular conditions such as epicondylitis may give rise to local tenderness or to poorly localised discomfort in the forearm.

Examination

Inspection. The elbow should be inspected for obvious deformity or swelling. The elbow often develops a flexion deformity in the presence of synovitis, erosive damage or degenerative change. An effusion may be apparent as a filling out of the hollow over the head of the radius and between the olecranon and lateral epicondyle with the arm slightly flexed.

Palpation. This is used to detect local tenderness over the epicondyles, and to define the nature and position of any swelling. Synovitis and effusion of the elbow may sometimes be more easily palpated than seen and is most obvious over the radial head and posterolateral aspect. An olecranon bursa should be readily distinguishable from a joint effusion by its superficial posterior position and consistency. If present the bursa should be palpated for the presence of nodules or fibrinous rice bodies.

Movement. The elbow should flex freely from neutral to 150°. In many normal individuals a few degrees of hyperextension will be evident. Movements may be restricted in the presence of synovitis, degenerative change and sometimes epicondylitis. If epicondylitis is suspected, further special tests should be performed as below.

Common syndromes

These comprise lateral and medial epicondylitis. In epicondylitis, tenderness is well localised to the origin of the common extensor tendon (tennis elbow) or flexor tendon (golfer's elbow). The pain of epicondylitis, which may radiate into the forearm, is exacerbated by actions which stretch the ligamentous attachment of the forearm muscles to the epicondyles.

Examination

Inspection
- ❏ Inspect both elbows from behind with both arms extended for deformity.

Palpation
- ❏ Palpate the elbow for bony contour, local tenderness, signs of inflammation, nodules or bursae.

Movement
- ❏ Compare the range of active flexion and extension.
- ❏ Perform supination and pronation of the forearm with the elbows flexed at 90° and with the elbows at the patient's side. (Failure to do this may give a misleading impression since pronation can be simulated by abduction and rotation at the shoulder.)
- ❏ Also palpate the elbow joint during flexion–extension and over the head of radius during supination–pronation to detect crepitus.
- ❏ Test the integrity of the collateral ligaments with the arm fully extended.

Testing for epicondylitis
- ❏ Ask the patient to grip tightly with the hand while the elbow is fully extended and then with the elbow partly flexed. If tennis elbow is present, the first manoeuvre will be painful and the second much less so or not at all. If the problem is severe, the patient may have difficulty extending the elbow even without clenching the hand.
- ❏ Place the patient's arm in the waiter's tip position (i.e. elbow fully extended, forearm pronated and wrist flexed) and then ask the patient to try to extend their fingers against resistance. This will exacerbate the pain at the extensor insertion.
- ❏ To test for medial epicondylitis place the patient's arm in the extended position with the forearm supinated and then ask the patient to try to flex the wrist or fingers against resistance. This will exacerbate the pain at the flexor insertion.

The shoulder

A number of pathological processes may affect the shoulder. Congenital dislocation is almost unknown, but in young adults dislocation readily occurs following injury and the tendency to recurrent dislocation is great. In adults, synovitis of the glenohumeral and sternoclavicular joints occurs in polyarthritides such as rheumatoid arthritis or polymyalgia rheumatica, but osteoarthritis is uncommon. Osteoarthritis may, however, affect the acromioclavicular joint. The glenohumeral joint also has a tendency to stiffen during middle age. This condition is known as frozen shoulder or adhesive capsulitis and may occur spontaneously or after trauma, immobility, myocardial infarction, hemiplegia or local radiotherapy. The humeral head, like the head of femur, is susceptible to osteonecrosis. The rotator cuff tendons and subacromial bursa are common sites of either degenerative change or synovitis which result in painful restriction of certain shoulder movements. Some of these problems are relatively common and require different therapeutic approaches. It is essential that they are distinguished by clinical examination.

Anatomy

Movement of the 'shoulder' is a complicated synthesis of movement occurring at four joints. The glenohumeral joint and thoracoscapular mechanism each account for about half the total range, whereas movements at the acromioclavicular and sternoclavicular joints are relatively small. With the scapula fixed, the glenohumeral joint permits flexion to 90°, abduction to 90°, extension to 30°, both internal and external rotation to 90°. Further range of movement requires movement of the scapula on the thorax – the thoracoscapular mechanism (Fig. 9.27). The overall range of movement varies with rotation of the arm. This can be shown with the elbow flexed to a right angle and the forearm acting as an indicator of rotation. Abduction can proceed little beyond 90° with the arm in neutral rotation. If the arm is then externally rotated, further abduction becomes possible. With the arm by the side in neutral rotation and the elbow flexed to 90° the forearm will be pointing medially by about 20°. Rotation to 90° in either direction should be possible from this position. In external rotation the forearm will not quite reach the coronal plane, but in internal rotation the patient should be able to touch the small of the back.

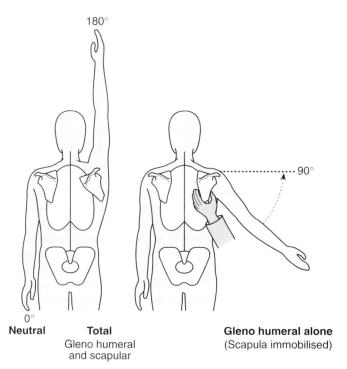

180°

90°

0°
Neutral **Total** **Gleno humeral alone**
Gleno humeral (Scapula immobilised)
and scapular

Fig. 9.27 Movements at the shoulder joint.

The rotator cuff comprises the conjoint tendons of the supraspinatus, infraspinatus and teres minor. Infraspinatus and teres minor externally rotate the humerus while supraspinatus initiates abduction. The cuff forms a hood-like structure covering the humeral head, holding it into the socket of the glenoid and initiating glenohumeral abduction. The cuff is separated from the inferior aspect of the acromion by the subacromial bursa. The rotator cuff, and especially supraspinatus tendon and related subacromial bursa, is the most common site of pathology in the shoulder.

Nerve supply. The spinal segments supplying the shoulder girdle also contribute to the phrenic nerve. Thus pain in areas supplied by the phrenic nerve (e.g. diaphragm or gall bladder) may be referred to the shoulder in the area of C4/5 dermatomes.

Special points in the history

Pain in the shoulder may be due to lesions in the neck, pleura, peritoneum and diaphragm. Referred pain is usually easy to distinguish from shoulder pathology since the former is not associated with restriction of, or pain on, shoulder movement. The picture in the elderly may be confused by the tendency to develop a frozen shoulder in response to referred pain.

Symptoms arising in the root of the neck tend to cause pain down the inside of the arm as in an apical bronchial carcinoma eroding the neck of the first rib and involving the T1 nerve root. Mid-cervical pain is usually referred to the upper border of the trapezius, superior aspects of the shoulder and into the upper arm.

True shoulder pain is usually referred to the upper arm around the insertion of deltoid and is not felt below the elbow. Many patients with painful pathology in the shoulder describe a tight band or bruised feeling in the upper arm and may have difficulty appreciating the true source of their pain. The pain may prevent them lying on the affected side at night.

Examination

The shoulder is a challenging joint to examine.

Inspection. Chronic restriction of movement of the glenohumeral joint from arthritic damage or an adhesive capsulitis (frozen shoulder) often results in marked disuse muscular atrophy. A synovial effusion in the glenohumeral joint is difficult to detect on inspection because of the overlying deltoid muscle, but it may bulge anteriorly. If substantial synovial swelling or effusion is present the whole shoulder may appear swollen like an American footballer's shoulder pad. When this occurs the effusion usually involves both the subacromial bursa and the glenohumeral joint.

Palpation. In rotator cuff syndromes local tenderness may be apparent over the tip of the shoulder and sub-acromial space (supraspinatus tendonitis), anteriorly over the bicipital groove (bicipital tendonitis) and sometimes over the anterior capsule if acute synovitis and effusion of the glenohumeral joint is present. There may be tenderness and a hard bony outgrowth directly over an osteoarthritic acromioclavicular joint. Synovitis of the sternoclavicular joint, which may occur in RA, polymyalgia rheumatica and the spondylarthropathies, presents with tenderness and palpable soft-tissue swelling directly over the joint.

Movement. Restriction of rotation of the gleno-humeral joint is virtually always due to pathology of the glenohumeral joint or its capsule. Restriction of other movements of this joint may be due to pathology of the glenohumeral joint, its capsule or the rotator cuff.

In synovitis of the glenohumeral joint without underlying joint damage, the range of active movement is much less than the range of passive movement and the latter will sometimes be almost normal. Following erosive damage to the cartilage, the range of passive movement will diminish. In contrast, from its onset, frozen shoulder (adhesive capsulitis) results in pro-gressive and equal loss of both active and passive movements with abduction and external rotation being the movements most obviously affected. Rotator cuff disease is principally due to supraspinatus pathology but the subaeromid bursa and the long head of biceps can also be involved. It tends to cause restriction of abduction or elevation of the shoulder and is often associated with a painful arc of movement (described below). Rotation is not usually affected

Examination

Inspection
- ❏ Inspect and compare the shoulders from the front and the back.
- ❏ Note any muscle wasting, soft-tissue swelling or difference in bony contour on the two sides.

Palpation
- ❏ Note any tenderness or swelling over the anterior aspect and tip of the shoulder, the acromio-clavicular joint and sternoclavicular joint.

Overall range of movement
- ❏ Stand behind the patient and observe the overall

range of movement by asking the patient to place the hands at the base of the neck with elbows pointing laterally and then to put arms down and to reach behind the back between the shoulder blades.
- ❏ Proceed with further examination only if pain, swelling, limitation or asymmetry of movement is present.
- ❏ Stand behind the patient and examine the range of rotation with the patient's arm by the side and elbow flexed to 90°. Note especially loss of external rotation which indicates glenohumeral joint pathology.

Glenohumeral joint movement
- ❏ Eliminate scapular movement on the thorax either by firmly holding the tip of the scapula or by placing a restraining hand over the top of the acromion. This will enable any movement of the scapula to be immediately felt during examination when the limits of movement of the glenohumeral joint are reached.
- ❏ With the arm by the side ask the patient to flex the shoulder forward; this should reach 90° if the range is normal.
- ❏ Now ask the patient to abduct the arm from the dependent position (normal range 90°).
- ❏ If abduction cannot be initiated, the test for rotator cuff rupture should be performed as described below.
- ❏ If active abduction is restricted, test whether further passive movement is possible and if this is painful (impingement pain).
- ❏ If 'impingement pain' is present the tests for painful arc syndrome should be performed (see below).

Common syndromes

These include the following.

Painful arc syndrome. When the rotator cuff is inflamed, shoulder movements are affected in a characteristic way, producing 'impingement pain' and the 'painful arc syndrome'. Attempts at active abduc-tion are usually limited by pain and the patient may, for example, describe pain on trying to reach up for things on a high shelf. This is because during abduc-tion and elevation the inflamed cuff is compressed under the acromion, producing 'impingement pain'. A 'painful arc' is present if the patient complains of pain as the arm moves through the mid arc of abduction (45°–140° approximately). Often the patient will lean sideways during the procedure to try to relieve the pain. In very acute cases it may not be possible to demonstrate a painful arc because the pain is too severe. However, even in these circumstances impingement pain can be demonstrated by rotation of the flexed arm. In the dependent position this will be full and painless, confirming that there is no glenohumeral pathology.

Demonstration of a painful arc or impingement pain is indicative of either an incomplete tear of the supraspinatus tendon, supraspinatus tendonitis or subacromial bursitis. These lesions may be associated with dystrophic tendon calcification or polyarthritides such as rheumatoid arthritis.

Rotator cuff rupture. When complete rupture of the supraspinatus tendon has occurred the patient is unable to initiate abduction of the arm from the dependent position. Attempts to abduct produce only a shrugging movement of the shoulder girdle as a result of deltoid muscle contraction.

Bicipital tendonitis. The long head of biceps may also be involved in rotator cuff lesions and give rise to shoulder pain. If the tendon is ruptured attempted contraction will cause the muscle to bunch like an egg just above the elbow.

Osteoarthritis of the acromioclavicular joint. This tends to occur in the middle-aged and elderly. The principal signs are bony swelling and tenderness over the joint, and sometimes pain on full elevation of the arm. This should not be confused with the painful arc syndrome.

Examination

Testing the rotator cuff

- ☐ Starting with arm by the side, ask the patient to abduct the arm against resistance. This may be painful if the supraspinatus tendon is inflamed. If the cuff is ruptured the patient will be unable to initiate abduction.
- ☐ If rupture is suspected, passively abduct the arm about 30° to 45° from the patient's side. The patient should now be able to continue active abduction from this position unaided.
- ☐ Next elicit 'impingement pain' by passively flexing the patient's arm to greater than 90° while restraining the shoulder girdle.
- ☐ Then rotate the shoulder internally in the 90° flexed position to exacerbate 'impingement pain'. (Hawkins sign.)
- ☐ Next assist the patient to bring the arm into full elevation and then ask the patient to lower it sideways in order to elicit a painful arc (Fig. 9.28).

To elicit the pain and tenderness of bicipital tendonitis

- ☐ Palpate the bicipital groove.

- ☐ Ask patient to flex elbow against resistance.
- ☐ Ask patient to supinate the forearm against resistance.

KEY POINTS

- The basic functions of the hand are to pinch and grasp.

- For normal daily activities it is necessary that the hand can be brought to the mouth, back of the neck and perineum. This depends on the normal functioning of each of the upper limb joints.

- Pain in the arm may be due to local pathology or may be referred from the cervical spine, root of neck or visceral structures.

- The symptoms of carpal tunnel syndrome may bear little relationship to the sensory distribution of the median nerve.

- Pain referred to the shoulder is not usually associated with restriction of shoulder movement.

- Restriction of movement or pain in the shoulder may be due to pathology of the glenohumeral joint, its capsule, the rotator cuff or the acromioclavicular joint.

EXAMINATION OF THE LOWER LIMBS

Like the spine the posture of the legs varies throughout life. Congenital abnormalities are more frequent in the lower than the upper limbs.

Abnormalities or deformities at any level in the lower limb may, by altering the patient's whole posture, cause biomechanical stresses and symptoms in other joints, including the spine. For example, a deformed stiff hip may cause backache from a secondary lumbar scoliosis.

The hip joint

This large ball and socket joint is vulnerable to disease. The hip joint may dislocate at birth, be the site of epiphysitis (Perthes' disease) or infection in childhood, may slip its femoral epiphysis at puberty, dislocate in the young adult, develop avascular necrosis or osteoarthritis in middle age and fracture in the elderly. It is also frequently damaged by synovitis in conditions such as rheumatoid arthritis, ankylosing spondylitis or psoriatic arthritis.

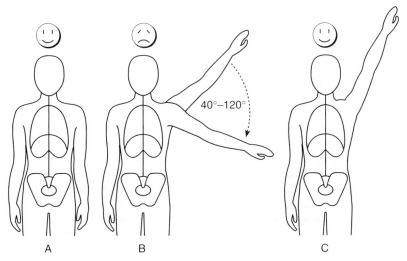

Fig. 9.28 Painful arc syndrome.

Anatomy

Owing to the depth of the normal acetabulum the hip is a stable joint. It is also remarkably mobile because the femur has a neck which is narrower than the maximum circumference of the head. In the adult the acetabulum faces outwards, downwards and slightly forwards. The neck of the femur is set on the shaft at an angle of 130° and is directed forwards or anteverted by some 30°. In the infant the acetabulum is directed forwards, the neck of the femur is set at a greater angle on the shaft, and is anteverted at least 70°. The infant's hip is therefore much more stable when flexed and abducted than when extended and abducted. In contrast, the adult hip is most stable when the femur is extended and is more liable to dislocate when flexed and adducted, the posture adopted when sitting. This accounts for the high incidence of posterior dislocation of the hip in car accidents when the front of the knee impacts against the dashboard.

As the hip is a ball and socket joint, flexion, extension, abduction, adduction, rotation and the combined movement of circumduction are all possible. The actual range changes throughout life, as does the posture of the joint. As age increases the first movements to decrease are extension and internal rotation followed by abduction.

The femoral and obturator nerves supply sensory branches to the hip and the knee joint, explaining the frequency of referred pain from the hip to the knee.

Special points in the history

Pain arising from the hip is most commonly felt in the groin, but may radiate to the anterior thigh and knee or be felt in the knee alone. Pain may sometimes be felt over the greater trochanter or in the buttock. Any patient who cannot accurately localise pain in the knee should be suspected of having a disorder of the hip, especially an adolescent, who may have a slipped femoral epiphysis.

Examination

This is normally performed in the erect and supine positions.

Inspection of the erect patient. *Gait.* The disability from a stiff hip may pass unnoticed unless the patient is lightly clad, when it should be apparent that the pelvis moves with the leg. A painful hip may produce an antalgic gait (p. 281). The 'Trendelenburg' gait of gluteal dysfunction is described below (p. 306).

Posture. Leg length inequality may be 'true', i.e. due to a short leg, or it may be 'apparent' as a result of hip deformity. If the hip is mobile but one leg is short, i.e. true shortening, the pelvis tilts down towards the shortened side and a scoliosis develops (Fig. 9.29A). Alternatively, the patient simply flexes the hip and the knee of the longer side to shorten this limb. A 'raise' under the short leg will correct the posture of the hips and the back (Fig. 9.29B).

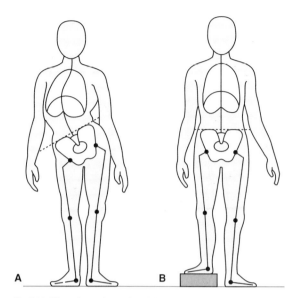

Fig. 9.29 Effect of true shortening of right leg on posture.

Osteoarthritis, synovitis or other pathology which damages the integrity of the hip may result in fixed deformity of the hip and 'apparent' inequality of leg length.

Fixed abduction deformity (Fig. 9.30A) causes apparent lengthening of the leg because the pelvis tilts down on that side to bring the legs parallel. (Fig.

9.30B) The patient can then adjust the posture by flexing the knee on the affected side in an attempt to shorten the limb (Fig. 9.30C), or by wearing a raise under the normal but apparently short limb (Fig. 9.30D). Either way the scoliosis remains uncorrected.

Fixed adduction deformity causes apparent shortening of the limb. The pelvis is elevated on that side to bring the legs parallel. Bending the other knee (Fig. 9.31A) or using a raise on the affected side does not correct the scoliosis (Fig. 9.31B).

Fixed flexion deformity will cause apparent shortening but the patient will be able to compensate by increasing the lumbar lordosis (Fig. 9.32B) and no scoliosis will occur. Raising the affected side will correct the lumbar lordosis (Fig. 9.32C).

A single deformity seldom occurs, the most common combination being flexion, external rotation and adduction of the hip.

Inspection of the supine patient. There are usually few external signs of hip disease on inspection, but any swelling, signs of inflammation, muscle wasting or sinus formation should be sought. When the patient lies on the examination couch it is often difficult to detect a deformity of the hip because the pelvis can tilt to compensate for a considerable malposition of the hip. The pelvis must first be positioned so that the pelvic brim is at right angles to the spine. Any fixed adduction or abduction will be revealed immediately. A flexion deformity will be masked partially or com-

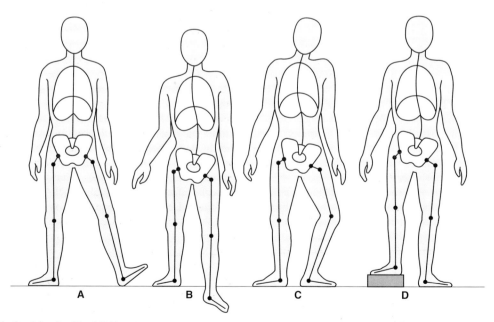

Fig. 9.30 Abduction deformity of the right hip.

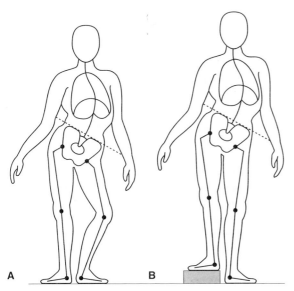

Fig. 9.31 Adduction deformity of the right hip.

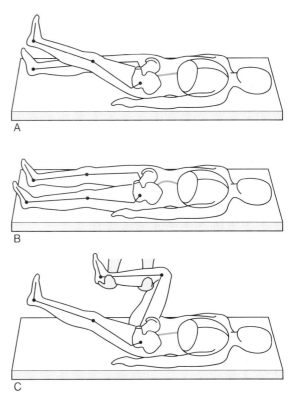

pletely by the patient tilting the pelvis forwards and increasing the lumbar lordosis (Fig. 9.33B). With a severe fixed flexion deformity of the hip, the knee will be flexed but can be passively extended, thus differentiating it from a fixed flexion deformity of the knee arising as a result of local knee pathology. The arthritic hip usually takes up a position at rest of flexion, external rotation and adduction.

Flexion deformity of the hip due to hip disease must also be distinguished from that due to femoral nerve

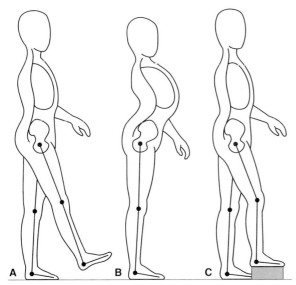

Fig. 9.32 Flexion deformity of the right hip.

Fig. 9.33 Flexion deormity of the left hip. Neutral position A. This may be masked by lumbar lordosis. **B.** and unmasked by full flexion of the right hip. **C.** (Thomas hip flexion test).

irritation (p. 289) or to psoas spasm. In psoas spasm the hip will be held flexed and attempts to straighten it passively are painful. Passive rotation with the hip flexed should be relatively pain free and unrestricted. This contrasts with hip disease, in which rotation and other movements are likely to be restricted and painful. Psoas spasm may be due to pathology in the lumbar spine (e.g. spinal abscess), abdomen (e.g. appendicitis) or pelvis (e.g. abscess or tumour), and these sites must therefore be carefully examined.

Measurement of leg length. Accurate measurement can be achieved only by special radiological techniques, but clinical examination gives a reasonable assessment. When a fixed flexion deformity of the hip joint is present the limbs will apparently be unequal in length when the legs are brought parallel (Fig. 9.34). The amount of apparent shortening is measured between a fixed point such as the xiphisternum or the umbilicus to the tip of the medial malleolus. True shortening is measured from the anterior superior iliac spine to the medial malleolus (Fig. 9.35), and to be accurate must be performed with the two limbs lying in a comparable position of adduction or abduction.

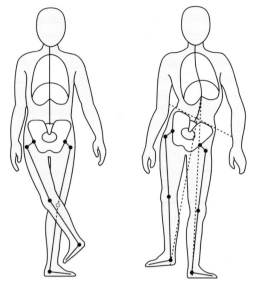

Fig. 9.34 Measurement for apparent shortening of the leg caused by adduction deformity of the right hip.

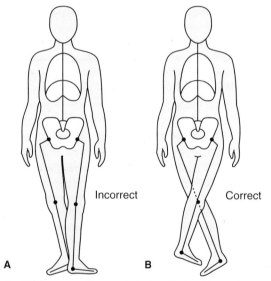

Incorrect   Correct

A   B

Fig. 9.35 Measurement for true shortening of the leg. **A.** Incorrect because legs are not in a comparable position **B.** Correct because the legs are in a comparable position of adduction.

Palpation. In adults it is difficult to detect anything other than gross swelling arising from the hip joint. Occasionally an iliopsoas bursa will point in the groin and may be associated with muscle spasm. Palpation can localise tenderness and so give some indication of the source of the symptoms. Tenderness over the lateral aspect of the greater trochanter may be due to trochanteric bursitis.

Movement. The pelvis must be immobilised during hip flexion by stabilising the iliac crest with one hand in order to be certain that the movement being measured is that of the hip alone and not also of the pelvis on the spine. During flexion any tendency for the hip to externally rotate should be noted since this is not uncommon where there is underlying hip disease; if this occurs in a teenager, a slipped epiphysis must be excluded by radiography. The Thomas test is carried out during examination of flexion to determine if a fixed flexion deformity is present.

During abduction and adduction, movements of the pelvis must again be eliminated by placing a hand on the opposite iliac crest. At each extreme the pelvis will be felt to tilt with the limb.

Rotation should be carried out with the hips first extended, and then with the hips and knees flexed at 90°. The accurate measurement of rotation is particularly relevant if a slipped upper femoral epiphysis is suspected. An increase in external rotation at the expense of internal rotation is one of the earliest clinical findings. The teenager complaining of pain around the hip or knee should be asked to lie supine and flex the affected limb at the hip and the knee, attempting to keep the knee in line with the ipsilateral shoulder while doing so. If the limb rotates externally while this is being attempted, then a slipped epiphysis must be excluded on radiographic examination. Congenital dislocation of the hip is accompanied by more internal than external rotation.

Examination

Inspection
- ❏ Observe the patient when standing and walking and note any abnormality of gait.
- ❏ Look for scoliosis and pelvic tilting which may conceal a hip deformity. If pelvic tilt is present, examination of leg lengths is essential.
- ❏ Inspect the patient supine, positioned so that the pelvic brim is at right angles to the spine.
- ❏ Inspect the posture of each leg and note any deformity, swelling or other signs of inflammation, muscle wasting, sinus formation or obvious asymmetry.

Palpation
- ❏ Palpate for local tenderness over the front of the hip and over the greater trochanter.
- ❏ Measure leg lengths as follows:
  - — With the legs lying parallel, the amount of any apparent shortening is measured between a fixed point such as the xiphisternum or umbilicus and the tip of the medial malleolus (Fig. 9.34).

— To measure true shortening place the normal limb in a comparable position of adduction or abduction to the abnormal limb. Measure from the anterior superior iliac spine to the medial malleolus (Fig. 9.35).

Movement

☐ With one hand stabilising the iliac crest, use the other hand to flex each hip and note the range of flexion (0–120°) (Fig. 9.36).

☐ Perform Thomas's test first on one side and then the other. Place one hand between the patient's lumbar spine and the examination couch. Obliterate the lumbar lordosis by flexing the unaffected hip to its limit and continuing to push to straighten the lumbar spine; this will squash the examiner's hand between the patient's spine and the examination couch. The opposite leg will remain flat on the couch if normal but will rise off the table if affected, revealing the amount of flexion deformity present (Fig. 9.33).

☐ Immobilise the pelvis by grasping the opposite iliac crest, then abduct (variable, minimum 45°) and adduct (25°) each hip, noting the range of movement (Fig. 9.37). At each extreme the pelvis will be felt to tilt with the limb.

☐ Roll each leg on the couch and measure the range of rotation using the feet as indicators (90° arc of movement).

☐ To measure rotation with the hip flexed, flex the hip and knee to 90° and use the tibia to assess the arc of rotation – internal rotation (30°) and external rotation (45°).

☐ Alternatively, and more accurately, lie the patient prone, flex either knee to a right angle and again use the tibiae to assess the arc of rotation.

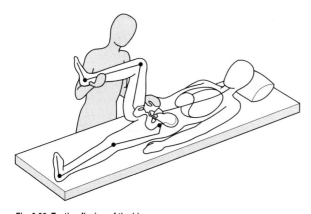

Fig. 9.36 Testing flexion of the hip.

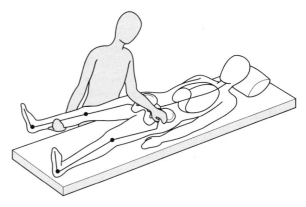

Fig. 9.37 Testing abduction of the hip.

Tests of the stability of the hip

Instability is encountered in congenital dislocation in infants, slipped epiphysis in adolescence, traumatic dislocations in adults, fractures of the neck of femur in the elderly, and in certain neurological and muscular disorders.

In *infancy and childhood* congenital dislocation of the hip must be diagnosed as soon as possible after the birth, certainly many months before the child walks. The three most obvious features are:

• Shortening and external rotation of the limb. The mother may remark that the child does not move the affected leg as much as the other.
• Asymmetry of the fine buttock folds.
• Limitation of abduction: 90° of abduction should be possible in both hips as an infant.

If any of these signs are present Ortolani's test should be performed (p. 352 and Fig. 10.13 p. 353). Indeed this test should be carried out on newborn infants as routine.

Telescoping of the limb occurs in established dislocation, and is therefore a late sign. The term vividly describes the sensation of the limb apparently sinking into the trunk as it pushed in the axis of the limb towards the trunk.

In *puberty and adult life* causes of instability are different in different age groups and are associated with characteristic postures:

• *Slipped upper femoral epiphysis.* This occurs at puberty. The limb is externally rotated, abducted and shortened.
• *Traumatic dislocation.*
  a. Posterior dislocation in which the limb is flexed, adducted and internally rotated, is the more common.

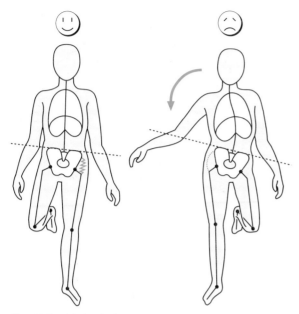

Fig. 9.38 Trendelenburg's sign.

b. In anterior dislocation the limb is flexed, abducted and externally rotated.
• *Fracture in the region of the neck of the femur.* This is common in the elderly, especially women. The limb is extended, externally rotated, adducted and shortened.

Trendelenburg's sign demonstrates that hip abductor function is deficient or absent. It is useful in the later stages of congenital dislocation of the hip when the patient is walking, in assessment of arthritis of the hip and to assess the disability in paralytic disorders, such as poliomyelitis, affecting the lower limbs. When the normal subject stands on one leg the glutei contract so that the opposite side of the pelvis is tilted up slightly to allow the leg to clear the ground during gait. If actions of the glutei are deficient, the opposite side of the pelvis will tilt downwards and the balance can only be maintained by leaning over towards the side of the lesion (Fig. 9.38).

When walking, the patient with lack of abduction compensates by leaning over to the opposite side so that the centre of gravity is moved over the affected hip. This causes the patient to dip or lurch towards the affected side; with bilateral abductor impairment the trunk leans from side to side producing a characteristic rolling gait.

Examination

Trendelenburg's sign
❏ Observe the patient from behind.

❏ Ask the patient to stand first on one leg and then the other while flexing the non weight-bearing leg at the knee to 90°.
❏ Observe any change in pelvic tilt on the non weight-bearing side.

The knee

The knee is particularly prone to injury or twisting because its stability through a full range of movement of 150° is entirely dependent on the control of muscles and ligaments. In addition, its position renders it liable to direct injury. Repeated kneeling can produce a traumatic bursitis, and there is risk of direct infection of the joint by puncture wounds. With advancing age, degenerative changes, especially in the medial joint compartment, are common. Inflammatory diseases such as rheumatoid arthritis, reactive arthritis or crystal related arthropathies also commonly affect the knee.

Anatomy

There is normally about 7° of valgus alignment of the tibia on the femur when the knee is fully extended. Because of the shape of the condyles of the femur, the tibia externally rotates on the femur during extension. This causes the collateral ligaments and the anterior cruciate ligament to become tight. In this position of full extension the joint is 'locked' and no abduction, adduction or rotation of the tibia on the femur is possible. This enables the individual to sustain the body weight using minimal muscle action. With a few degrees of flexion, external rotation is undone, the ligaments are relaxed and it is now possible to abduct, adduct and rotate the tibia on the femur or vice versa.

The semilunar cartilages, or menisci, are mobile structures and are attached by their periphery to the capsule. Although very resistant to compression forces they are very sensitive to movements involving flexion and rotation whilst taking the body weight, e.g. changing direction while running or twisting to kick a ball or rotating in a squatting position. Under these circumstances the cartilages may be sucked between the bones to produce a variety of cartilage tears. The anterior or, more commonly, the posterior horn may be caught momentarily between the tibia and the femur to produce a 'parrot beak' tear. The patient is aware of a sensation of the knee giving way. Sometimes a longitudinal tear of a meniscus will occur resembling a 'bucket-handle'. The 'bucket-handle' fragment may displace medially and comes to lie between the condyles of the femur. The knee is then said to be 'locked' because full extension is obstructed.

The quadriceps is the most important group of muscles controlling the knee both in maintaining an upright posture and in engaging the locking mechanism. When these muscles contract they tend to pull in a straight line from the trochanter to the tibial tubercle. Because of the normal valgus angle of the knee this tends to displace the patella laterally. This tendency, however, is counteracted by the important action of the obliquely disposed vastus medialis muscle.

Special points in the history

The precise history of the mechanism of any injury of the knee is important.

- When the ligaments are tight in full extension they are particularly liable to injury.
- The knee responds differently according to the degree of injury. Severe violence results in bleeding within the joint. Seventy per cent of patients with haemarthrosis have ruptures of the anterior cruciate ligament. Some of the remainder may have fractures, and in these circumstances aspiration reveals fat globules within the bloody aspirate. Very severe violence will also rupture the collateral ligament. The blood will escape from the joint and present as swelling and bruising about the damaged side of the joint itself.
- The history will often differentiate between a large effusion and a haemarthrosis, as an effusion takes some hours or even a day to develop, while a haemarthrosis accumulates quickly.
- Effusions tend to develop in relation to damage to avascular structures such as the menisci.
- The menisci are liable to be torn by twisting injuries, especially when playing football. A careful examination of the knee is required when there is a history of locking. When its occurrence is unpredictable, locking is likely to be due to loose bodies. Under these circumstances the knee often unlocks very quickly as the loose body moves to the wider channels of the joint.
- In females, possibly because of the greater valgus angle at the knee, lateral dislocation of the patella is not uncommon, and may be followed by spontaneous reduction. The history may be identical to that of a medial cartilage injury and the diagnosis may depend on the clinical or radiological demonstration of patellar instability.

Arthritis is common in the knee joint and the pain

and stiffness after sitting may be described as 'locking' by the patient. This underlines the importance of finding out exactly what the patient means by this description and not accepting such terms uncritically. Popliteal bursae (Baker's cysts) may form in association with arthritis. They are produced by fluid being forced under high pressure in the joint through a valve in the posterior capsule into the bursa. If these rupture the signs and symptoms produced may be mistaken for deep vein thrombosis (p. 131).

Pain may be referred to the knee, notably from the hip, and in these circumstances the patient is often unable to indicate its site accurately.

Examination

Examination of the ambulant patient starts as soon as the patient walks into the consulting room.

Inspection. The characteristic gait of a stiff knee is immediately evident (p. 281). Provided there is reasonable control of the hip or foot, the patient can walk even when all the controlling muscles in the knee are paralysed, because of the locking mechanism achieved by bracing the knee into extension as the hip is extended.

Abnormalities of posture are most evident from the patient's stance. Sometimes the most difficult problem is to determine when the degree of deformity becomes abnormal. Knock knee, for example, is common in young children but in the majority the deformity corrects spontaneously by the age of 6–8 years. Thenceforth significant valgus deformity is unlikely to correct. Asymmetrical genu valgum is abnormal at any age. In the adult genu valgum deformity may develop secondary to erosive arthritis such as rheumatoid arthritis, while genu varum is often associated with osteoarthritis. Either deformity may be secondary to bony or ligamentous damage in either medial or lateral compartments.

Wasting of the muscles and any swelling of the joint can be more easily assessed in the supine patient.

A large effusion can be observed as a 'horseshoe' swelling immediately above the patella. This delineates the outline of the suprapatellar pouch as it extends a hand's breadth above the upper border of the patella.

Palpation. Tenderness must be accurately localised. Tenderness over the joint lines suggests intra-articular pathology.

Sometimes a loose body can be felt, especially in the suprapatellar region of the joint.

Movement. The normal range in the adult is 0–150° of flexion. In some subjects a few degrees of hyperextension is possible. This is more frequent in females.

An inability to fully straighten the knee joint may occur as a result of quadriceps muscle weakness resulting from wasting secondary to knee pathology.

In its early stages this deformity can be passively corrected by the examiner and is referred to as an *extensor lag.*

A fixed (i.e. irreducible) flexion deformity is referred to as a *flexion contracture* and may occur as a result of an intra-articular block to extension by a torn cartilage or loose body. Sometimes a long-standing extensor lag may be converted into a fixed deformity by the secondary contracture of the posterior capsule and hamstring muscles.

Care must be taken to detect even a few degrees of limitation of extension because this can seriously impair the stability of the joint. When a 'bucket-handle' cartilage tear is displaced, active and passive extension of the knee is blocked. The sensation is of pushing against a firm rubber stop and the knee recoils as soon as the pressure is released. Sometimes difficulty can be encountered in distinguishing between a mechanical intra-articular block and an apparent loss of extension due to spasm of the hamstrings. With the patient prone and the legs projecting over the end of the examination couch, in a true block one heel remains higher than the other whereas with muscle spasm both heels eventually come to adopt the same position (Fig. 9.39).

Effusions. A large effusion can be distinguished from synovial thickening by squeezing the swelling while palpating each side of the patella. This will demonstrate a fluid thrill over an effusion. Furthermore, synovitis usually produces a more boggy thickening associated with local increase in skin temperature.

With a moderate effusion there is sufficient fluid to 'float' the patella off the femur allowing it to be tapped against the underlying condyle. (Fig. 9.40).

A trace effusion cannot be detected in this way but may be demonstrated by the 'massage test' (Fig. 9.41).

Examination

Inspection
❏ Inspect the limb alignment, bony contour and muscle development with the patient erect and

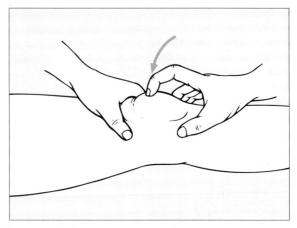

Fig. 9.40 Testing for an effusion by the patellar tap.

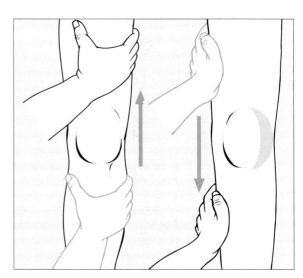

Fig. 9.41 Testing for an effusion by the massage test.

supine. Note signs of erythema and swelling.
❏ In the presence of muscle wasting, record muscle girth at a selected level above the patella (say 10 cm).

Palpation
❏ Palpate the soft tissues, including the full extent of both collateral ligaments, and define any area of tenderness.
❏ With the knee flexed find the medial and lateral joint lines anteriorly and palpate posteriorly throughout their length, noting any tenderness.
❏ Measure genu valgum by recording the distance between the medial malleoli with the patient standing and knees just touching. With genu varum

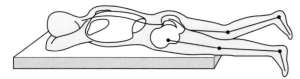

Fig. 9.39 Locked right knee.

measure the gap between the medial condyles of the femur with the feet together.

Movement

❑ With one hand placed on the knee to detect crepitus, ask the patient to flex the knee fully. At the limit of movement check the range of passive movement.

❑ Note any flexion contracture or extensor lag on straight leg raising. To assess any minor limitation of full extension, lie the patient prone with legs supported on the thighs and projecting over the end of the examination couch and observe the level of the heels.

Patellar tap

❑ With the knee extended, empty the suprapatellar pouch by pressure with the palm of the examiner's hand. The increased fluid pressure lifts the patella off the underlying femoral condyle.

❑ With the fingers of the opposite hand, press the patella sharply against the femur to produce a tapping sensation (Fig. 9.40).

Massage test

❑ With the knee straight and the quadriceps relaxed, massage any fluid in the anteromedial compartment of the knee into the suprapatellar pouch.

❑ Then firmly stroke the lateral side of the joint and the suprapatellar pouch with the back or palm of the hand to push the fluid back into the anteromedial compartment (Fig. 9.41).

❑ Observe any fluid impulse on the medial side of the joint.

Tests of stability of the knee

To test the *collateral ligaments* the knee must be fully extended. In this position there is normally no abduction or adduction. A small amount of movement becomes apparent once the knee is slightly flexed and 'unlocked'. When a ligament is strained no movement occurs but pain is localised over the damaged ligament when it is stretched. When a ligament is lax the knee 'opens' when pushed from the opposite side and is felt to close when pressure is released. Lateral instability may also be apparent in an arthritic joint as a consequence of significant erosion of the cartilage.

The *cruciate ligaments* are tested with the knee flexed to a right angle. In this position there is normally a little anteroposterior glide of the tibia on the femur. Movement in excess of this is abnormal. Excessive anterior 'glide' or 'draw' is due to the laxity of the

anterior cruciate, and posterior displacement is associated with laxity of the posterior cruciate ligament.

Gross instability is usually due to laxity of one of the collateral ligaments and vice versa. When there is an isolated tear of a cruciate ligament, with intact collateral ligaments, it is rarely possible to demonstrate an abnormal 'draw sign'. In these circumstances the Lachman test may detect the instability. This test is difficult to perform by those who have small hands, and it is not always possible to say precisely in which direction the laxity is occurring.

Rotary instability. It is now recognised that there are various forms of complex rotary instability of the knee which can develop subsequent to injuries to the cruciate and collateral ligaments. Of these the most common follows rupture of the anterior cruciate ligament. In these circumstances the lateral tibial plateau is subluxed anteriorly beneath the lateral femoral condyle. At about 30° of knee flexion a sudden posterior shift of the tibia occurs with a palpable and often visible reduction of anterior tibial subluxation. This can be demonstrated by a useful test known as

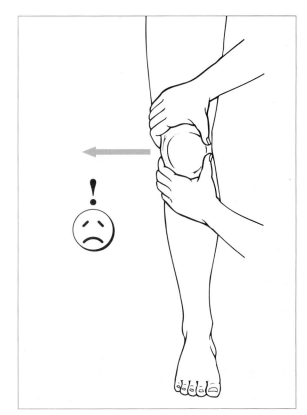

Fig. 9.42 Patella apprehension test.

the lateral pivot shift test or jerk test.

Stability of the patella. Recurrent subluxation of the patella may be associated with genu valgum, joint hypermobility or trauma with wasting of the vastus medialis. Mobility of the patella is best tested with the knee relaxed and flexed to about 30°. If the patella has previously dislocated, the patella apprehension test is usually positive. The attempted lateral displacement of an unstable patella causes the patient great apprehension, and they actively resist further flexion, fearing that it may dislocate (Fig. 9.42).

Stability of menisci. The most commonly performed and best-known test of cartilage integrity is the McMurray test. Although often applied generally to diagnose cartilage lesions, it was specifically intended to diagnose lesions of the posterior horn of the medial meniscus.

Examination

Testing the collateral ligaments
- ❏ With the knee fully extended hold the patient's ankle firmly between the examiner's elbow and side.
- ❏ Use both hands to attempt to abduct and adduct the femur while keeping the knee straight (Fig. 9.43).

Cruciate ligament test
- ❏ Flex the knee and maintain the position by sitting on the patient's foot (Fig. 9.44).
- ❏ With both hands first check that the hamstrings are relaxed, otherwise the test is invalid.
- ❏ Test the anterior cruciate ligament by grasping the tibia below the knee and drawing it forward.
- ❏ Test the posterior cruciate by pushing backwards.
- ❏ Compare the degree of movement in the normal knee with the abnormal side.

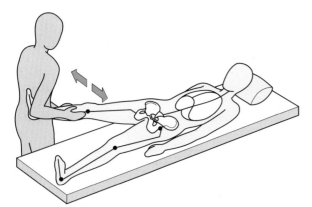

Fig. 9.43 Testing the collateral ligaments of the knee.

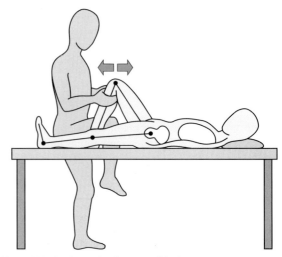

Fig. 9.44 Testing the cruciate ligaments of the knee.

Lachman test
- ❏ Flex the knee to 20°.
- ❏ Firmly grasp the lower end of thigh in one hand and the upper end of tibia with the other.
- ❏ Push the lower thigh in one direction and pull the tibia in the opposite direction, then reverse the direction of action and assess any increased mobility between tibia and femur; (Fig. 9.45).

Pivot shift test
- ❏ Hold the patient's hind foot with one hand.
- ❏ Fully internally rotate the foot and tibia while simultaneously applying valgus stress to the knee joint.
- ❏ Flex the knee from 0° to 30° to detect any palpable or visible reduction between femur and tibia (Fig. 9.46).

Patellar apprehension test
- ❏ With the patient supine and the knee in extension apply pressure against the medial border of the patella.
- ❏ Maintain the pressure while slowly passively flexing the knee to about 30° and assess the degree of lateral patellar movement and note any patient apprehension (Fig. 9.42).

McMurray test
- ❏ To examine the knee, stand on the right side of the couch, if right-handed, with the patient's hip and knee flexed to 90°.
- ❏ Grasp the patient's heel with the right hand and steady the knee with the left hand.

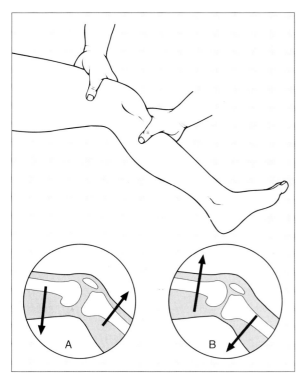

Fig. 9.45 Lachman's test. Showing **A.** No laxity in the anterior cruciate ligament **B.** Posterior cruciate ligament rupture.

☐ Slowly extend the knee with the right hand while palpating the joint line with the left hand, first with the tibia in external rotation then in internal rotation. If positive, a 'clunk' is felt over the

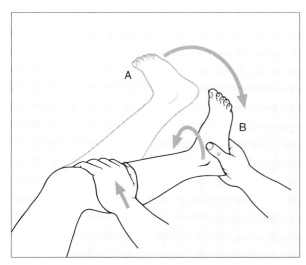

Fig. 9.46 Pivot shift test. While applying an abduction force at the knee and with the ankle internally rotated, flex the knee from A to B.

displacing cartilage and the patient experiences some discomfort.

The leg, ankle and foot

Congenital deformities in the feet are common. Acquired problems also occur frequently. The feet have often to bear the stress of the body weight on hard unyielding surfaces, and may be cramped and confined by fashionable footwear. For these reasons problems are frequently encountered in the feet. Congenital or postural abnormality of the feet may also give rise to altered gait and symptoms at higher levels.

Anatomy

For convenience the foot may be divided into three regions: the hind foot (talus and calcaneus), mid-tarsals (navicular, cuboid and cuneiforms) and forefoot (metatarsals and toes).

The feet placed side by side resemble an inverted soup plate, each foot corresponding to half a plate. The inner border of the foot is raised to form the longitudinal arch. The outer border, corresponding to the rim of the plate, lies on the ground. When the feet are placed together an arch lying across the mid-tarsal region is formed. When not weight bearing a further, but lesser, transverse arch lies under the metatarsal heads. The arches of the feet and their associated ligaments and soft tissues act as shock absorbers when the feet take the weight of the body and give spring to the gait. The flattened outer border gives stability when standing. When the patient is standing the long axis of the talus, navicular, medial cuneiform and first metatarsal normally lie in a straight line.

Normal function of the foot requires a sequence of complex integrated movements at each level; for simplicity of description the major movements are:

- Ankle dorsiflexion and plantar flexion.
- Subtalar joint supination (inverting the calcaneum) and pronation (everting the calcaneum).
- Mid-tarsal joint (talonavicular and calcaneocuboid) supination and pronation. Supination brings the sole of the foot medially and pronation laterally. During supination of the subtalar joint, the mid-tarsal joints become locked and the interosseus ligament of the subtalar joint is tightened. This converts the foot into a rigid lever for propulsion. On pronation of the subtalar joint, the mid-foot can move freely, allowing adaptation of the sole of the foot to the ground.
- Inversion of the whole foot brings the sole of the

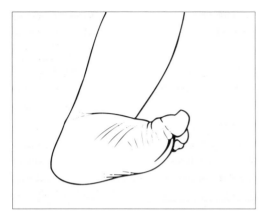

Fig. 9.47 Talipes calcaneus.

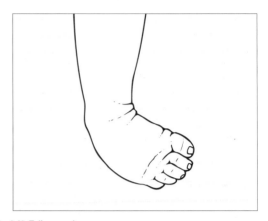

Fig. 9.48 Talipes equinovarus.

foot medially and involves a combination of supination, adduction of the forefoot and plantar flexion. Eversion pronates, abducts and dorsiflexes the foot.
- Forefoot (metatarsophalangeal joints) flexion and extension.

Terms used to describe deformity of the foot and ankle

Talipes is derived from the words talus and pes, implying that there is a deformity involving the ankle and foot, and must be further qualified to have any meaning. *Talipes calcaneus* indicates that the heel is dorsiflexed (Fig. 9.47). *Talipes equinus* means the foot and ankle are plantar flexed, like the foot of a horse which walks on the tip of one 'finger'.

Talipes equinovarus deformity means that in addition the hind foot and mid-tarsal joints are supinated (Fig. 9.48). This is the typical club foot deformity.

Talipes calcaneovalgus, the other common congenital foot deformity, means that the hind foot and mid-tarsal joints are pronated. Valgus deformity may also be acquired (Fig. 9.49).

Pes planus and *pes cavus* are the respective terms used to describe loss and exaggeration of the long arch of the foot. Pes implies deformity of the foot only and that the ankle posture is normal. In practice, pes planus is often associated with pronation of the whole foot (i.e. a talipes calcaneovalgus planus deformity) and pes cavus is usually associated with varus deformity (talipes equinovarus cavus).

Hallux valgus is probably the most common foot

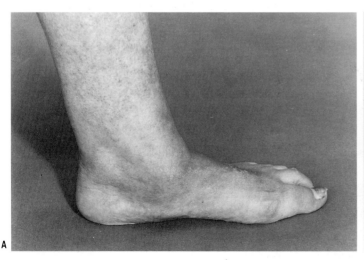
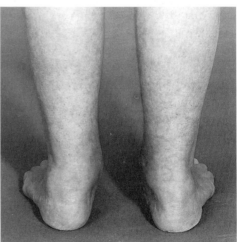

A   B

Fig. 9.49 Pes planus and hind foot valgus deformity in a patient with rheumatoid arthritis.

deformity. In addition to valgus deformity of the phalanges the first metatarsal is often shorter than normal and deviated in the opposite direction, *metatarsus primus varus et brevis*. In *hallux rigidus* the big toe is often longer than the other toes, and because of this develops degenerative change or osteoarthrosis in the metatarsophalangeal joint. Extension is diminished, giving pain and difficulty with 'toe-off' while walking. In extreme instances the toe may become permanently fixed – *hallux flexus*.

Special points in the history

In children, pain in the feet directly related to the musculoskeletal structures is not common. When there is no obvious deformity or inflammatory changes, the cause is usually epiphysitis involving the calcaneum (Sever's), navicular (Köhler's) or the metatarsal head (Freiberg's).

In the adult, pain in the foot or lower leg usually arises locally but may be referred, for example in sciatica. Pain arising in the foot may also be referred up the leg. Special enquiry should be directed at the condition of the feet in elderly patients as severe but remediable disability can be caused by minor abnormalities such as callosities or overgrowth of nail (onychogryphosis).

Osteoarthrosis has the familiar pattern of pain and stiffness after rest which is relieved temporarily by activity. Pain which gets gradually worse the longer the patient is standing suggests chronic ligamentous strain or a postural abnormality of the foot. Inflammatory arthropathy will cause typical early morning exacerbation of stiffness and pain which tends to ease with use. Pain related to ischaemia of the feet may be claudicant in nature and induced by exercise, but ischaemia can also cause distressing rest pain at night (p. 126).

Metatarsalgia (pain in the forefoot). This is a common symptom in any inflammatory arthropathy affecting small joints. The patient often describes the pain as walking on pebbles or on glass. With persistence of joint inflammation, as in rheumatoid arthritis, typical forefoot deformities develop, including hallux valgus, spreading of the forefoot, clawing of the toes and callosities under the metatarsal heads. The callosities develop because the fibro-fatty pad normally present under the metatarsal head is pulled forward under the toes, leaving the metatarsal heads unprotected. Other causes of metatarsalgia are stress fractures (march fractures of the metatarsal shafts) and epiphysitis of the second metatarsal head in adolescence (Freiberg's disease). A pain of burning, tingling character radiating

into the third and fourth toes of the foot suggests a digital neuroma in the cleft between these toes. The patient notices that removing the shoe relieves the pain and on examination there is tenderness between the third and fourth metatarsal heads and sensation is diminished between the toes.

Examination

It is convenient to examine the leg, ankle and foot together.

Inspection. *Footwear.* An abnormality of gait may be suspected or confirmed by irregularities in the pattern of wear on the soles or heels of the shoes or boots; unless patients visit the doctor wearing their newest footwear.

Gait. Stiffness without pain causes little alteration in the gait. Some characteristic locomotor gaits due to foot pathology are shown in Table 9.9.

If hallux rigidus is present, great toe dorsiflexion is restricted and the patient will be unable to toe-off. The patient walks on the outer border of the foot to relieve pain. As a result secondary calluses may develop on the outer border of the foot or lateral metatarsal heads.

Posture. In the presence of a significant equinus deformity the patient may be unable to stand in bare feet without a heel support. This may be because of neurological or muscle disease but occasionally it is simply a result of contracted calf muscles in an individual who normally wears very high-heeled shoes.

Varus deformity of the hind foot may be seen in club foot (talipes equinovarus), juvenile chronic polyarthritis and occasionally in adults with erosive polyarthritis.

Valgus deformity of the hind foot is not uncommon and is associated with pes planus and abduction of the forefoot. Often idiopathic, it also occurs in patients with erosive polyarthritis such as rheumatoid arthritis.

Hallux valgus (Fig. 9.50) will be obvious and may be associated with metarsus primus varus, pes planus and hind foot valgus. If clawing of the toes is present (e.g. as in rheumatoid arthritis) (Figs. 9.50 and 9.51) the toes may fail to make any useful contact with the floor and will be functionally useless. There may also be secondary calluses over the dorsum where the toes

Table 9.9 Some locomotor gaits

Paralytic foot drop	High stepping and flapping
Fixed equinus deformity	High stepping and fixed
Talipes calcaneus	'Peg-leg' – lacking in spring
Hallux rigidus	Foot inverted and supinated
Stiff painful hind foot and fore foot (e.g. RA)	Slow, flat-footed and springless

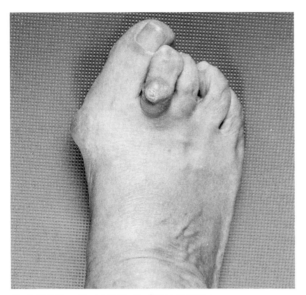

Fig. 9.50 Hallux valgus and clawing of the second toe.

Table 9.10 Some causes of heel pain

- Bruised or jogger's heel
- Plantar fasciitis
- Rheumatoid nodule
- Achilles tendonitis or enthesitis
- Retrocalcaneal bursitis
- Subtalar joint synovitis

joint line. Tendon sheath synovitis is apparent either in the retromalleolar areas or over the anterior aspect of the ankle.

If heel pain is present careful palpation will be required to locate the site of maximum tenderness. There are a number of possible causes (see Table 9.10).

Movement. Movements of the ankle, subtalar joints, mid-tarsal and forefoot joints are examined in sequence to identify whether there is restriction, instability or pain on movement.

Special problems

Achilles tendon. Diagnosis of a ruptured Achilles tendon may be missed because of the pain and swelling at the time of injury and because the foot can still be plantar flexed by the long toe flexors. The signs are:

- A palpable gap in the tendon about 5 cm above the heel
- An inability to stand on tiptoe on the affected foot alone
- A positive calf squeeze test. This is a particularly valuable sign as it is independent of the degree of pain and swelling (Fig. 9.54).

The calf squeeze test also differentiates a ruptured tendo-Achilles from another common calf injury, avulsion of the medial head of the gastrocnemius muscle. If the latter is present, the squeeze test causes local tenderness in the muscle and plantar flexion of the foot. Partial tear of the tendon will be associated with local swelling and tenderness and careful palpation may reveal a small defect in the tendon at the site of the tear.

are rubbing on the shoes. Other deformities include mallet toe (Fig. 9.52), which is due to flexion deformity of the DIP joint of the toe, and hammer toe (Fig. 9.53), in which there is hyperextension of the MTP joint and flexion deformity of the PIP joint of the toe. Mallet toe results in a very painful callus over the tip of the toe and hammer toe causes callosity over the dorsum of the PIP joint.

Indeed the site of any callosity on the sole or dorsum may provide an indication of abnormal pressure.

Palpation. Synovitis of the MTP joint may result in puffiness over the dorsum, splaying of the toes and forefoot and sometimes swelling of the bursae under the metatarsal heads. Compressing the MTP joint will elicit tenderness in the presence of joint synovitis. Generalised swelling of individual toes (dactylitis or sausage digit) is typically seen in psoriatic arthritis and the spondylarthropathies. Mid-tarsal joint synovitis bulges over the dorsum of the foot, subtalar joint synovitis bulges laterally through the sinus tarsi and synovitis of the ankle joint points anteriorly over the

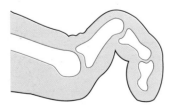

Fig. 9.51 Claw toe.

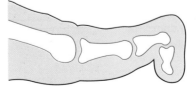

Fig. 9.52 Mallet toe.

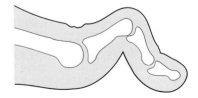

Fig. 9.53 Hammer toe.

Lateral ligament of the ankle. The lateral ligament of the ankle is commonly damaged as a result of an inversion injury. It may be partially or completely torn. It is important to differentiate between these two types of injury because inappropriate treatment of a complete tear may lead to long-term instability of the ankle joint. A complete tear is usually associated with more pain, swelling and bruising than the incomplete lesion. Tenderness in both instances is found over the ligament itself rather than over their proximal or distal bony attachments, which helps in differentiating the injury from a fracture. Stressing the ligament during inversion may reveal increased joint laxity indicating complete rupture (p. 279). The examination may be inhibited by pain, and satisfactory demonstration of abnormal joint laxity usually requires radiography.

Examination

Inspection

❑ Inspect the patient walking.
❑ Inspect the standing patient's feet and ankles.
❑ From behind, note if the calcaneum is in a neutral position with the Achilles tendon in a vertical line, or if there is valgus or varus deformity.
❑ Note the long arch and whether there is pes cavus or pes planus.
❑ If there is pes planus, ask the patient to try to stand on the ball of the feet to determine whether it is correctable.
❑ Note the posture of the toes from the front.

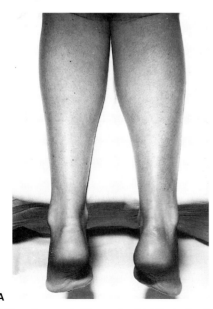

❑ With the patient supine, note the general appearance of the feet, the condition of the nails and skin, the site of any callosities and the presence of swelling.

Palpation

❑ Palpate the hind foot and mid-foot and accurately localise any tenderness.
❑ Palpate the forefoot to localise any tender areas in relation to the MTP and IP joints or the interdigital clefts. Gently compress the forefoot to exacerbate pain arising from these areas.

Movement

❑ Note whether active or passive movements of the ankle or foot joints elicit pain. Examine both feet and note any differences in the range of movement.
❑ Note the active and passive range of movement of the ankle (normally dorsiflexion 10° and plantar flexion 30°).
❑ If dorsiflexion is reduced, eliminate calf tightness as a cause by flexing the knee and re-examining the range of dorsiflexion (Fig. 9.7).
❑ To examine the subtalar joint hold the calcaneum in the neutral position and then passively invert and evert the calcaneum. Fig. 9.56A and B.
❑ To examine the midfoot joints, immobilise the heel with one hand and rotate the forefoot with respect to the hindfoot. Fig. 9.56A and B.
❑ Assess the composite range of movement of the subtalar and midtarsal joints. This is normally 30° of inversion (supination) and 20° eversion (pronation) with 80% of the movement occuring at the subtalar joint.
❑ Note the range of passive extension and flexion of the toes as a group.
❑ Carefully identify any restriction of movement in individual toes (e.g. hallux rigidus).

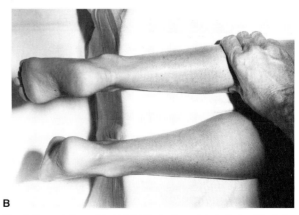

A   **B**

Fig. 9.54 The calf squeeze test for a ruptured Achilles tendon. A. The control position. **B.** Demonstrating an intact left Achilles tendon and plantar flexion of the foot. The apparent wasting is due to compression.

Calf squeeze test

❏ Carefully palpate the Achilles tendon and gastrocnemius muscle and note the presence of tenderness, swelling or any defect in the tendon.

❏ With the patient prone or kneeling, gently squeeze the calf just distal to its maximum circumference. Note whether plantar flexion of the foot occurs. If it does not, the tendon is ruptured (Fig. 9.54).

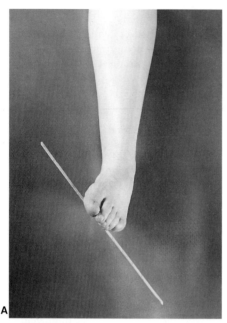
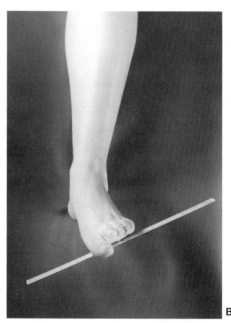

Fig. 9.55 Examining movements of the midtarsal and subtalar joints.   A. Inversion (supination). **B.** Eversion (pronation)

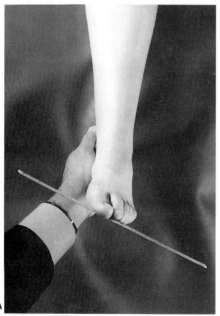
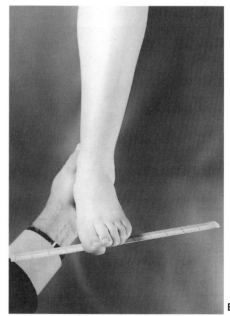

Fig. 9.56 Examining movements of the midtarsal joints.   A. Examiner holds the patient's heel to block subtalar joint inversion. The reduced rate of inversion is due to midtarsal movement. **B.** The examiner holds the patient's heel to block subtalar eversion. The reduced range of eversion is due to midtarsal movement.

KEY POINTS

- Hip disease may present with anterior thigh or knee pain.

- Sacroiliac or spinal disease may present with buttock or posterior thigh pain.

- Flexion deformity of the hip is easily missed unless the Thomas test is performed.

- The commonest hip deformity is flexion, external rotation and adduction.

- Flexion deformity of the hip due to hip disease must be distinguished from that due to femoral nerve irritation or psoas spasm.

- Increase in external rotation at the expense of internal rotation is an early sign of slipped epiphysis of the hip.

- Rotational injuries of the knee are often associated with meniscal tears.

- Asymmetrical genu valgum is abnormal at any age.

- The point of maximal tenderness is important in the localisation of pathology in the knee.

- If a rupture of the Achilles tendon is suspected, the 'calf squeeze test' must be performed.

SCREENING HISTORY AND EXAMINATION

A rapid screening history and examination of the locomotor system can be performed which will identify those joints where a more detailed regional examination is needed.

History

Two simple screening questions are:

- Do you suffer from pain or stiffness in your arms, legs or spine?
- Do you have any difficulty with your normal daily activities such as washing, dressing or walking?

If the answer to either question is yes then further information must be obtained as outlined above (p. 274).

Examination

Gait
- ☐ Observe the patient's gait for rhythm and symmetry on entering the clinic room.

Spine and posture
- ☐ Observe the standing patient's spine and posture from behind and the side. From behind note abnormalities such as spinal scoliosis or valgus deformity of the hind foot, and from the side abnormal kyphosis or lordosis or flattening of the longitudinal arch of the foot.
- ☐ Standing behind the patient and holding the shoulders, ask the patient to look right, left, and then tilt the head sideways aiming to touch each ear on the shoulder.
- ☐ Ask the patient to try to touch the toes without bending the knees and to tilt sideways from the vertical to try to touch the sides of the knees.
- ☐ Note whether a smooth spinal curve develops during these movements or whether there is restriction, protective spasm or scoliosis.

Peripheral joints
- ☐ Examine the upper limb joints with the patient sitting or standing, and the lower limb joints with the patient comfortably supine.
- ☐ Observe right and left limbs simultaneously to provide control comparison.

Upper limbs
Inspection
- ☐ Inspect the hands and upper limb joints for deformity, swelling or other signs of joint disease.

Palpation
- ☐ Palpate the upper limb joints for tenderness or increased warmth.

Movement
- ☐ Ask the patient to open and spread the fingers, close the fingers (power grip), and then to pinch the tip of index finger and thumb (precision pinch) (Fig. 9.57).
- ☐ Compare active with passive if active range limited, and feel power grip and fine pinch.
- ☐ Ask the patient to put their hands together in the position of prayer and then to lower the hands keeping the palms together (Fig. 9.57). This demonstrates the range of dorsiflexion of the wrists.
- ☐ Ask the patient to place the backs of their hands together and to raise their arms upwards. This demonstrates the range of flexion of wrists.
- ☐ Instruct the patient to bend and straighten both elbows simultaneously (0–150°), then with elbows flexed to 90° to turn hands palm up (supination 0–90°) and then palms down (pronation 0–90°).
- ☐ Ask the patient to put both hands behind the head with elbows pointing laterally (abduction and external rotation), then to put the arms down and

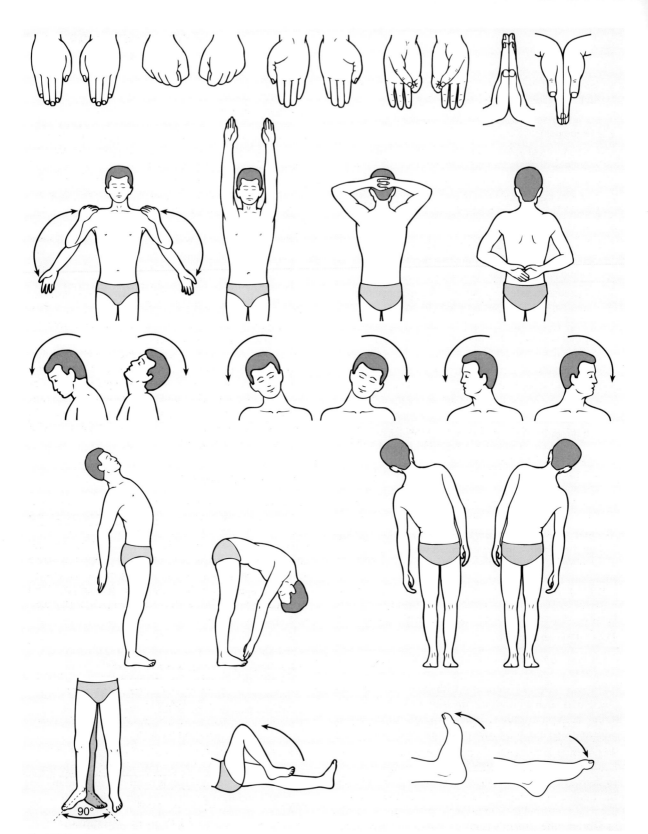

Fig. 9.57 Examination of active movements.

reach up behind the back (extension, adduction and full internal rotation) (Fig. 9.57).

Lower limbs
Inspection
- Inspect the legs and lower limb joints for deformity, swelling or other signs of rheumatic disease. Note the presence of muscle wasting or obvious asymmetry such as leg length inequality.

Palpation
- Palpate the lower limb joints for tenderness or increased warmth.

Movement
- Rotate the hips with the legs extended using the foot as an indicator (90° arc of movement) (Fig. 9.57).
- Ask the patient to flex each knee in turn and observe the range of movement (0–150°) and any signs of pain.
- With the hip and knee at 90° check the range of internal (30°) and external rotation (45°) of the hip.
- Complete hip flexion noting the range (0–120°).
- As the patient straightens each knee place a hand on the knee to feel for crepitus.
- Ask the patient to abduct (variable, minimum 45°) and adduct (25°) the hip.
- Ask the patient to dorsiflex (20°) and plantar flex (30°) each ankle (wide range of normal).
- Passively evert (10°) and invert (20°) the subtalar joints with the ankles in neutral.
- Flex and extend the MTP joints.

If a significant abnormality (i.e. tenderness, pain on movement, swelling, restriction or deformity) is found in any joint, a careful detailed regional examination should be performed.

FURTHER INVESTIGATIONS

In the majority of patients the diagnosis or differential diagnosis will be apparent from the clinical findings. Any further investigations should be carefully selected and interpreted in the light of these findings and used to help to confirm or refute a diagnosis. For example, the finding of a positive rheumatoid factor does not of itself indicate rheumatoid arthritis, and may occur in a variety of other inflammatory or infectious diseases or may be associated with complete normality.

Investigating common syndromes

The acute hot joint

The main differential diagnosis, in the absence of trauma, lies between gout, sepsis, pseudogout and occasionally reactive arthritis. Psoriatic or rheumatoid arthritis should be considered with more chronic and subacute presentations but may also have an acute onset. The most likely diagnosis should be apparent from the clinical information.

The single most useful test is examination of a synovial fluid aspirate for cell count and differential, presence of crystals under polarising light microscopy, or for infection by Gram stain and culture. Radiographs of the joint may provide useful information (see Table 9.11) but degenerative changes may be a coincidental finding and must not deter careful search for other diagnoses (see Table 9.11).

Acute-phase reactants (ESR and CRP) and full blood count will help with the assessment but are not diagnostic. A raised serum urate is suggestive but not diagnostic of gout. Likewise, a normal serum urate does not exclude gout. Abnormal renal function must be identified since it may be the cause of gout or may complicate its management.

Acute or subacute oligoarthritis

Common causes include reactive arthritis or spondylarthritis, psoriatic arthritis and crystal arthritis. Blood count, ESR and CRP will confirm the presence of inflammation, and tests for rheumatoid factor and antinuclear factor will normally be negative. If reactive arthritis is suspected triggering organisms should be sought using serological tests for Chlamydia and Yersinia or stool culture for Salmonella, Campylobacter and Shigella organisms.

Table 9.11 Radiological features in the acute hot joint

Gout	Punched-out juxtarticular erosion only when disease chronic or tophaceous
Pseudogout	Chondrocalcinosis in typical sites (e.g. menisci of knees, triangular cartilage of wrists)
Septic arthritis	Initially normal, later periostitis or bone change due to adjacent focus of osteomyelitis, progressive periarticular osteoporosis, rapid cartilage loss and eventually joint destruction
Trauma	Evidence of recent fracture
Reactive arthritis	Initially normal, later periostitis, and may occasionally progress to cartilage erosion

Polyarthritis

The differential diagnosis is considerable, but the common diagnoses include seropositive or seronegative RA, psoriatic arthritis, SLE and viral arthritides. Blood count and ESR will give a guide to the presence and severity of the inflammatory response, but normal results do not exclude polyarthritis. Radiographs of hands, wrists and feet should be performed to identify whether there is an erosive process (e.g. rheumatoid arthritis). Radiographs are useful even in early disease since they provide a baseline for future comparison and may also reveal unsuspected erosive changes, especially in the feet. Serological tests for rheumatoid factor and antinuclear factor will also assist with diagnosis but must be interpreted in the light of the clinical picture. When the clinical picture suggests SLE, or one of its variants, a number of other investigations including tests for serum complement levels, antibodies against DNA and extractable nuclear antigens may be required.

Low back pain

In patients with chronic low back pain and stiffness of an inflammatory character, ankylosing spondylitis should be considered. Radiographs of the pelvis and lumbar spine should be performed to identify sacroilitis, syndesmophytes and other typical changes. The ESR may be raised or normal. The HLA-B27 tissue type is sometimes performed when the clinical and radiographic findings are equivocal. Absence of the HLA-B27 tissue type makes the diagnosis highly unlikely, but its presence, although suggestive, is *not* diagnostic.

In patients with back pain of a mechanical nature with evidence of nerve root compression, imaging techniques which delineate soft tissues as well as bone may be required. These include myelography or computed axial tomography (CAT) scanning. Although widely used, plain radiographs of the lumbar spine are of limited value.

Commonly used investigations

Plain radiographs

Radiological examination plays a very important part in the further investigation of abnormalities involving the locomotor system. Noteworthy points include the following:

- Radiography is essential for clinical and medicolegal reasons if a fracture is suspected.
- Two views must be taken in planes at right angles to each other to demonstrate the position of the bone fragments.
- Two views may fail to show a crack fracture.
- Fracture of the scaphoid is notoriously difficult to demonstrate even with four views. If clinically suspected, a plaster should be applied and radiography repeated 2 weeks later. The alternative is to carry out a radionuclide bone scan before committing the patient to treatment.
- In children the epiphyseal cartilage may be confused with a fracture, especially in the elbow. Comparable views of the normal joint will help to clarify the situation.
- The extent of injury to soft tissues can be demonstrated by special radiological techniques. For example, if the lateral ligament of the ankle is ruptured, an anteroposterior view of the ankle with the foot held in forced inversion will show the talus to be tilted within the ankle mortice as compared with the normal side. This may have to be performed under anaesthesia.
- If loose bodies are suspected in a joint, special views will often be required, e.g. intercondylar views of the knee.
- Special oblique views may be required for the demonstration of certain joints, particularly in the spine, e.g. the sacroiliac joints in the early stages of ankylosing spondylitis, or to show defects in the pars interarticularis if spondylolysis is suspected.

Synovial fluid examination.

Examination of synovial fluid is helpful in the diagnosis of infective or crystal-induced arthritis or traumatic lesions. The aspirate should be inspected for the colour, turbidity and viscosity.

- Frank haemarthrosis will be obvious and the aspirate may clot.
- Bleeding secondary to inflammation produces a uniformly blood-stained fluid which does not clot and whose colour will depend on how recently the bleeding has occurred.
- Purulent effusions due to infection or other cause of intense acute inflammation will be yellow or green–yellow and opaque.
- Less acute effusions tend to be opalescent and yellow or straw coloured.
- Non-inflammatory effusions are usually pale straw coloured and translucent.

Viscosity can easily be assessed by allowing a drip of synovial fluid to fall from the tip of the hypodermic needle. Low-viscosity inflammatory synovial fluid drips

Table 9.12 Examples of the application of specialist investigations

Damage to intra-articular structures	Arthrography, arthroscopy, MRI
Ruptured Baker's cyst	Ultrasound, arthrography, MRI
Prolapsed intervertebral disc, spinal stenosis, spinal tumours	Myelography, CT scan, MRI
Undisplaced fractures (e.g. scaphoid, neck of femur, stress fractures) or inflammation (e.g. osteomyelitis)	Bone isotope scan
Avascular necrosis of bone	MRI, bone isotope scan
Bone tumours	Bone isotope scan, MRI, CT scan

like water, while high viscosity non-inflammatory fluid forms a long hanging string of syrupy fluid. The synovial fluid should be examined by ordinary light microscopy to obtain a differential white cell count and by polarising light microscopy to identify urate or pyrophosphate crystals, and should be submitted for bacterial culture.

Specialist tests

A detailed discussion of more specialised investigation is outwith the scope of this textbook, but some indications are summarised in Table 9.12. A range of options is available for investigating different conditions and the choice of investigation will depend both on the details of the individual case and on the availability of each technique and local expertise.

METHODS IN PRACTICE

Backache

This example has been chosen mainly because it illustrates one way in which an examination sequence can be integrated in order to cause the patient the minimum inconvenience and to economise on the clinician's time.

History and examination

The characteristics of the backache should be established with particular reference to its site and radiation, any associated symptoms suggesting nerve root compression, exacerbating or relieving factors – especially the effect of rest or activity and any diurnal variation – and impact on activities of daily living. This information should allow distinction to be readily made between inflammatory problems such as ankylosing spondylitis and mechanical backache due to prolapsed

disc or degenerative disease. For example, a young man who complains of chronic low backache radiating to either buttock, with exacerbation of morning stiffness lasting an hour or more, and whose pain is eased by activity is much more likely to have sacroiliitis or early ankylosing spondylitis than a prolapsed lumbar disc. In contrast, the latter condition would tend to cause episodic back pain which is eased by rest, exacerbated by activity and associated with pain or radicular symptoms radiating to one leg.

After taking the history it is necessary to undertake a comprehensive examination to include posture, gait, spinal movements and neurological findings. One effective sequence in a patient with suspected lumbar disc prolapse is described below. When positive findings are encountered the examination should be expanded as appropriate.

Examination

- ❏ Inspect the posture of the patient anterioly, posteriorly and laterally.
- ❏ Check the spinal movements by assessing flexion, extension, lateral flexion and rotation.
- ❏ Observe the gait as the patient walks to the examination couch.
- ❏ With the patient lying supine, stress the sacro-iliac joints and test rotation of the hips (p. 289).
- ❏ Perform straight leg raising, the ankle dorsiflexion test and the posterior tibial nerve stretch test (p. 288).
- ❏ Test the knee and ankle reflexes (p. 231) and observe the plantar response (p. 235).
- ❏ Test sensation from thigh to foot (p. 240).
- ❏ Assess dorsi and plantar flexion of the foot (p. 316).
- ❏ Palpate the pedal pulses (p. 218).
- ❏ Measure the girth of calf and thigh for wasting (p. 307).
- ❏ Observe the patient rolling into the lateral and then prone position.
- ❏ Palpate the spine in the midline for centre and local tenderness. Palpate the asymptomatic and then the painful side for areas of tenderness (p. 287).
- ❏ Perform the femoral nerve stretch test either in the lateral position or preferably with the patient prone (p. 289).
- ❏ Only if necessary, check the authenticity of the sciatic stretch test by asking the patient to sit on the side of the couch and perform a flip test (p. 289).
- ❏ Check for muscle weakness by asking the patient to walk on heels and then tip-toes.

❏ Perform a general medical examination looking for relevant features such as for lymphadenopathy and for signs of malignancy. Perform a rectal examination to assess anal sphincter tone and to exclude local neoplasia (p. 186).

Interpretation of the findings

The history combined with the clinical signs will establish the diagnosis or indicate what further investigations are required. In the majority there may be few or no positive findings, for example in osteoarthritis, spondylolistheses, spinal stenosis, early ankylosing spondylitis and early malignancy. In the minority there may be a plethora of clinical signs, for example in the presence of a prolapsed intervertebral disc, an abscess or an advanced malignancy. They will each present a consistent and anatomical pattern.

In all cases the probable diagnosis should dictate the appropriate investigations to be performed, if any. For example while plain radiographs and the ESR are helpful in ankylosing spondylitis, CT scan or myelography will be needed in spinal stenosis, or radionuclide bone scan and calcium biochemistry in suspected malignancy.

The psychologically distressed patient or the malingerer may also produce a wealth of clinical signs, often easily recognised by their bizarre nature and inconstant and non-anatomical pattern. The affect of the patient with hysterical conversion is one of indifference while the malingerer is on the defensive and often aggressive. In the latter the typical history is one of prolonged continuous pain, even at rest, unaccompanied by any deterioration in general health.

H. Simpson

10

The infant and child

General considerations

In previous chapters the emphasis has been on the acquisition of history-taking and examination skills in the adult. It is usually easier to learn standard methods of approach in adults and then to adapt or modify them to take account of differences and variations that occur within infancy and childhood. Some of these are listed in Table 10.1.

In this chapter it is assumed that preliminary experience has been gained with adults. The main emphasis will be placed on differences in approach to history-taking and eliciting physical signs peculiar to, or of special significance in, infancy or childhood.

Age periods

It is convenient to divide infancy and childhood into the following age periods:

Infancy	First year of life
Neonatal period	First month of life
Childhood	1–18 years
Pre-school child	1–4 years
Schoolchild	5–18 years

INTERVIEW SETTING

The introduction made to the parents and the child is important. A warm and friendly greeting does more than anything else to allay anxiety and promote confidence. A complimentary remark and a few words of conversation appropriate to the child's age, about school, sports, hobbies, etc., may help achieve the empathy essential for cooperation in the physical examination. Young children are usually eager to look at picture books or play with the toys which should be available in the interview room. The history may then be obtained without too much interruption.

Older children may give the history unaided but they also often prefer to let a parent (usually mother) give the history and contribute only when questioned directly or if they disagree with the account.

The limitations of obtaining a history through an intermediary must be appreciated.

- Parents may describe their interpretation of events rather than what occurred.
- They may also fail to recognise misinterpretations which children put on words. For example, a young child may generalise from past experience and use a phrase such as 'sore tummy' to describe any pain or discomfort.
- Misunderstandings may be created by previous medical advice. For example, a fever may have been attributed to 'otitis' or 'tonsillitis'. Parents may thereafter regard all other pyrexias as due to these causes, even when unsupported by other features.

It is easier to see how misunderstandings arise than it is to prevent them. Uncritical acceptance of a parent's interpretation of the child's symptoms must be avoided.

Careful questioning and a shrewd appreciation of the degree of insight which parents have into the child's symptoms will enable the doctor to place such information in the appropriate perspective.

THE HISTORY

The following approach is directed mainly towards infants and young children. It may require to be modified as appropriate for the age and sex of the patient and for the reason for seeking medical advice.

Begin by noting the child's age, date of birth and sex and the source of referral. These details have usually been entered in the hospital records. Record also the name and status of the informant (mother, father, relative, social worker, etc.) and, where appropriate, any help required from an interpreter.

Presenting complaint and present history

The parent should be encouraged to tell the story without unnecessary interruption. The history may be initiated by such questions as 'When did Mary's problem start?' followed by 'Tell me what has happened since then'. If difficulties arise in dating the onset it may be helpful to ask 'When was she last completely well?' and to proceed from there.

Obtaining a thorough chronological account of

Table 10.1 Some aspects of history-taking and examination peculiar to children

- The history is generally obtained from a second person
- The cooperation of the child cannot be taken for granted
- The predominant impact of disease may be on growth and/or development
- The expression of disease may be influenced by the child's growth and developmental status
- Clinical norms may be different from those in adults
- Clinical signs of disease may differ from those in adults with respect to occurrence, interpretation and significance

events without interruption is ideal but seldom possible. Intrusions may be necessary to avoid overemphasis on one aspect of the history or to clarify parental interpretation of events.

Once the account of the illness has been obtained, further specific questions may be required to amplify and clarify the parents' description. For example, if vomiting has occurred its amount and frequency should be ascertained. Is it effortless, forceful or projectile? Is it bile or blood stained?

Similarly, when pain is the dominant symptom, enquiry must be made about its characteristics (p. 29). The younger the child, the less precise the details will be concerning the location, nature and severity of pain. An inconsolable infant with episodic screaming should be suspected of being in pain although the site may not be apparent. Ask about associated symptoms; otherwise associations and important negative information may be missed. For example, the diagnostic possibilities are influenced by whether or not abdominal pain is an isolated symptom or is associated with vomiting, diarrhoea, constipation or abdominal distension. Enquiry should also be made about similar symptoms or illnesses affecting other family members or children in the same class at school.

Systemic enquiry

A brief system review will ensure that relevant information has not been overlooked. Its nature depends in part on the age of the child concerned. It is always useful to enquire about:

- general activities
- appetite and bowel habit
- micturition
- sleep routine
- behaviour.

The child's behaviour and ability to relate to peers, siblings and other family members may be extremely relevant. When the main problems are behavioural or emotional, it may be best to first discuss sensitive issues in the child's absence.

The nature and extent of systemic enquiry will depend on individual circumstances. It is helpful to consider symptoms in relation to the various body systems:

1. Alimentary:
   - appetite, feeding, vomiting
   - diarrhoea, constipation
   - screaming attacks (or abdominal pain)
   - jaundice, weight loss

2. Respiratory:
   - discharge from nose, eyes or ears
   - sore throat or earache
   - cough and its nature
   - respiratory noises (wheeze, stridor, grunting, snoring)
   - apnoeic or cyanotic episodes
3. Cardiovascular:
   - breathlessness
   - tiredness and lethargy
   - slow feeding, poor weight gain
   - pallor or cyanosis
4. Genitourinary:
   - urinary incontinence (having previously been dry)
   - increased urinary frequency
   - pain on micturition, abdominal pain
   - change in odour and appearance of urine
   - urine stream in boys
   - fever
5. Central nervous:
   - changes in activity, mood, behaviour
   - school performance
   - headaches or disturbance of vision
   - abnormalities of posture, gait or coordination
   - 'fits' (include a detailed description)

Previous history

The child's age and presenting symptoms will influence the emphasis placed on different aspects of the previous history. In general this will include the following.

Mother's health during pregnancy. The maternal account may require to be supplemented from the general practitioner's and antenatal records. Relevant points include:

- illness or accident suffered during pregnancy
- threatened miscarriage
- contact with rubella or other infections
- medication, drugs, smoking and alcohol consumption
- nature of employment
- genetic counselling
- screening or diagnostic procedures undertaken (chorionic biopsy, amniocentesis, ultrasound examination)
- toxaemia and antepartum haemorrhage.

The manner of birth. This may have a profound effect on subsequent health and development. Mothers may not remember exact details and precise information may have to be obtained from the obstetric records regarding the following:

- the nature and duration of labour
- mode of delivery
- need for resuscitation at birth
- gestation and birth weight.

Neonatal period. Information should be sought about the neonatal period. Relevant points include:

- breathing difficulties and blueness
- feeding difficulties, vomiting, jaundice
- convulsions, or any other specific symptoms
- admission to a neonatal intensive care unit (NICU) for mechanical ventilation, parenteral nutrition, etc.
- special treatment required, for example antibiotics, oxygen therapy or phototherapy
- vitamin K prophylaxis; include the dose given and the route.
- weight gain.

Post-neonatal. Relevant points relating to feeding problems in the early months include:

- breast, bottle or both
- type, composition, volume and frequency of artificial feeds
- the age at which solids were introduced
- age of full mixed feeding
- use of vitamin supplements or a special diet
- problems relating to appetite, feeding and growth.

Previous illnesses. In addition to asking about the nature, date, duration and severity of any previous illnesses or operations, specific enquiry should be made about the following:

- previous measles, rubella, pertussis, mumps and chicken pox
- recent contact with infectious illnesses
- history of allergic disease and details of any suspected allergic response to drugs, for example penicillin.

Immunisations. Procedures (primary and boosters) should be recorded, referring when necessary to pre-school health surveillance records.

Residence abroad.. A history of periods of residence abroad or of recent travel introduces the possibility of imported diseases including tuberculosis, malaria and typhoid fever.

Developmental milestones. Knowledge of normal developmental milestones is important in the diagnosis and evaluation of suspected neurodevelopmental disorders. Enquiry will depend on the background history, the child's age and individual circumstances. If there are no apparent problems, simple questions may suffice:

- Has there been admission to a special care baby unit (SCBU)?
- Has there been concern about early development, school placement and progress?

If neurodevelopmental delay is suspected from the history, more detailed questions are required relating to gross motor development, vision and fine movement, language and social/adaptive functioning. Enquiry should be made about the ages at which the following skills or milestones of development were attained:

- smiling, head control, fixing and following
- sitting alone, crawling, standing, walking
- the result of the 8-month hearing test
- utterance of single words and hearing ability
- ability to use a cup and spoon
- ability to comprehend and obey simple commands
- undressing without help
- ability to identify different parts of the body.

Between 2 and 4 years speech facility increases, motor function develops more fully, e.g. walking up and down stairs, and the ability to dress with supervision and to give name and sex is attained. The ages at which the child became invariably dry by day and during the night should be noted. Similar information is required for bowel control and any special difficulties in toilet training. Progress at school, including the child's ability to mix with other children, academic ability and any special aptitudes are also relevant.

Family history

Ascertain the ages, present state of health, past health and possible consanguinity of the parents. With adopted children any available medical history of the natural parents should be obtained as this may be very relevant (e.g. epilepsy or tuberculosis). Illness in other close relatives should also be noted. The ages and sexes of other children in the family and the occurrence of any stillbirths or miscarriages should be noted. The past and present illnesses of siblings and any deaths that have occurred may provide important clues (see Table 10.2).

It is helpful to construct a family tree that includes first-degree relatives, namely parents and siblings

Table 10.2 Some examples of relationships between death of siblings and illness

Genetic conditions	Cystic fibrosis
	Inborn errors of metabolism
	(may present as 'cot deaths')
	Immune deficiency states
	Muscular dystrophy
	Neurodegenerative disease
Infections	Tuberculosis
	HIV
Social	Child abuse
	Drug abuse
	Malnutrition from poverty

(Fig. 10.1). In genetically determined conditions, specific enquiries about second- and even third-degree relatives may be necessary.

Social history

This embraces the home, the school and the provision for play and recreation. It is frequently the most important part of the history, particularly in infants and pre-school children and in those with chronic disease or handicap. Adverse factors influence the life of the child and the family. Social problems should be identified and also the level of support available. The parents' occupations, smoking and other habits, attitudes to each other and to their children, domicile, neighbourhood, financial means, whether living together or apart and whether isolated or supported may all be relevant. Equally important may be the care for the child if the parents work, the size and conditions of the home and the number of occupants and any special environmental circumstances of possible physical or psychological significance, e.g. parental smoking, dampness or frequent changes of domicile.

A knowledge of pets in the home and recent contact with animals may be relevant, for example asthmatic attacks may be precipitated by inhaled animal dander, and lymphadenopathy or unexplained fever may be due to toxoplasmosis.

Many disorders of the child have a psychological basis, commonly but not exclusively related to poverty or deprivation. An appreciation of the financial and other stresses at home and school, the ability of the parents to cope, and the child's intelligence and capacity for survival are all relevant. Certain provoking situations occur (see Table 10.3).

Summary

It is helpful to précis the main points in the history at this stage, taking account of any concerns about the intelligence and reliability of the informant. These impressions guide the approach to the clinical examination. For example:

Informant – mother: well informed and perceptive:

Helen is a 3-year-old girl with a history of recurrent cough and wheeze from the age of 6 months, when she was admitted to hospital with a severe chest 'infection'. Her symptoms are usually precipitated by upper respiratory infections and tend to be worse at night-time and in the winter months. She has been admitted to hospital twice in the past 3 months with severe wheeze and breathlessness. These symptoms have usually responded to treatment with beta-2 agonists. Her father has asthma, an older sibling hay fever and a 6-month-old brother infantile eczema. In other respects she has been healthy. Birth, history, growth and developmental progress have been normal and she has been fully immunised. There are no adverse social factors.

Impression: Bronchial asthma. The original illness may have been acute bronchiolitis.

Table 10.3 Examples of stress-provoking situations

- A new baby in the home
- The death of an immediate relative
- Absence of one or other parent
- First attendance at school
- Change of school class or new teacher
- Bullying at school
- Change of residence to another district
- Learning difficulties
- Lack of, or excessive, parental control

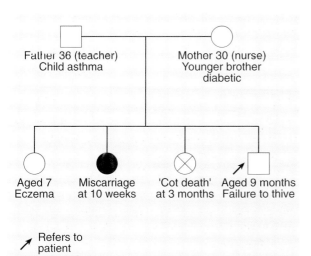

Father 36 (teacher)
Child asthma

Mother 30 (nurse)
Younger brother diabetic

Aged 7
Eczema

Miscarriage
at 10 weeks

'Cot death'
at 3 months

Aged 9 months
Failure to thrive

Refers to patient

Fig. 10.1 A family tree.

KEY POINTS

- The potential limitations of obtaining a history through an intermediary should be appreciated.

- The younger the child the less precise will be the description of symptoms, e.g. the nature, location and severity of pain.

- Knowledge of normal developmental milestones is important in evaluating a history. It is part of the history when neurodevelopmental disorders are suspected.

- The social history is frequently the most important part of the history, particularly in pre-school children and in those with chronic disease or handicap.

THE PHYSICAL EXAMINATION

GENERAL APPROACH

The scheme of examination of children is broadly similar to that adopted in adults in spite of the difficulties and differences peculiar to infants and young children. There is no all-embracing technique appropriate to every situation. The patient may be an inconsolable infant, a toddler clinging to his mother and burying a tearful face in her lap at the slightest approach of the examiner, a defiant 5-year-old boy who will resist all attempts to remove any clothing, particularly trousers, a hyperactive child intent on destroying toys and furniture or an apprehensive schoolgirl who just retains her self-control during questioning but recoils in terror when a sphygmomanometer or ophthalmoscope is produced. In contrast, many children cooperate fully without being alarmed in any way. Understanding, sympathy, patience, and at times finesse and subtlety, enable most problems to be overcome. Adolescents should be treated sensitively and their desire for privacy fully respected.

GROWTH MEASUREMENTS

The most useful measurements of physical development in infancy and childhood are weight and height. Accurate measurements and precise recording are essential as clinical impressions can be misleading. Recording these measurements on centile charts provides information on whether height and weight are within the normal range for age and sex. Special charts are available for children aged 0–1 (Fig. 10.2A), 1–3 (Fig. 10.2B), and 5–18 (Fig. 10.3). When a problem with growth is suspected, measurements noted in the Child Surveillance records will often indicate the previous pattern of growth – further sequential measurements provide additional information about natural growth or the effects of treatment.

Weight

A comparison between actual and expected weight should be routine in any examination. Expected weight according to age can be roughly estimated in a number of ways, or may be determined more accurately from tables. In the early weeks of life the average infant should gain approximately 30 g per day after the tenth day, at which time the birth weight should have been regained. Thus at 6 weeks the expected gain in weight would be almost 1 kg. By 5 months of age the birth weight should have doubled, and by a year it should have trebled (Fig. 10.2). For the next few years the expected weight in kilograms can be estimated from the formula: age in years plus 4, multiplied by 2. However, the average is not necessarily the normal; the normal weight for a child of small parents may be well below the average. Changes in weight of the individual child are more significant.

Length

Length is the other valuable parameter of growth. It can be measured as standing height in toddlers and older children and as crown-heel length in infants. Average heights from birth to 18 years are shown in Figures 10.2 and 10.3. The same considerations concerning 'normal' and 'average' apply as with weight.

A correlation normally exists between height and weight. A knowledge of the expected weight for any particular height and any dissociation between these measurements may be important. In hypothyroidism, for instance, height may be reduced and weight normal. In a malnourished child height may be normal or reduced to a lesser degree than weight, whereas in obesity due to an excessive calorie intake both height and weight are increased.

Head size

The occipitofrontal circumference is recorded routinely

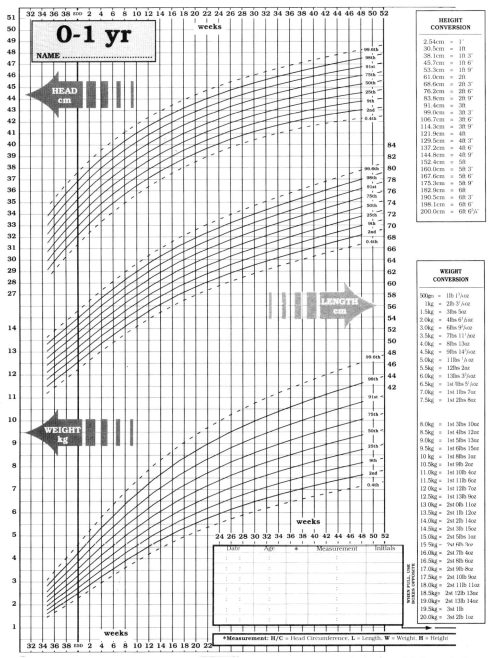

Fig. 10.2A Charts for recording length in cms, weight in kgs and head circumference in cms (or boys aged 0–1 years). The measurements for girls are also available and are very similar (By permission of the Child Growth Foundation).

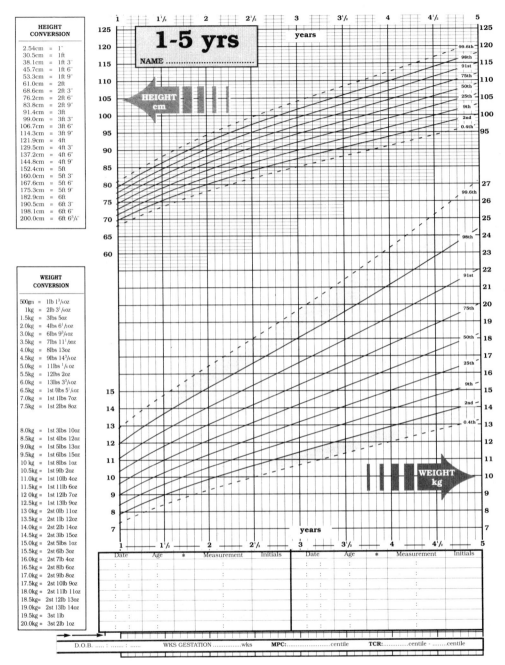

HEIGHT CONVERSION

2.54cm	= 1"
30.5cm	= 1ft
38.1cm	= 1ft 3"
45.7cm	= 1ft 6"
53.3cm	= 1ft 9"
61.0cm	= 2ft
68.6cm	= 2ft 3"
76.2cm	= 2ft 6"
83.8cm	= 2ft 9"
91.4cm	= 3ft
99.0cm	= 3ft 3"
106.7cm	= 3ft 6"
114.3cm	= 3ft 9"
121.9cm	= 4ft
129.5cm	= 4ft 3"
137.2cm	= 4ft 6"
144.8cm	= 4ft 9"
152.4cm	= 5ft
160.0cm	= 5ft 3"
167.6cm	= 5ft 6"
175.3cm	= 5ft 9"
182.9cm	= 6ft
190.5cm	= 6ft 3"
198.1cm	= 6ft 6"
200.0cm	= 6ft 6³/₄"

WEIGHT CONVERSION

500gm	= 1lb 1³/₄oz
1kg	= 2lb 3¹/₄oz
1.5kg	= 3lbs 5oz
2.0kg	= 4lbs 6¹/₂oz
3.0kg	= 6lbs 9³/₄oz
3.5kg	= 7lbs 11¹/₂oz
4.0kg	= 8lbs 13oz
4.5kg	= 9lbs 14³/₄oz
5.0kg	= 11lbs ¹/₄oz
5.5kg	= 12lbs 2oz
6.0kg	= 13lbs 3³/₄oz
6.5kg	= 1st 0lbs 5¹/₄oz
7.0kg	= 1st 1lbs 7oz
7.5kg	= 1st 2lbs 8oz
8.0kg	= 1st 3lbs 10oz
8.5kg	= 1st 4lbs 12oz
9.0kg	= 1st 5lbs 13oz
9.5kg	= 1st 6lbs 15oz
10 kg	= 1st 8lbs 1oz
10.5kg	= 1st 9lb 2oz
11.0kg	= 1st 10lb 4oz
11.5kg	= 1st 11lb 6oz
12 0kg	= 1st 12lb 7oz
12.5kg	= 1st 13lb 9oz
13 0kg	= 2st 0lb 11oz
13.5kg	= 2st 1lb 12oz
14.0kg	= 2st 2lb 14oz
14.5kg	= 2st 3lb 15oz
15.0kg	= 2st 5lbs 1oz
15.5kg	= 2st 6lb 3oz
16.0kg	= 2st 7lb 4oz
16.5kg	= 2st 8lb 6oz
17.0kg	= 2st 9lb 8oz
17.5kg	= 2st 10lb 9oz
18.0kg	= 2st 11lb 11oz
18.5kg	= 2st 12lb 13oz
19.0kg	= 2st 13lb 14oz
19.5kg	= 3st 1lb
20.0kg	= 3st 2lb 1oz

1-5 yrs

years

NAME ....

HEIGHT cm

WEIGHT kg

years

Date	Age	*	Measurement	Initials	Date	Age	*	Measurement	Initials

D.O.B. ..... : ..... : .....   WKS GESTATION ....wks   **MPC:**.....................centile   **TCR:**............centile - ....centile

Fig. 10.2B Charts for recording height in cms and weight in kgs for boys aged 1–5 years. The measurements for girls are also available and are very similar. (By permission of the Child Growth Foundation).

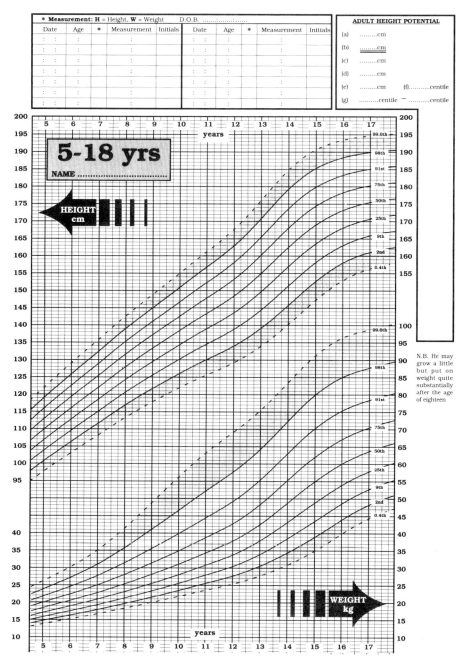

Fig. 10.3A Chart for recording height (in cm) and weight (in kg) for boys aged 5–18. (By permission of the Child Growth Foundation).

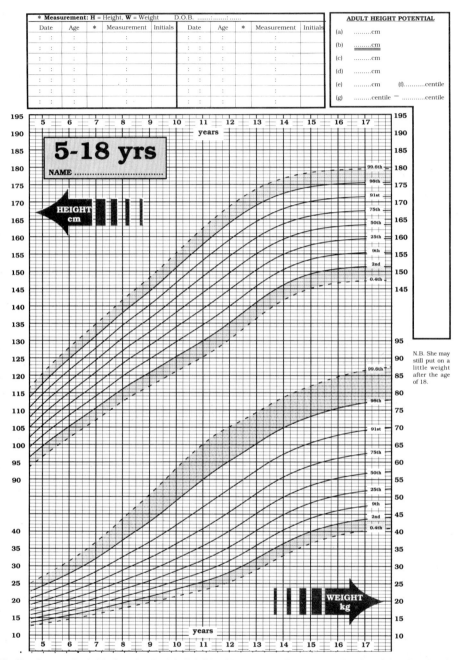

Fig. 10.3B **Chart for recording height (in cm) and weight (in kg) for girls aged 5–18.** (By permission of the Child Growth Foundation).

in infants and young children. It is measured by a non-stretch tape from the frontal bones (just above the eyes) in a horizontal plane. Variations in this, above and below normal, may have considerable significance in respect of childhood disease. Values for different ages are given in Table 10.6.

Pubertal development grading

This is not assessed routinely but may be of crucial importance when problems of growth and maturation are suspected in later childhood. The stages of physical sexual development, related to age and sex, are given in Table 10.4. For each of the indices considered, stage 1 is fully infantile and stage 5 fully adult. Only stages 2, 3 and 4 need be remembered.

PRELIMINARY OBSERVATIONS

The examination starts with the first contact with the child and parent(s). These impressions are reinforced during history-taking by observation of the child's appearance, general demeanour, state of alertness, play activities, speech, posture and perhaps gait. The interaction between child and parent should be observed. Some parents dominate the situation and may constantly correct the child or demand inappropriately high standards of conduct and behaviour. At the opposite extreme, others make no attempt to control their child's actions. By the time the history has been completed, most children should have accepted the examiner's presence and may be showing signs of trust and friendship.

Guidelines

1. Allow young children, particularly toddlers, time to take stock of their surroundings. If kept occupied and interested while the history is being taken, they are usually ready for attention when it has been completed.
2. Establish rapport with the mother before starting the examination. Children are quick to sense any lack of empathy between parent and doctor.
3. Infants under 6 months may be examined lying supine. Those over 6 months and very young children are best examined sitting or lying on their mother's laps.
4. Many pre-school children are happy to be examined standing or lying supine. The mother should remain in close attention if the child shows any signs of apprehension.
5. Undressing may require to be gradual and staged. It is not appropriate to undress children completely as a preliminary step.
6. A relaxed unhurried approach is essential. Let the child handle instruments, such as the stethoscope, or 'blow out' the oroscope light, to distract attention from the examination.
7. Examine with warm hands. If necessary, also warm the head of the stethoscope before applying it to the child.

General examination

Certain observations are made without disturbing the child. The facies and expression may reveal whether the child is well or ill, relaxed or apprehensive, at ease or in pain. An impression is gained about the child's growth, development, nutritional status and hydration. The breathing rate is best counted by observing movements of the abdomen and the pulse rate counted at the wrist while the child holds the parent's hand. Table 10.5 lists some additional information that may be gained by careful observation of the head and face (see also Figs. 10.4 and 10.5). The presence of bruising, skin rashes or blemishes, e.g. *café au lait* spots may also be apparent.

A systematic approach to examination is seldom possible in very young or ill children. Information is gleaned as the opportunity presents, and examination proceeds from one area to another without rigorous adherence to 'system'. During examination the following guidelines are helpful:

- Observation always precedes palpation, percussion and the use of the stethoscope.
- Speak quietly to the child before touching and explain what you are doing.
- Examine by region and not by system.
- Talk to, and indicate how, the parent may help.
- Be gentle at all times.
- Be continually aware of the child's response.
- Pause immediately if the child becomes upset or cries.
- Improvise when necessary to ensure cooperation.
- Do not lose the opportunity to examine the sleeping infant or young child.
- Leave any uncomfortable procedures until the end. These include examination of the ears, mouth, throat and hips.
- Be prepared to postpone the examination in fractious children.

Table 10.4 Physical sexual development: centile distribution of ages at which the stages of puberty occur (2+ indicating that stage 2 is reached but not yet stage 3). The centile values are the reverse of what might be expected. Thus the 97th centile represents the early age limit at which only 3% of children will show this feature and 97% have yet to do so. (Courtesy of Dr John Buckler)

Boys: genital development
Stage 1 Preadolescent: the testes (< 3 ml), and proportions as in early childhood.
Stage 2 Enlargement of the scrotum and testes (> 5 ml). Skin of scrotum reddens and changes in texture. Little or no enlargement of penis.
Stage 3 Lengthening of the penis. Further growth of the testes and scrotum
Stage 4 Increase in breadth of the penis and development of the glans. The testes and scrotum are larger; the scrotum darkens.
Stage 5 Adult.

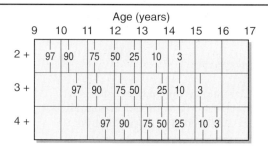

Boys: pubic hair
Stage 1 Preadolescent
Stage 2 Sparse growth of slightly pigmented downy hair chiefly at the base of the penis.
Stage 3 Hair darker, coarser and more curled, spreading sparsely over junction of pubes.
Stage 4 Hair adult in type, but covering a considerably smaller area than in the adult. No spread to the medial surface of the thighs.
Stage 5 Adult.

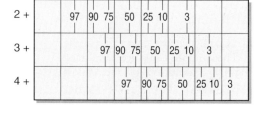

Girls: breast development (See Fig. 3.41, p. 80)
Stage 1 Preadolescent: elevation of papilla only.
Stage 2 Breast bud stage. Elevation of the breast and papilla as a small mound. Enlargement of the areola diameter.
Stage 3 Further enlargement and elevation of the breast and areola, with no separation of their contours.
Stage 4 Projection of the areola and papilla above the level of the breast.
Stage 5 Mature stage, projection of the papilla alone due to recession of the areola.

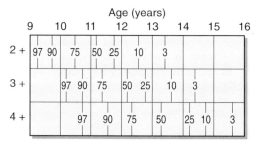

Girls: pubic hair
Stage 1 Preadolescent.
Stage 2 Sparse growth of slightly pigmented downy hair chiefly along the labia.
Stage 3 Hair darker, coarser and more curled, spreading sparsely over junction of pubes.
Stage 4 Hair adult in type, but covering a considerably smaller area than in the adult. No spread to the medial surface of the thighs
Stage 5 Adult.

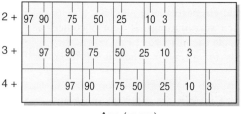

Menarche

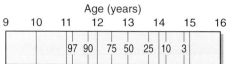

Table 10.5 Head and neck

Area	Observation	Abnormality	Associations
Cranium	Size and shape	Plagiocephaly Microcephaly Brachycephaly Scaphocephaly Oxycephaly Hydrocephalus	Prematurity Mental retardation Down syndrome Sagittal suture stenosis Coronal suture stenosis Neural tube defect
	Hair	Loss Coarse, plentiful Dry, brittle Low line posteriorly White forelock	Acrodermatitis entero- pathica Mucopolysaccharidosis Hypothyroidism Turner syndrome Waardenberg syndrome
	Fontanelles	Delay in closure Premature fusion Depression Tense, bulging	Raised intracranial pressure Rickets Impaired brain growth Dehydration Meningitis
	Sutures	Premature fusion Separation	Craniostenosis Raised intracranial pressure
	Bones	Bossing Craniotabes Maxillary prominence Bruit	Rickets Prematurity Thalassaemia major A–V malformations
Ears	Setting	Low set	Pierre Robin syndrome
	Development	Dysplastic	Potter syndrome
	Configuration	Malformations Tags	Renal abnormalities, hearing defects Treacher Collins syndrome
Face	Expression	Anxiety, fear 'Dead pan'	Emotional status Neuromuscular abnormality
	Movements	Asymmetrical Involuntary	Facial nerve palsy Tics
	Appearance	Characteristic grouping of abnormalities	Down syndrome
	Forehead	Prominent, narrow receding, bossed	Varied

Table 10.5 (cont'd)

Area	Observation	Abnormality	Associations
Eyes	Setting	Mongoloid slant Ante-mongoloid slant	Down syndrome Treacher Collins syndrome
	Interpupillary Distance	Hypertelerism	Oesophageal abnormality
	Lids	Epicanthic folds Periorbital oedema	Down syndrome Nephritis, nephrosis
	Conjunctiva	Colour	Jaundice, osteogenesis imperfecta
	Iris	Aniridia	Wilms' tumour
	Lens	Opacification	Galactosaemia
	Cornea	Cloudiness	Mucopolysaccharidosis
	Movements	Squint	Raised intracranial pressure Intraocular diseases
Nose	Shape	Depressed ridge	Hypothyroidism
	Alae nasi	Movements	Chest infection
	Nostrils	Discharge	Infection
	Mucosa	Pallor	Allergy
Lips	Appearance	Swelling Fissuring, ulceration	Allergy Infection, e.g.candidiasis
	Colour	Pale Blue	Cyanotic congenital heart disease Anaemia
Jaw	Size	Small	Cleft palate
Mouth	Size and shape	Small oral cavity	Dehydration
	Mucosa	Dryness Ulceration Adherent 'curd' Koplik spots	Down syndrome Herpes simplex infection Candidiasis Measles
	Tongue	Macroglossia	Glycogen storage disease
	Gums	Bleeding	Gingivitis
	Teeth	Number, shape, size, colour, caries	Various
	Tonsils	Redness	Tonsillitis
	Oropharynx	Swelling and redness	Pharyngitis

Table 10.6 Average head circumference

Age	Cm	Inches	Age	Cm	Inches
Birth	35.0	13.8	6 years	51.2	20.2
3 months	40.4	15.9	7 years	51.7	20.3
6 months	43.4	17.1	8 years	52.0	20.4
9 months	45.2	17.8	9 years	52.2	20.6
12 months	46.4	18.3	10 years	52.5	20.7
18 months	47.7	18.8	11 years	52.9	20.8
2 years	49.0	19.3	12 years	53.4	21.0
3 years	49.6	19.5	13 years	53.8	21.2
4 years	50.0	19.7	14 years	54.1	21.3
5 years	50.7	20.0	15 years	54.8	21.6

One standard deviation from these averages is approximately ± 2¹/₂%

KEY POINTS

- The most useful measurements of physical development in infancy and childhood are weight and height. A comparison between actual and expected weight should be routine in any examination.

- An opportunistic approach to examination in very young or ill children is often necessary. Examine by region rather than system.

- Leave any uncomfortable procedures until the end of the examination.

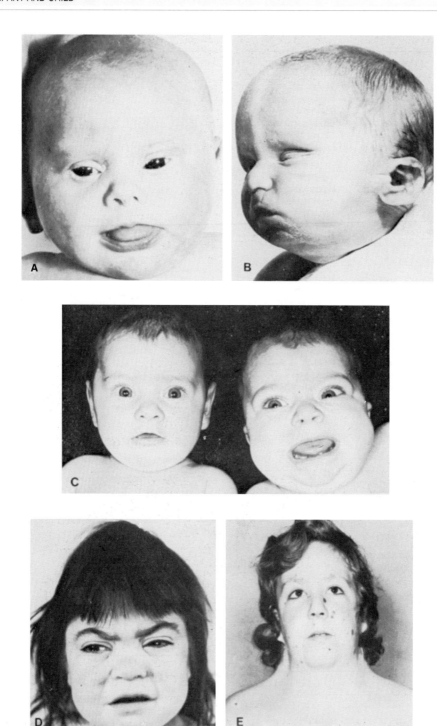

Fig. 10.4 The face as a diagnostic aid. A. Down syndrome – palpebral fissures sloping laterally upwards and elongated prominent protruding tongue associated with a small mouth. **B.** Renal agenesis – small jaw, flattened nose, low-set ears. **C.** Cretin right with normal twin left – large tongue, coarse features, bloated cheeks and double chin due to myxoedematous change. **D.** Mucopolysaccharidosis – wide nose with depressed bridge, prominent supraorbital ridges and eyebrows. **E.** Webbing of the neck in Turner's syndrome. Pigmented naevi are also present.

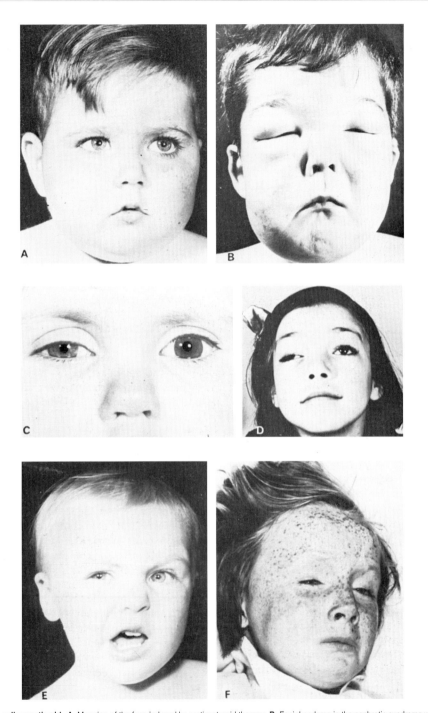

Fig. 10.5 The face as a diagnostic aid. **A.** Mooning of the face induced by corticosteroid therapy. **B.** Facial oedema in the nephrotic syndrome with periorbital involvement almost preventing opening of the eyes. (Courtesy of Professor Gavin Arneil.) **C.** Right-sided Horner's syndrome – smallness of the pupil (miosis), enophthalmos and a narrow palpebral fissure. **D.** Ptosis (more marked on the right side) in myasthenia gravis. **E.** Left-sided facial palsy. **F.** Risus sardonicus in tetanus; marked freckling of the skin.

EXAMINATION OF SYSTEMS

Although the examination may have been opportunistic the presentation should be orderly, beginning with general observations.

For ease of presentation, the examination of the various systems is described separately although the physical examination is often undertaken on a regional basis.

Cardiovascular system

Infants and young children are best examined sitting on their mother's knees. Significant heart disease is usually associated with failure to thrive. Many children with Down syndrome have congenital heart disease, and some other syndromes are associated with specific cardiac lesions (see Table 10.7).

General inspection

Questions to consider on general inspection include:

- Does the child look ill or undersized?
- Is the breathing rate increased?
- Is there grunting or wheezing?
- Is the child blue around the lips or the extremities? Is central cyanosis present?
- Is there flushing of the face, sweating or clubbing of the fingers and toes?

Clubbing may not be apparent before 6 months of age even when cyanosis has been obvious since birth.

Inspection of the chest

Inspection of the chest may be very valuable. For example:

- Asymmetric prominence of the left anterior chest wall may indicate cardiac enlargement.
- A thrusting apical impulse is characteristic of left ventricular hypertrophy.
- Pulsation at the lower left sternal border or xiphisternum suggests right ventricular hypertrophy.

Table 10.7 Various syndromes with specific heart disease

Turner syndrome	Coarctation of the aorta
Noonan syndrome	Pulmonary stenosis
Williams syndrome	Aortic stenosis and pulmonary stenosis
Down syndrome	Atrial septal defect, ventricular septal defect, etc.

- A right thoracotomy scar is often due to a previous shunt procedure with an accompanying continuous murmur and weak brachial pulse on the same side.
- A left thoracotomy scar may be a sequel to previous correction of coarctation, ligation of a patent ductus arteriosus, banding of the pulmonary artery or a more complex procedure.
- A midline incision is evidence of previous cardiac bypass surgery.

Palpation

Up to the age of 3 the apex beat is usually palpable in the fourth left interspace just outside the mammary line. Thereafter it is within the mammary line in the fifth or sixth interspace. The apex may not be palpable in infants and young children unless the heart is enlarged. Sometimes one or both heart sounds are also palpable. A palpable second sound in the pulmonary area suggests increased pulmonary arterial pressure. A systolic thrill at the lower left sternal edge suggests left ventricular septal defect, at the apex mitral incompetence, at the upper right sternal edge aortic stenosis, and at the upper left sternal edge pulmonary stenosis or patent ductus arteriosus. A thrill in the suprasternal notch may accompany aortic stenosis or less often pulmonary stenosis or coarctation of the aorta.

Auscultation

Provided the room is quiet and the child reasonably still, the heart sounds are easily heard. The first heart sound is single and the second is generally split, with widening of the two components during inspiration and narrowing during expiration. The two components are usually of equal intensity. Splitting is best heard at the second left intercostal space. A third heart sound at the apex may be common in normal infants and young children. The presence of murmurs – site, timing and quality, intensity, propagation and variations with positional change – should be noted. Most murmurs in children are innocent; they are not accompanied by thrills and tend to disappear more readily with changes of position than organic murmurs. In distinguishing between innocent and organic murmurs, account must be taken of the child's overall state of health and other physical findings. There are several varieties of innocent murmurs:

- Still's murmur: a musical vibratory low-pitched systolic murmur, best heard at the mid- or lower left sternal edge.

- A basal ejection systolic that is high-pitched and blowing at the upper sternal border (left or right). This usually disappears when the patient is upright.
- Carotid bruit: a short high-pitched blowing systolic murmur heard in the neck and confined to early systole.
- Peripheral pulmonary artery branch stenosis murmur: a blowing high-pitched ejection systolic murmur audible in the early months of life in the pulmonary area and over the back.
- Venous hum. In the sitting or erect position it is a low-pitched humming systolic/diastolic murmur in the infraclavicular area (right > left). It is usually absent in the supine position and is abolished by occluding the veins in the neck.

Over 90% of pathological murmurs are attributable to relatively few cardiac conditions. The characteristics of murmurs associated with common congenital heart defects are summarised in Table 10.8. Any propagation to the axilla (mitral incompetence), neck (aortic stenosis) or back (coarctation of the aorta, pulmonary stenosis) should be noted.

Percussion

Percussion of cardiac borders is sometimes useful in children in determining heart size but does not distinguish between left and right ventricular hypertrophy. An increased area of cardiac dullness indicates cardiac enlargement or a pericardial effusion.

Examination

Inspection
- ☐ Look for visible pulsations, chest deformities and scars.
- ☐ Locate the apex beat with the child sitting and leaning forward.

- ☐ Confirm the presence of left or right ventricular heaves.
- ☐ Identify its nature and note any palpable heart sounds.
- ☐ If a thrill is palpable localise its site of maximum intensity using light pressure with the palm of the hand or fingertips.

Auscultation
- ☐ Auscultate early in the examination while the child is cooperative.
- ☐ Use the technique described for adults (p. 103).

Pulses

Many normal children have sinus arrhythmia, and sometimes extrasystoles. The average resting pulse rate ranges from about 120/min in infants to 80/min in older children. There is a wide variation in normal values at all ages. In suspected congenital heart disease the pulses should be palpated for rate, rhythm, quality and amplitude.

- The brachial pulses are best palpated simultaneously using the thumbs.
- The femoral arteries are most easily felt if the hips are abducted and extended.
- Brachial and femoral pulses should be palpated simultaneously; absence, weakness or delay in femoral pulsation suggests coarctation of the aorta.

Arterial blood pressure

Blood pressures should be measured at the arms and, when appropriate, the legs. The auscultatory method is usually easy in children over the age of 3. Cuff dimensions are important – a ratio of 2:3 (cuff width to upper arm length) is necessary. A cuff that is too narrow will produce spuriously high blood pressure and vice versa (Table 4.23 p. 97).

Table 10.8 Murmurs associated with some congenital heart defects

Lesion	Nature of murmur	Maximum site	Other features
Ventricular septal defect (VSD)	Harsh Pansystolic	Lower left sternal edge	Mid-diastolic mitral valve flow murmur
Pulmonary stenosis (PS)	Harsh Ejection systolie	Second left intercostal space	Ejection click may be present
Aortic stenosis (AS)	Harsh Ejection systolie	Second right intercostal space or apex during early childhood	Ejection click Radiating to neck
Atrial septal defect (ASD)	Blowing Ejection systolie	Second left intercostal space	Parasternal lift Fixed splitting S2 Mid-diastolic tricuspid valve flow mumur
Patent ductus arteriosus (PDA)	Continuous	Second left intercostal space and under left clavicle	Collapsing peripheral pulses

In infants palpation of the pulse distal to the occluding cuff provides an approximation of the systolic pressure. The flush method is useful in small infants.

Examination

The flush method

☐ Apply a cuff of appropriate size round the upper arm or thigh.
☐ Blanch the area distal to the cuff by squeezing or by wrapping an elastic bandage around it.
☐ Inflate the cuff then release the compression of the limb.
☐ Deflate the cuff slowly; flushing corresponds to a value approximately that of the mean systolic pressure.

The Doppler ultrasonic method is now widely used. This combines a small ultrasound transducer with earphones and a sphygmomanometer. Cuff dimensions remain critical.

Average blood pressure readings (mmHg) in infants and children are as follows:

> Newborn 60 (flush method)
> Infancy 80/55 (auscultation)
> Pre-school child 90/60 (auscultation)
> Schoolchild 100/65 (auscultation).

Venous blood pressure

The level of the distended jugular vein above the suprasternal notch when the child is at a 45° angle is a measure of venous pressure in older children. In infants and young children the neck tends to be short and fat and the method unhelpful. Cannon waves may be seen in the neck in infants with congenital heart block, and excessive pulsation when tricuspid incompetence is present.

Extremities

- Central cyanosis is usually indicative of cyanotic congenital heart disease.
- Oedema of the legs is characteristic of right ventricular heart failure in older children and adults.
- In infants and young children, peripheral oedema is more likely to affect first the face, then the presacral area and eventually the legs.

In common with liver and splenic enlargement, limb oedema is a late sign of cardiac failure in infancy and childhood and is usually preceded by wheezing, grunting, tachypnoea or tachycardia.

KEY POINTS

- General observations provide crucial information about growth, nutrition and signs of respiratory distress.
- In potentially fractious young children auscultate the praecordium when the opportunity arises.
- Most murmurs in children are innocent.
- A cuff that is too narrow will produce spuriously high blood pressure and vice versa.
- Enlargement of the liver and peripheral oedema are late signs of right heart failure in infants and young children.

Respiratory system

General considerations

- Age, behavioural state (sleep/wakefulness), level of cooperation and posture are important considerations in evaluating the respiratory system in children.
- At birth the chest is roughly circular in cross-section. The ratio of the anterior to the transverse diameter falls gradually to the adult value of 0.75 by the age of 3 years.
- Breathing movements are mainly abdominal in infants and young children, with little apparent chest movement. Abdominal distension may cause considerable respiratory embarrassment by restricting the movement of the diaphragm.
- In young infants breathing may be somewhat irregular and periodic in pattern with apnoeic pauses up to 10 seconds a normal occurrence.
- The average sleeping respiration rate varies widely, falling from about 45 per minute in the newborn to 30 per minute at a year, 20–25 between 1 and 5 years and 20 by the age of 10.

Inspection

The younger the child the more one is likely to gain from observation than from percussion and auscultation.

Palpation

Tracheal deviation is unreliable as a clinical sign in young children.

Examination

☐ Before examining the chest, note any pallor, flushing or cyanosis. Remember that cyanosis is a late sign of hypoxaemia during the course of acute respiratory illnesses.

☐ Count the respiration rate by watching abdominal movements and observe the pattern of breathing.

☐ Look for conjunctival suffusion, any discharge from the nose or ears, and listen carefully for respiratory 'noises' (wheeze, stridor, grunting, snoring), and cough.

☐ Note any signs of respiratory distress – increased respiration rate, head bobbing, flaring alae nasi, difficulty in speaking, restlessness and anxiety, use of accessory muscles in the neck and indrawing (suprasternal, supraclavicular, intercostal and subcostal).

☐ Note any chest deformity (pectus carinatum, funnel chest, Harrison's sulci or scoliosis), hyperinflation or asymmetry of chest movements.

☐ Check the degree and symmetry of chest movements, and for palpable wheeze.

☐ Identify the apex beat and the position of the trachea in older children.

Auscultation

The technique for auscultation is similar to that in adults (p 155). Normal breath sounds in infants and children are often more intense and expiration more prolonged than in adults, giving the mistaken impression of bronchial breathing. They are often described as bronchovesicular. In young children with lower respiratory tract infection, for example pneumonia, the sequence is also different. Instead of the adult respiratory cycle (inspiration, expiration, pause) expiration is followed immediately by inspiration and then the pause (inspiration, pause, expiration). Confusion in timing may arise unless the abdominal inspiratory movements are observed during auscultation.

• If breath sounds are harsher on one side of the chest than the other, the harsher side is probably normal.

• Accompaniments related to localised pathology may be heard on both sides as sound is readily transmitted through the chest wall of the young child.

• Do not confuse any localised sounds present with transmitted noises from the upper respiratory tract.

• Note any area of bronchial breathing and the nature of any accompaniments (crepitations, wheeze, pleural rub).

• Check vocal resonance, especially when consolidation, collapse or pleural effusion is suspected.

Remember that extensive lung disease may be present in infancy without obvious chest signs on auscultation.

Percussion

In young children it is sometimes less disturbing to auscultate before percussing the chest. Percussion requires familiarity with the surface markings of the lungs and their lobes. It may be helpful in detecting diminution of cardiac dullness when the chest is overinflated, or dullness due to consolidation, collapse or a pleural effusion.

KEY POINTS

• Observation is very important at all ages.

• Tracheal deviation is unreliable as a clinical sign in young children.

• In young or ill children it is sometimes less disturbing to auscultate before percussing the chest.

• If breath sounds are harsher on one side of the chest than the other, the harsher side is probably normal.

• Extensive lung disease may be present in infancy without obvious chest signs on auscultation.

Alimentary system

In young children it is best to leave the examination of the mouth, tongue, teeth and gums to the end. Abdominal examination is usually carried out when the patient is supine and relaxed. This may not always be possible. The young infant may be examined on mother's lap, while feeding or sucking the teat. In the toddler age group the abdomen may be examined for tenderness and masses while the child sits facing mother with the legs straddling her lap. Alternatively, many young children cooperate best when placed supine with the head and body on mother's lap and the legs supported by the examiner seated facing the mother (Fig. 10.6). The abdomen can then easily be examined and in addition the genitalia, perineum, anus and even the lower back inspected simply by flexing the hips and exposing the child's bottom. In fractious infants do not lose the opportunity to examine the abdomen if the child is lying temporarily quiet in the prone position. This may provide the only opportunity to confirm the diagnosis of intussusception. The abdomen cannot be examined adequately while a child is crying.

Inspection

Examination

❏ Observe the size and contour of the abdomen. It may be distended or scaphoid.
❏ Note movements with respiration, the state of the skin, the presence of visible peristalsis, umbilical hernia (common in the first 2 years of life), sepsis, distended veins and any groin swelling.
❏ Inspect the genitalia.

Palpation

Remember:

• If abdominal pain has been present the child should be asked to point to the area most affected and to indicate whether the pain has moved.

• Position yourself at the appropriate level, either by kneeling or sitting, at the cot-side. Place a hand (previously warmed) flat on the abdomen.
• Light palpation, especially for the spleen, is more informative than deep palpation.
• Start remote from the site of any pain.
• Look at the child's face during palpation.

The technique of palpation does not differ from that in the adult (p. 175–180). The liver is normally palpable 1–2 cm below the right costal margin in the first 2 years of life. In older children an enlarging spleen becomes palpable in the left hypochondrium and enlarges towards the right iliac fossa, while in infancy it is more laterally placed and enlarges towards the left iliac fossa. The kidneys can sometimes be felt by bimanual palpation in normal children and especially in the newborn. The bladder, when distended, is felt as a rounded pyriform swelling in the suprapubic region. A full bladder can interfere with palpation (Fig. 10.7). Other masses of varying size, site and consistency may also be felt. Faeces may be palpable along the descending colon. Mesenteric nodes may be felt. Tumours, such as those due to neuroblastomas and Wilms' tumour, are likely to be easily felt. The soft sausage-shaped tumour of an intussusception in the right upper quadrant may be difficult to feel. It may be associated with a detectable emptiness in the right iliac fossa.

When congenital hypertrophic pyloric stenosis is

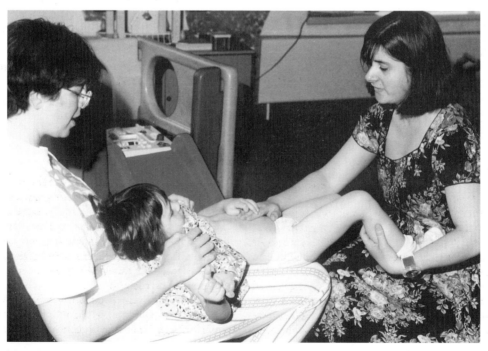

Fig. 10.6 A useful examination position.

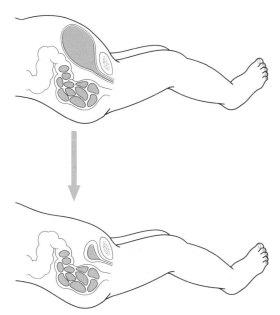

Fig. 10.7 Palpation of the abdomen Other structures may be rendered inpalapable by a full bladder.

suspected a pyloric tumour must be sought. The infant is best examined when feeding though the tumour may be most easily felt when the stomach is empty immediately after vomiting.

Examination

Pyloric tumour
- Sit on the infant's left.
- Place the left hand flat on the abdomen, the fingers directed towards the right hypochondrium with the tips below the liver edge and lateral to the rectus muscle.
- The tumour, which tends to harden intermittently, can be felt by gentle depression of the tips of the fingers.

For swellings in the groin, it is important to distinguish between herniae, lymph glands, cryptorchidism and hydrocele in boys.

In examining for suspected maldescent of the testes, start in the inguinal area and work downwards towards the scrotum. This avoids the testes being pushed upwards during examination or being retracted due to a brisk cremasteric reflex. Note any abnormalities of the penis but remember that the foreskin may not be retractile before the age of 2–3 years. In females any vaginal discharge, labial adhesions or hypertrophy of the clitoris should be noted. The need for more detailed examination will depend on clinical circumstances. In both sexes pubertal changes may be apparent.

Percussion

Light percussion from tympanic to dull areas may help to confirm enlargement of liver and spleen and define the nature of any abdominal mass present. It is essential in detecting shifting dullness (p. 180).

Auscultation

Tinkling or cracking bowel sounds are normal. They will be accentuated when there is increased peristalsis and diminished or inaudible in the absence of peristalsis. It is unnecessary to perform rectal examination routinely. It is, however, essential in children with acute abdominal pain and in any cases of suspected sexual abuse. Observation may reveal irritation, fissuring or prolapse of the anus. When indicated, rectal examination should be performed by slowly inserting the little finger and then noting muscle tone, character of stools, tenderness or the presence of masses.

KEY POINTS
- The abdomen cannot be examined adequately while a child is crying.
- Always enquire about pain before palpating the abdomen.
- Look at the child's face while examining the abdomen.
- Remember to examine the hernial orifices when intestinal obstruction is suspected.
- In boys check that the testes are in the scrotum.

Nervous system

Examination of the nervous system in cooperative school-age children can be conducted with the same precision as in the adult (Ch. 7). In infants and young children the central nervous system has not fully developed and full cooperation is not possible. Eliciting neurological signs requires a modified and flexible approach which makes demands on the examiner's patience, sensitivity and skill.

It is conventional to document the findings starting with general observations and then in turn the cranial nerves, motor and sensory function and tendon and superficial reflexes. In practice, the procedure may have to be varied as circumstances permit.

Inspection

During history-taking, unobtrusive observation of the young child's activities, alertness, attention span, creativity and demeanour provide clues about intelligence, development status and emotional maturity.

General inspection may also help in other respects. Abnormalities of growth, head size or shape may provide important clues of neurological abnormality. Observation of the hair, nails and skin can sometimes give diagnostic information, for example depigmented areas of skin in tuberous sclerosis. Similarly, disturbance of breathing rate or pattern may indicate brainstem abnormalities or neuromuscular weakness. Asymmetry of growth or hemihypertrophy suggests the presence of neurological disorder.

Posture and movements

Relevant questions include:

- What position does the child adopt voluntarily?
- Is posture appropriate for age?
- Is there local or general limitation or asymmetry of movements? Clear hand or foot preference before the age of 3 may indicate a defect on the other side.
- Is there obvious peripheral nerve damage – facial palsy, wrist drop of Erb's palsy?
- Are there involuntary movements of the trunk, limbs, face or eyes?
- Is there unsteadiness while sitting or walking and any incoordination in reaching for toys?
- Is the gait abnormal – broad-based and unsteady (ataxic), stiff-legged (spastic), scissoring (diplegic) or accompanied by an outward fling of the leg with paucity of ipsilateral arm movements (hemiparetic)?

Cry and speech

The cry may be high-pitched, as in cerebral birth injury or meningitis. Delay in the onset of speech may indicate deafness, lack of stimulation or educational subnormality. The intelligibility and quality of speech should be noted. The range of vocabulary and language and the reading and writing ability give further indication of mental and cerebral function status.

Conscious level

This may be impaired in such disorders as meningitis,

encephalitis, post-epileptic states and cerebral palsy. Assessment of the unconscious child is similar to that in adults .

Cranial nerves

The cranial nerves can be examined with reasonable thoroughness even in very young children.

Cranial nerve I. Specific appreciation of smell does not develop until later childhood.

Cranial nerve II. Vision is probably present at birth.

- At about 4 weeks infants will watch their mother.
- By 6 weeks they will follow moving objects but the arc of visual movement will not be more than 90°.
- By 8 weeks they will fix, converge and focus.
- By 12 weeks the arc of movements will be approximately 180°.

Thus, by 6–8 weeks defects in visual perception and from 12 weeks disordered eye movements begin to be evident. The ability of the young child to follow or pick up very small objects is a rough indication of visual acuity. Visual fields are more difficult to test – a rapidly approaching object (the examiner's hand) from either side at eye-level will elicit a blink if the temporal fields of vision are normal. In 4- to 5-year-olds finger counting can be used: the child is asked to hold up the same number of fingers as the examiner. After that age quantitative perimetry may be used to define any defect present. Examination of the fundus may reveal a wide range of disc and retinal abnormalities (optic atrophy, retinopathy of prematurity, haemorrhages, etc.) (see p. 267–9).

Cranial nerves III, IV and VI. A full range of eye movements depends on the integrity of these nerves. In infancy, horizontal and vertical movements can be assessed by spinning the infant through 360° of arc and by tilting the vertically held infant in a semiprone position. In late infancy, the ability to follow attractive objects in vertical, horizontal and diagonal directions can be tested, and the presence of nystagmus noted.

Strabismus (Squint). Squint is a common problem. A certain amount of transitory squinting occurs in the early weeks of life. Squinting after that age is always significant.

- Paralytic (non-concomitant) squint. The paralysed eye will constantly fail to move in one or more directions when a slowly moving light is being followed. Thus, the angle between the axes of the eyeballs will vary according to the direction in which the child is looking. For example, in paralysis of the right VI nerve, the squint will be evident on looking to the right and will disappear when looking straight ahead or to the left.

- Non-paralytic (concomitant) squint. Here the two eyes maintain the same relative position in whatever direction the child looks. Squinting is not necessarily persistent and may be more obvious at the end of the day when the child is tired.
- Convergent or divergent squint. Ocular alignment can be assessed from the relationship of the pupillary light reflection to the centre of the pupil.

The light reflections are normally symmetrical and placed slightly nasal to the centre of the pupils. With a convergent squint the light reflection is displaced slightly temporal to the centre of the pupil on the affected side – displacement is nasal with a divergent squint. The most accurate test to measure defects in alignment of the eyes is the cover test (p. 262). The pupillary response depends on the integrity of the II and III cranial nerves.

Cranial nerve V. Facial sensation can be tested in infants and children. Light touch and response to pain can be tested using a silver of cotton wool and the straight end of a paper clip (not a sharp pin) respectively. The corneal reflex may be elicited as in adults (p. 216) or by blowing gently into the child's eyes. Its absence may result from sensory (cranial nerve V) or motor (cranial nerve VII) deficit. Testing in the latter situation results in lacrimation. Muscle power (temporalis, masseter, pterygoids) is easily tested in older children.

Cranial nerve VII. Facial symmetry is not uncommon in young children but may indicate weakness of the VII cranial nerve. In cooperative children, test as in adults (p. 218).

Cranial nerve VIII. Testing of hearing is vital in early infancy as corrective measures at that stage can result in normal speech development. Hearing can be assessed crudely in early infancy by observing the response to a loud auditory stimulus presented to one or other ear. In the newborn period hearing loss may be detected using an acoustic cradle which measures the motor responses of the baby to auditory stimuli. It is not yet a routine screening method but can be applied to babies at high risk of deafness. These include:

- positive family history
- low birth weight
- birth asphyxia or severe neonatal jaundice
- intrauterine infection
- malformation of ears or face.

The *distraction test* is a screening procedure carried out in 7- to 8-month-old infants by health visitors (Fig. 10.8).

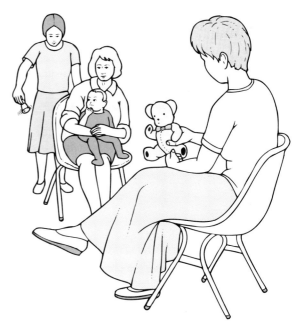

Fig. 10.8 The distraction test to assess hearing.

Examination

Distraction test

- ❑ Sit the child on the mother's knee, with the distractor in front of the child, and a third person who performs the test standing behind the child.
- ❑ Engage the child's attention by holding up an attractive object.
- ❑ Make a test sound about 3 feet from the baby at the same level as the ear while the distractor notes the child's reaction.
- ❑ Repeat the test on each side using high- and low-frequency sounds.

A variety of performance tests can be used in children who either fail the distraction test or are judged to be at increased risk of deafness, for example post meningitis or head injury. In a young child the ability to repeat numbers whispered close to each ear separately indicates at least some hearing ability. At school entry, the 'sweep' test is widely used for auditory screening. Parents' views on children's hearing ability may be very valuable.

In testing vestibular function check carefully for nystagmus. Avoid lateral extremes of gaze; the object to be followed should be held at 30° from the midline on each side.

Cranial nerves IX and X. When these nerves are intact there will be normal palatal movements and an intact gag reflex; swallowing will be normal. Inspiratory stridor may be a sign of peripheral nerve damage to the X cranial nerve, causing weakness of vocal cord abduction.

Cranial nerve XI. An asymmetrical head posture may indicate unilateral weakness of the sternomastoid muscle. The head will tilt away from, and the face towards, the affected side.

Cranial nerve XII. The movement of the tongue and any associated fasciculation, wasting or tremor may be observed directly.

KEY POINTS

- Clinical observation is of crucial importance in detecting neurological dysfunction.
- Early detection of squint is a prerequisite to successful corrective measures.
- Testing of hearing is vital in infancy as corrective measures at this stage can result in normal speech development in the deaf.

Motor system

Muscle tone. Posture may suggest abnormal muscle tone, particularly in infants, for example the frog-like position in generalised hypotonia. Hypotonia will be indicated by softness of the muscles, floppiness on handling or excessive joint laxity, or by hand flapping to assess 'passivity'. With hypertonia excessive firmness of the muscles and stiffness in movements of the limbs may be apparent, for example thigh adductor spasm in spastic diplegia.

Muscle power. Muscle power may be inferred by observing children at play. Loss of power is deduced from lack of activity or limitation of movement without obvious cause. In cooperative children, power can be assessed systematically in the limbs, neck and trunk.

Examination

Testing tone
- ❏ Handle the child to obtain a general idea of muscle tone.
- ❏ Stretch the muscles slowly to detect rigidity, i.e. an increased tonic stretch reflex, and then more quickly to detect spasticity – an increased phasic stretch reflex.

Testing power
- ❏ Start by inspecting for any wasting, asymmetry or hypertrophy.
- ❏ Compare one side with the other.
- ❏ Allow the child to make the movement that requires testing, then try to overcome it.
- ❏ Grade any weakness detected using the MRC scale (Table 7.16, p. 231).

In young children a simple screening assessment includes wheelbarrow manoeuvres to assess proximal upper limb power, or a 'tug-of-war' competition to assess more distal power. For the lower limbs, walking on toes or heels tests may detect distal impairment; proximal weakness is tested by stepping, hopping or Gower's sign. This is positive when the child is unable to rise from the floor without 'climbing up' the lower limbs.

Movements. These can be assessed actively and passively. Careful examination of infants and children while they are relaxed and quiet and again when they are moving will help to differentiate various forms of movement disorders. In general, spasticity becomes more marked when a child runs, whereas extra-pyramidal signs lessen. A decreased swing of an arm may indicate a mild hemiparesis. A waddling gait may be due to weakness of the pelvic girdle musculature, and disinclination to walk a sign of pain.

The ability to maintain a stable postural base depends on normal extrapyramidal function and can be tested by asking the child to stand with the feet together, hands outstretched and fingers separated. Involuntary movements (tremor, choreoid, athetoid) may be obvious and may be exacerbated by closing the eyes or opening the mouth. Dinner fork posturing of hands, hyperpronation of forearms extended above the head, and trombone-like movements of the tongue may be observed in Sydenham's chorea. The Fog test is useful in demonstrating associated movements – walking with both feet in the varus position may be associated with supination of the upper limbs, while walking on the heels may lead to dorsiflexion of the upper limbs.

Fine movements can be tested by asking the child to carry out specific tasks, for example picking up small objects, rapidly alternating pronation and supination of the hands, or making piano-playing movements of the fingers.

Cerebellar function. This can be assessed by looking for:

- *Ataxia.* Test the ability to walk in a straight line.
- *Intention tremor.* Revealed by finger-to-nose testing.

- *Nystagmus.* Accompanied by muscular hypotonia.
- *Reduced reflexes.*

Sensation

Conditions associated with sensory impairment in childhood include peripheral neuropathy, meningomyelocele and Friedreich's ataxia.

- Sensation is difficult to test reliably and consistently in infants and young children.
- Most children over 3 years will cooperate for testing of peripheral modalities including light touch, temperature, pinprick, vibration and movement of the joints.
- Testing of cortical function becomes possible in children over 5.

Reflexes

Tendon reflexes. Tendon reflexes may be elicited at all ages. Care must be taken in positioning the limbs correctly with some muscle stretch (p. 231). Any increase or decrease in resting muscle tone will influence reflex responses. In assessing reflexes in infants, posture should be symmetrical and the head in midline. In older children the same rules apply as in adults. Corresponding reflexes on each side may be compared using reinforcing techniques when necessary. Clonus and a crossed adductor response of the lower limbs may be seen in patients with an upper motor neurone lesion.

Superficial reflexes. Many superficial reflexes are present from birth.

- The *abdominal reflexes* show the adult pattern of response throughout childhood.
- A *plantar flexor* response is seen in children over 1 year of age. Under this age, an equivocal response with fanning of the toes is normally obtained.
- The *anal reflex* consists of constriction on stroking the perianal skin. In certain disorders, for example meningomyelocele, it may be lost.
- The *cremasteric reflex* is active in boys from the age of 6 months.

So-called *'infantile' reflexes* are normally present in young infants during the early months of life. With cortical development they are progressively inhibited; persistence beyond the normal time of disappearance suggests diffuse cerebral dysfunction. They include the following.

Sucking and swallowing reflexes. These are present in all normal full-term infants and persist until voluntary control of these activities is achieved.

Rooting reflex. When light contact is made with the infant's cheek, the infant turns towards the point of contact. This reflex is present in normal infants and helps them to find the mother's nipple.

Grasp reflex. This is elicited by placing the examiner's forefingers in the palm of the infant's hand. The baby's hand closes around the examiner's finger.

Tonic neck reflex. This is elicited with the baby in the supine position. Rotation of the head to one side produces increased tone and partial extension of the arm of the same side accompanied by flexion of the knee on contralateral side.

Moro reflex. The reflex involves rapid abduction of the arms which then come together in an embracing movement.

Examination

Moro reflex

- ❑ Hold the infant in the supine position with the shoulders, back and buttocks supported by the examiner in one hand and arm.
- ❑ Support the head (occiput) in the other.
- ❑ Allow the head to fall back about an inch while the body remains supported.

Cranium and spine

Any abnormality of shape or size of the head and the measurement of its occipital frontal circumference should be noted (Fig. 10.9). Specific considerations include:

- The condition of the fontanelles may be open or closed. The anterior fontanelle usually closes between 15 and 18 months. It may be large, small, bulging in raised intracranial pressure or depressed with dehydration.
- Midline defects over the cranium, spine and lumbosacral area include encephalocele, meningocele, dermoid cysts and dermal sinuses.
- Venous distension over the scalp or a crackpot sound on percussion may indicate raised intercranial pressure.
- Transillumination of the infant's skull may help in indicating focal or diffuse abnormalities of the brain.
- Cranial bruits are not uncommon in healthy infants and children. They sometimes indicate an underlying vascular malformation.

Note the spinal contour, particularly any exaggeration of the lumbar lordosis or thoracic scoliosis. Localised tenderness over the spine may indicate infection of the epidural or intervertebral disc spaces.

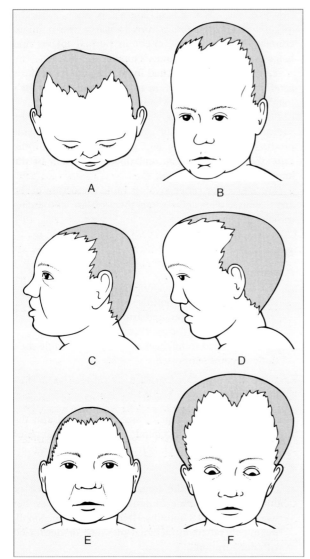

Fig. 10.9 The cranium as a diagnostic aid. A. Plagiocephaly – asymmetrical skull. **B.** Okycephaly or turricephaly – elongated skull with prominent vortex. **C.** Brachycephaly – short cranial vault. **D.** Scaphocephaly – long narrow skull. **E.** Microcephaly – small cranial vault. **F.** Hydrocephalus – large cranial vault due to enlarged ventricles.

Tests of meningeal irritation

Neck stiffness and a positive Kernig's sign may be present (p. 206) in meningitis. In infants neck stiffness can be detected by passively flexing the neck with a hand held behind the occiput. The child may then resist flexing and cry. Alternatively, with one hand behind the head and the other behind the upper trunk both head and trunk can be raised slightly off the bed

and the trunk lowered gently: any neck stiffness is then readily apparent. The absence of neck stiffness in young infants does not exclude meningitis.

KEY POINTS

- Sensation is difficult to test reliably and consistently in children and young infants.
- Under the age of 1 the plantar response is normally equivocal with fanning of the toes.
- Persistence of infantile reflexes beyond the normal time of disappearance suggests diffuse cerebral dysfunction.
- The absence of neck stiffness in young infants does not exclude meningitis.

Developmental diagnosis

The progressive acquisition of the various body movements and motor skills which characterise normal development is closely related to the maturation of all systems, and especially to that of the nervous system. A knowledge of how children develop and of the normal variations that occur is necessary to identify those in whom development is delayed or deviant. The recognition of such children is an important activity of community child health services.

In assessing development, motor, linguistic, social and adaptive achievements are considered. Clinically, a convenient sequence is to observe in turn:

- posture and gross body movements
- visual perception and fine motor movements
- speech and hearing
- social adaptation and play.

A summary of age-related developmental attainments is given in Table 10.9. It is no more than a general guide as the age at which normal infants acquire individual skills varies widely. Sequential observations over a period of months are often more informative than a single evaluation. The assessment of developmental progress is now incorporated in an integrated child health surveillance programme utilised throughout the UK with minor local differences. Table 10.10 (p. 354) gives a summary of an integrated programme now carried out largely in general practice. Details of assessments that should be made at each visit are beyond the scope of this book. Examination of gross motor development in infants provides an

Table 10.9 Some developmental attainments

12 months	Walks with support
	Says 1–3 words
	Precise pincer grip
	Waves goodbye
15 months	Walks unsupported
	Says 3–6 words
	Uses cup and spoon
	Helps undress
18 months	Walks upstairs, one hand held
	Says 4–10 words
	Builds 3–4 blocks
	Identifies parts of the body
2 years	Climbs steps holding rail
	Says 50 or more words and short phrases
	Builds 6–8 blocks
	Feeds self well; indicates toilet needs
3 years	Pedals tricycle, stands on one foot
	Speech 50% intelligible; can give name and sex
	Copies ○
	Toilet trained
4 years	Hops on one foot
	Counts from 1 to 10; names 3–4 colours
	Copies ○, +
	Dress-up play

example of how knowledge of normal development can be applied in routine clinical practice.

Gross motor development in infants

Examination

❏ Observe the infant's posture while lying supine. The normal posture is one of semiflexion of the arms and legs.
❏ Assess head control by means of the 'pull to sit' manoeuvre – the head may move in unison with the trunk, lag behind or precede it depending on the infant's age and developmental status.
❏ Next observe the posture of the infant when lying prone. Vertical suspension with the infant held prone may yield additional information on the distribution of muscle tone and power.
❏ Support the infant standing and note the posture adopted and ability to weight support.
❏ Test the forward and lateral parachute responses.

Knowledge of normal development is necessary to interpret the findings (see Table 10.9).

Locomotor system

In children any examination of the nervous system will inevitably involve some examination of the locomotor system. More specific examination may reveal other defects. Congenital and inherited defects and growth disturbances of the musculoskeletal system figure more prominently in children than in adults. The possibility that bony injuries are non-accidental must be considered (Fig. 10.10).

Generalised skeletal disorders

These conditions are rare and are usually recognised soon after birth. Infants with the severe type of osteogenesis imperfectica present with recurrent fractures and develop bony deformities and growth retardation. In Klippel–Feil syndrome, the neck is short and stiff, the hairline low and the ears often low-set. Multiple spinal abnormalities may be present with hemivertibrae and scoliosis. A high scapula (Sprengel's deformity), renal anomalies and deafness are common associated defects. Conditions such as achondroplasia and osteochondrodystrophy are readily recognised by their characteristic skeletal effects.

Deformities of trunk and neck

Examine for scoliosis, kyphosis or lordosis with the child standing erect. Torticollis, suspected by the characteristic tilting of the neck to one side and slight turning of the head to the other, is excluded by checking the range of head movement. In the lumbosacral area, a tuft of hair may be visible overlying a spina bifida occulta.

Deformities of the limbs

In the upper limbs a variety of deformities may be evident. These include:

• an increased carrying angle at the elbow, as seen in Turner's syndrome
• severe flexion and lateral twisting of a hand at the wrist in the absence of the radius
• absence of part of the arms or fingers
• extra digits (polydactyly)
• fusion of digits (syndactyly).

Functional deformities may also be elicited, such as the dinner fork deformity at the wrist with the hands outstretched (as in chorea).

In the lower limbs examples of deformity include absence of part of the limbs, talipes equinovarus (club foot), matatarsus varus, shortening or unequal development, for example hemiatrophy or hemihypertrophy.

Pes planus is best observed with the child standing.

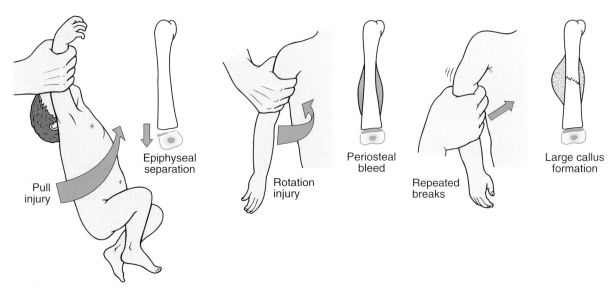

Fig. 10.10 Examples of non-accidental bone injuries.

Eversion of the foot and flattening of the normal plantar arch will be evident.

Muscles

The muscles may show evidence of general or local wasting or absence of individual muscles. e.g. pectoralis major. Enlargement of the calves may be noted in Duchenne muscular dystrophy and in the less severe Becker's muscular dystrophy.

Joints

Examination of joints has been described in Chapter 9. Always enquire about the presence of pain before touching or moving the joint. Swelling may be seen in a variety of conditions, e.g. of the large joints in haemophilia and of the small joints in juvenile rheumatoid arthritis. The diagnosis of congenital dislocation of the hip in the newborn is described on page 352.

Growth disturbances

Idiopathic scoliosis is about five times more common in girls than in boys. Its presentation and assessment have been described (p. 282). Remember to examine the back in adolescents presenting for routine physical examination at school.

Slipped femoral epiphysis must be considered in otherwise healthy children who present with a painful limp. Pain is often referred to the knee. It is important to examine the hip joint in any child complaining of knee pain, particularly in adolescence. Physical examination reveals limitation of internal rotation. This condition should be distinguished radiologically from transient synovitis of the hip.

Other conditions – genu varum (bow legs), genu valgum (knock-knees), tibial torsion, femoral anteversion and a range of foot problems (flat foot, claw toes, etc.) – are not uncommon in young children. Diagnosis and treatment demand a knowledge of the normal changes that occur during growth.

Fractures

These may be suspected because of bony deformity, local pain and tenderness on attempted movement. Crepitus may be present but should never be actively elicited. In non-accidental injury a range of bony injuries may occur (Fig. 10.10).

KEY POINTS

- Age-related developmental attainments are only a general guide as the age at which normal infants acquire individual skills varies widely.

- The possibility that bony injuries are non-accidental must always be considered, particularly in children under two years old.

- Idiopathic scoliosis is about five times more common in girls than in boys; remember to examine the back in adolescents presenting for routine physical examination.

POTENTIALLY UNCOMFORTABLE EXAMINATIONS

Procedures that are likely to be disturbing or uncomfortable should be left until the end of the examination. These include examination of the ears, mouth, neck and hips.

Ears

Infection in the ears is common in childhood, and auriscopic examination is important (Fig. 3.17).

Examination

☐ Hold the child as shown in Figure 10.11.
☐ Use a speculum appropriate to the size of the auditory canal.
☐ Note wax or purulent discharge and also any other obstruction such as a boil.
☐ If necessary, remove wax by a loop, or discharge by dry mopping with cotton wool on an orange stick.
☐ Examine the drum for colour, bulging, retraction and perforation.

The drum will appear dusky and injected in the

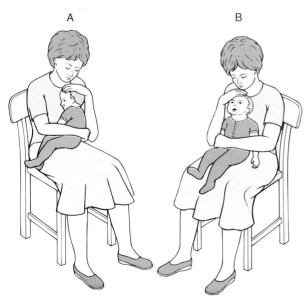

Fig. 10.11 Positions for inspection of the ear.

presence of acute infection and there may be distortion of the cone of light normally extending forward from the tip of the handle of the malleus. A bulging drum appears to be displaced towards the examiner and the light reflex is usually lost. With retraction, the malleus is unduly prominent. Perforation may occur in any part of the drum but is more likely to present in the upper part.

Mouth

A child may open the mouth voluntarily. Refusal is likely where there is too much display of shiny instruments and too obvious an intent to use them. Most children will react more willingly to the request to 'Let me see your teeth' than to 'Open your mouth' or 'Show me your throat'. The demonstration of the teeth is more likely to be a matter of some childhood pride. Physical force should be avoided as it breaks the confidence built up between patient and doctor and will make subsequent examinations very difficult.

With a willing child, inspection of the mouth should include the following:

- *State of the mucosa* – dryness, abnormal colour, ulceration, purpura; the white adherent curd-like lesions of thrush which leave bleeding points when scraped off; Koplik's spots in measles, and disorders of the gums.
- The *teeth* for number, whether of the primary or secondary dentition, size and shape, caries and enamel defects, and discoloration. Yellow discoloration may occur in the primary dentition of prematurely born children who have suffered from neonatal jaundice, or in children whose mothers have been given tetracycline during pregnancy. The time of eruption of the teeth may be an index of development.
- The *palate* for defects.
- The *tongue* size (large in cretinism), shape (elongated and thin in Down's syndrome) and surface appearance.
- The *tonsils* for size (varying with age and maximal at the age of 7–8 years), colour, exudate or pitting, and the peritonsillar region for swelling and inflammation.
- The *posterior pharyngeal area* for inflammation, swelling, postnasal discharge and the presence of lymphoid tissue.
- *Oropharynx.* Some children in saying 'Aah' will depress the tongue sufficiently to visualise the oropharynx. In others a spatula will have to be used.

Sometimes examination of the mouth will have to be performed in a child who remains uncooperative in spite of coaxing.

Examination

The cooperative child

- ❏ In order to see the throat clearly, as the child says 'Aah', place the spatula on the back of the tongue.
- ❏ If the child continues to cooperate, depression of the tongue will reveal the oropharynx.
- ❏ If tense or actively resistant, the child will arch the tongue and defy depression of it.
- ❏ At this point, only if necessary, elicit the gag reflex by advancing the spatula to touch the posterior wall of the pharynx. As gagging is induced the posterior part of the tongue will be actively depressed and the throat visualised. One gag should be enough, as repetition will upset the child.

The uncooperative child

- ❏ Seat the infant or toddler either on the knee of the assistant or lay the child on a couch.
- ❏ Prevent movement of the arms by wrapping the child in a blanket.
- ❏ If the child is held on the knee, the assistant places one arm around the child's body to prevent movement of the arms and trunk and the other round the head, holding the forehead. If the infant is examined supine, the assistant supports both the child's head and arms as shown in Figure 10.12.
- ❏ Introduce a wooden spatula between the teeth at the side of the mouth and advance it slowly by

gentle levering towards the posterior pharynx. It is possible to do this through clenched teeth.

- ❏ When the tip of the spatula reaches the posterior pharyngeal wall the child will open the mouth and gag. In this brief moment, unless the procedure is repeated, observe all the features of the mouth.

Neck

Limitation of flexion (neck stiffness or rigidity) may be an important sign of meningeal irritation due to infection or haemorrhage. It can be tested passively as described on page 206. An older child may be asked to bend forward with the knees drawn up and asked to kiss mother's hand placed on the knee.

Abnormal swellings such as enlarged lymph nodes should be sought in the anterior and posterior cervical triangles and over the occipital region. Cystic hygromata are soft and transilluminable, while abnormal thyroid swellings are confirmed by palpation and by observing movement on swallowing. A sternomastoid tumour is a firm nodule or swelling in the sternomastoid muscle seen in infancy. Branchial cleft remnants may also be found.

When cervical lymph glands are enlarged, other groups should be palpated. In palpating the axillary lymph nodes the child's arm should first be held at right angles to the trunk to allow adequate access of the fingers to the axilla, and with the fingers in position the arm returned to a position beside the trunk. In generalised lymphadenopathy the epitrochlear, inguinal and femoral lymph glands may be enlarged. The significance of enlarged lymph nodes is influenced by the findings on examination of the skin, liver and spleen.

Hips

The treatment of congenital hip dislocation is most effective when diagnosis is made in the newborn. This depends upon demonstrating instability of the joint.

Examination

- ❏ Place the infant supine on a hard surface.
- ❏ Place the examining forefingers over the greater trochanters and the thumbs over the inner aspect of both thighs.
- ❏ Flex both hips to 90° and then slowly abduct from the midline.
- ❏ With gentle but firm pressure attempt to lift the greater trochanters forward. A feeling of slipping as the femoral head goes into the acetabulum is a sign of instability (Ortolani's test, Fig. 10.13).

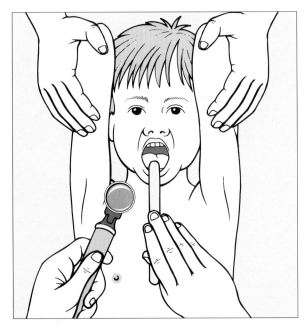

Fig. 10.12 Examining the mouth using restriction. The infant is placed supine with both the arms and the head supported by the assistant.

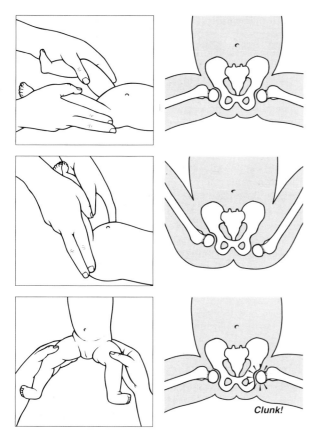

Clunk!

Fig. 10.13 Ortolani's test.

purposes skin temperature is adequate, but the site selected should not have been unnaturally cooled by exposure or heated by artificial means. The accepted dividing line between normal and abnormal temperatures, namely 37°C, is appropriate for infants and children when a skin temperature is taken. The rectal temperature is normally about 0.25°C higher. Somewhat lower temperatures are normal in premature infants.

- Rectal temperature is usually recorded in infants.
- In young children the groin is probably the best site with the thigh held flexed on to the abdomen.
- In older children the axilla is more suitable.

When there is any possibility of hypothermia, for instance in so-called neonatal cold injury, special low-reading thermometers covering the range from 30 to 40°C should be used.

KEY POINTS

- Leave all potentially disturbing or unpleasant examinations to the end.
- Treatment of congenital hip dislocation is most effective when the diagnosis is made in the immediate newborn period.

EXAMINATION OF THE NEWBORN INFANT

All newborn infants should be medically examined. It is especially important to identify those conditions that are amenable to prompt and effective treatment, e.g. choanal atresia or congenital dislocation of the hip. However, clinical examination at this age has limitations. For example, a gross congenital cardiac defect may be present without murmur, signs of cardiac failure or cyanosis; mental defect may be impossible to recognise and genetic disorders such as cystic fibrosis may be present without physical signs. The physical examination of the newborn is usually performed in hospital. It is the first step in infant and child surveillance programmes (Table 10.10) that embrace care in hospital, community and general practice.

The history

Routine examination of the apparently normal full-term newborn infant is usually carried out without the benefit of a detailed history, though this information becomes essential if any abnormality is detected. It may include details concerning the following.

⎦ If the hips appears to be stable, reapply downward pressure with thumbs on the medial side of the thighs as they are again adducted (Barlow's sign). A positive finding is a palpable 'clunk' on entry, or exit of the femoral head over the acetabular ring.

These signs of instability are the most reliable criteria for diagnosing congenital dislocation of the hip in the newborn period. They become less obvious in the subsequent weeks of life. Limitation of abduction of the hip then becomes the main sign of abnormality. Normally the hip should abduct fully to 90° on either side during the early months of life. When testing for symmetry of abduction the pelvis should be held level. If dislocation remains undetected until the child walks a painless limp may be present with a lurch to the affected side. In bilateral dislocation the gait is waddling.

Temperature

When there is constitutional upset temperature is one of the most common observations made. For most

Pregnancy

The history of the pregnancy should include the following:

- maternal diet, smoking and alcohol consumption;
- complications of pregnancy such as vaginal bleeding, hypertension, hydramnios or prolonged leaking of liquor;
- maternal diseases such as rubella, cytomegalovirus infection, toxoplasmosis or HIV infection during pregnancy, which have potentially profound effects on the fetus;
- drugs administered early in pregnancy that may cause congenital abnormalities, for example phenytoin.

The labour and birth

The birth history should include information about the following:

- fetal distress, e.g. slowing of the heart rate, meconium staining of the liquor
- early rupture of the membranes
- induction and duration of labour
- difficulties of delivery – forceps delivery or caesarean section
- maturity, birth weight and birth rank
- asphyxia such as that associated with delayed onset of respiration
- respiratory distress with increased respiratory effort (grunting or irregular respirations)
- twitching and convulsions or disturbances of consciousness
- jaundice, pallor or cyanosis.

Previous obstetric history

The mother's previous obstetric history may include miscarriages or stillbirths or indicate recurrent factors such as prematurity or post-maturity. There may be a history of difficult delivery or the need for intervention or caesarean section. Age may be important, e.g. Down syndrome is more common in the elderly mother.

Family history of disease

It is important to establish if there is any family history of disease or congenital abnormality. Examples include a range of haematological and endocrine disorders, history of deafness or blindness, congenital abnormality of the hips, heart, palate, bones, etc., and any chromosomal abnormalities. There may be a strong family background of atopy or previous cot deaths. Any previous genetic counselling or diagnostic tests carried out during pregnancy (chorionic biopsy, amniocentesis, ultrasound) should also be known.

A parent may have a history of recurrent or chronic illness including diabetes, epilepsy, heart disease, recurrent urinary infection or inherited disorders such as thalassaemia. Rubella status and occupation during pregnancy may also be relevant.

Table 10.10 Integrated child health surveillance programme

Antenatal	Health promotion The personal child health record will be given to parents
Birth	Statutory notification – NHS number generated in 0–6 weeks G.P. and H.V. informed Child registered with GP
0–5 days	Neonatal examination
6 days	PKU, TSH blood tests by midwife
0–7 days	BCG injection to 'at-risk' groups
11+ days	Home visit by HV Discussion of immunisation Surveillance visits agreed
7–14 days	Examination by GP
1 month to 6 weeks	Visit to CHC Seen by HV
6 weeks to 2 months	Examination by GP Discussion about immunisation
2–6 months	Three visits to CHC at monthly intervals Immunisations given: diphtheria, tetanus polio, pertussis H. influenza 'B'.
7½–10 months	Visit to CHC Hearing test by HV
12–15 months	Visit to CHC Immunisation for measles, mumps and rubella
18 months to 2 years	Visit to CHC Clinical examination by GP Discussion with parents
3–3½ years	Visit to CHC Examination by GP Discussion with parents
4½–5 years	Booster immunisation for diphtheria, tetanus and polio
5 years	School entry – results of pre-school surveillance available to school nurse Hearing and vision tests Results to GP

Personal child health record is completed after each CHC visit. The form is returned to the community unit after the following assessments: 2–6 months; 7½–10 months; 18 months to 2 years; 3–3½ years.
G.P. = General Practitioner   H.V. = Health Visitor
C.H.C. = Child Health Centre.

Before examining the baby ask the parents about any concerns that they may have. This may help to allay undue anxieties or reveal important information in the family history or problems that have arisen during the pregnancy or birth. Enquire about the feeding method and if any problems have arisen. Mothers will usually know whether baby boys have passed urine with a good stream and in both sexes whether meconium has been passed. Unusual problems such as apnoeic episodes, cyanosis, choking or sweating during feeds may also have been observed.

Examination

The examiner should know the infant's birthweight, length (crown–heel) and head circumference. If available, the weight charted from the time of birth is also valuable. The examination should be carried out in a warm room, free from draughts, with the infant fully undressed and lying on a nappy.

General inspection

Rapid assessment can usually be made of the baby's posture and movements, general appearance, awareness, responsiveness, cry, and how the mother handles the infant.

The following are examples of abnormalities which will usually be obvious:

- Defects of body covering, for example meningomyelocele or gastroschisis.
- Abnormalities in cranial shape and size such as hydrocephalus, caput succudaneum, excessive moulding or cephalohaematoma.
- Abnormal facies, as in Down syndrome, or the flattened nose and low-set ears of renal agenesis.
- Deformities of the limbs such as talipes equinovarus or hemimelia (arm ends abruptly above or below elbow).
- Abnormalities of extremities, for example absent or supernumerary digits.
- Tumour masses such as sacrococcygeal teratoma.
- Areas of local swelling such as an umbilical hernia or a cystic hygroma.

Skin

The skin is elastic and pink in the healthy infant. Some abnormalities that may occur are shown in Table 10.11.

The character of the umbilical cord and the presence of umbilical bleeding or infection should be noted.

There may be skin rashes such as erythema toxicum, haemangiomas or Mongolian blue spots, usually over the buttocks or lumbosacral area, skin defects or areas of fat necrosis (hard subcutaneous plaques) where there has been previous trauma, e.g. forceps blades. Examine the breasts for redness, swelling and discharge. If the skin feels cool check the temperature with a low-reading rectal thermometer.

Cranium

Obvious abnormalities will have been apparent.

Examination

- Record the size and tension of fontanelles, the degree of separation or overriding of sutures and the presence of defects or areas of thinning and softening of the skull (craniotabes).
- Examine the eyes for abnormalities of size or shape, discharge and cataracts. An increase in size and haziness of the iris may be due to congenital glaucoma, and absence of the red reflex to retinoblastoma.
- Hold the stethoscope under the nostrils; misting of the shiny end suggests that the nares are patent.
- Examine the mouth to exclude an isolated cleft palate, drying of the mucous membrane, ulceration and infection.
- Assess the size of the mandible; if it is small, consider the Pierre Robin syndrome.
- Note the setting, size, shape and symmetry of the ears and examine the external canals for patency.

Spine and limbs

The entire midline including the cranium and pos-

Table 10.11 Abnormalities that may be observed in the skin following birth

Appearance	Cause
Cracked and parchment-like	Placental insufficiency
Abnormally pallid	Fetal exsanguination
Cyanosis	Asphyxia or cyanotic congenital heart disease
Jaundice	Hepatobiliary and haemolytic disorders
Loose and inelastic	Prematurity
Dry and inelastic	Dehydration
Blemished	Superficial angiomata or milia*
Pustule formation	Infection

*Milia are pinpoint white spots due to retention of sebaceous material.

teriorly is examined for the presence of a cyst, naevus, dimple or hairy patch. Check carefully for scoliosis. Agenesis of the lumbosacral area may occur in infants of diabetic mothers. Look at the limbs for any positional deformities such as varus and valgus positions of the ankles. Count fingers and toes. Examination of the hips is left to the end (p. 352).

Central nervous system

The initial assessment includes the infant's posture and the state of consciousness. The unresponsiveness of severe apnoea or the open eyes and hyperactivity of cerebral irritation may be evident. The response to stimuli such as pinching of the skin may be abnormal. The amount of spontaneous movement may be significant. Convulsive movements where present may be localised or generalised. There may be paresis, for instance, on one side of the face in facial palsy or of legs in the presence of spina bifida. The hemi syndrome is characterised by diminished movement on one side of the body. The Moro and grasp reflexes may be absent in the presence of acute cerebral injury. The character of the cry may be helpful – the high-pitched cry of cerebral irritation or the 'cri du chat' syndrome. Muscle hypotonia or hypertonia frequently indicates cerebral disturbance.

The performance of certain basic activities in the newborn, such as sucking, swallowing and crying, and a normal sleep pattern (about 20 hours of sleep and 4 hours awake) is dependent on the integrity of the nervous system. Any deficiency in these activities or disturbances of pattern raise the question of brain damage. Examination should include observation of the infant's ability to suck and swallow and an appreciation of the pattern of sleep and wakefulness.

Abdomen

The normal abdomen in the newborn often seems protruberent but is not taut or overdistended. A scaphoid appearance suggests herniation of the abdominal contents into the chest, or high bowel atresia. Peristaltic waves may be obvious in intestinal obstruction.

Examination

- ☐ Palpate the abdomen for enlargement of the liver, spleen, kidneys and bladder and for abnormal masses.
- ☐ Feel for inguinal herniae and examine the anus for position and patency.

- ☐ Examine the genitalia: in the male for conditions such as hydrocele, undescended testes and hypospadius; in the female for labial fusion and clitoral enlargement as in adrenogenital syndrome.
- ☐ Watch the infant while feeding for vigour and coordination of sucking and character of swallowing.

Meconium and urine

Enquire about the passage of meconium and whether urine has been passed. The character of stools passed subsequently should be noted. Where indicated, urine is examined chemically and bacteriologically.

Respiration

The shape of the chest, the respiration rate, the pattern of respiration, the presence of grunting or indrawing, mucus at the mouth and abnormalities in auscultation may all be important. There are many causes of tachypnoea, including respiratory distress syndrome, meconium aspiration, cardiac failure, hypovolaemia, anaemia, neurological dysfunction and metabolic acidosis.

Heart

Examination

- ☐ Examine the heart for its position, for the presence of any abnormal precordial pulsation and for murmurs.
- ☐ Palpate the brachial and femoral pulses and, if indicated, measure the blood pressure in the arms and legs (Doppler method).

Screening investigations

Screening tests for phenylketonuria (Guthrie test) and hypothyroidism (TSH) are carried out in all infants after feeding has been established. Screening tests for cystic fibrosis, HIV infection and other inherited metabolic defects are also available. Additional investigations – haematological, biochemical, bacteriological and radiological – are seldom indicated in the absence of symptoms. These investigations are frequently performed in intensive care neonatal units together with repeated estimations of blood gas tensions and pH, and ultrasound examination of the head to detect intracranial bleeding.

KEY POINTS

- All newborn infants should be medically examined.
- Part of the examination involves taking an appropriate history.
- Before examining the baby enquire about any parental concerns.
- Examination should include observing the infants ability to suck and swallow and an appreciation of the pattern of sleep and wakefulness.
- Symptoms are less specific in infancy than in later childhood and all infants who appear unwell should be examined in detail.
- Potentially devastating conditions, such as meningitis, must be excluded in infants with non-specific symptoms.

Summary

The following provides a summary of the neonatal examination:

- Record weight and length.
- Inspect the cranium and face – head circumference, excessive moulding, fontanelle tension, ears, nostrils, palate.
- Inspect the eyes, e.g. for signs of infection; check the red reflex.
- Inspect for obvious malformation, e.g. club foot, scoliosis.
- Check for congenital dislocation of the hips.
- Palpate the femoral pulses.
- Inspect the skin, including breasts.
- Examine external genitalia and anus.
- Check for herniae.
- Examine heart, lungs, abdomen and central nervous system.
- Ensure that the blood has been taken for 'Guthrie' test at least 48 hours after a full protein feed.

The examination of the newborn is the first step in childhood surveillance, now largely conducted in a general practice or community setting. Early diagnosis leading to immediate and effective treatment is essential if potentially disastrous delays are to be avoided.

The manifestations of systemic disease in the newborn period may be different from those found later. Symptoms tend to be less specific, and all infants who appear unwell should be examined in detail. Potentially devastating conditions such as meningitis must be

Table 10.12 Average daily urine output at different ages

Age	Volume (ml)
1–2 days	30–60
3–10 days	100–300
10 days to 2 months	250–450
2 months to 1 year	400–500
1–5 years	500–700

considered and excluded in any infant with non-specific symptoms – fever, poor feeding, irritability or unexplained vomiting. To delay investigations such as lumbar puncture until more definite conventional signs appear could be a grave error.

COLLECTION OF BIOLOGICAL SAMPLES

Time is well spent explaining to the parents and the child why any diagnostic or therapeutic procedure requires to be performed and what is involved. Encouragement and reassurance help to allay anxiety and fear and greatly increase the likelihood of success. Patience, adequate preparation and proper positioning and restraint during the procedure are essential. This section describes important differences in performing common procedures in infants and young children.

Urine

The average daily output of urine at different ages is shown in Table 10.12. In infants it is normal practice to collect urine samples into a bag.

Even with careful cleansing before application, culture is frequently positive because of contamination. A midstream urine sample may be needed for bacteriological purposes. This method can be obtained in toilet-trained children but is also available in infancy provided the attendant has the time and patience to wait!

In selected cases suprapubic percutaneous bladder aspiration is indicated when it is essential to obtain an uncontaminated urine sample. It is particularly valuable in the newborn infant in whom the bladder is high and easily accessible.

Potential dangers include the introduction of infection, transient haematuria and puncture of the bowel.

Examination

Normal procedure

❑ Use a plastic bag with a round opening surrounded by an adhesive surface that adheres to the skin. In boys place the penis in the plastic bag and apply adhesive surface to the surrounding skin; in girls

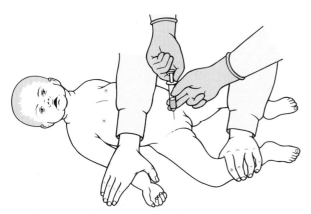

Fig. 10.14 Suprapubic aspiration of the bladder.

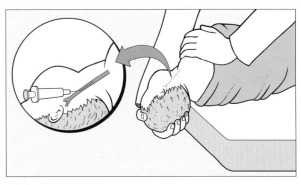

Fig. 10.15 Jugular venepuncture.

place the opening of the bag around the external genitalia.

❑ After voiding remove the bag and empty the urine.

❑ Use bags with a catheter outlet from which urine may be periodically removed for collection of 24-hour urine specimens.

Bladder aspiration

❑ Confirm a full bladder by palpation or percussion before any attempt is made to aspirate urine.

❑ Ask an assistant to hold the child in the frog-leg position (Fig. 10.14).

❑ Prepare the skin carefully with an antiseptic solution. Insert a sterile needle (22- or 25-gauge) through the skin and abdominal wall at the midline 1–2 cm above the pubic symphysis with the needle at right angles to the skin.

❑ Gently withdraw the plunger while advancing the needle. The appearance of urine in the syringe indicates a successful tap.

❑ Withdraw the needle swiftly and cover the area with a dressing.

Blood samples

Venepuncture is more difficult in infants than in older children because of the plumpness of the limbs and the small size and greater mobility of the veins. If available, use the antecubital vein or the superficial dorsal veins of the hand or wrist; alternatively, a puncture of the external jugular vein is a safe procedure in infancy.

As an alternative capillary blood may be obtained from a fingertip or heel in small infants. The earlobe is a less satisfactory site as excessive bleeding is more likely to occur.

Femoral vein puncture and internal jugular vein puncture are not recommended.

Examination

❑ Wrap the infant in a sheet securing the arms. Ask the assistant to hold the child on one side with the neck flexed laterally. This brings the external jugular vein into prominence as it crosses the sternomastoid; its distension will be increased by crying.

❑ Insert the needle at an angle nearly parallel to the skin (Fig. 10.15).

Capillary blood

❑ Warm the skin and cleanse with alcohol.

❑ Make a stab with a lancet.

❑ Collect free-flowing blood into capillary tubes or an appropriate container.

❑ Apply pressure with sterile cotton-wool to ensure haemostasis but check the site periodically in case of persistent oozing.

Nose, throat and lower respiratory tract secretions

Nasopharyngeal secretions are collected for virological studies in respiratory tract infections. An ordinary polyvinyl feeding tube attached via a sterile container to a syringe is introduced into the nostril and naso-pharynx and gentle suction applied with the syringe.

A *throat swab* may be obtained by visualising the oropharynx and swabbing the tonsils and pharynx.

Sputum is more difficult to obtain as it is generally swallowed and not expectorated.

Gastric aspiration is not a routine procedure but early morning gastric washings may be of value when tuberculosis is suspected.

Gastrointestinal secretions

In babies it is easy to pass a fine polythene tube into the stomach through the nose or mouth as active swallowing is not necessary. In infants and unco-operative older children, restraint in the supine position may be required to pass a nasogastric tube. The posture selected for gastric aspiration depends on the circumstances. When there is danger of pulmonary aspiration place the patient with the head dependent. When consciousness is impaired, tracheal intubation with a cuffed tube should precede gastric aspiration.

Faeces

Specimens of faeces should be collected in sterile containers using a spoon or spatula to transfer the specimen from the pot or the nappy. Where a speci-men is not obtainable a rectal swab may be taken for bacteriological examination. An ordinary throat swab is introduced gently into the anus for about an inch for this purpose.

Cerebrospinal fluid

Lumbar puncture. The procedure is performed as in adults. Points to note, however, are:

• Meningitis may be present even in the absence of signs of meningism.
• Raised intracranial pressure may exist in the absence of the usual features.
• The infant or young child must be properly restrained (Fig. 10.16).
• The characteristic 'give' felt when the dura is pierced may not be appreciated in the newborn or young infants.

Bone marrow aspirate

The indications for this procedure are broadly similar in children and adults as is the technique. Points to remember include the following:

• The anterior and posterior iliac crests may be used at any age, the tibia or femur up to 2 years.
• Place the child supine when performing anterior iliac crest aspiration.
• Sedation is usually necessary, and in children who require repeated bone marrow aspirations general anaesthesia may be preferred.

Sweat

The diagnosis of cystic fibrosis depends almost entirely on the accuracy with which sweat tests are carried out.

The collection and analysis of sweat is now a specialised laboratory procedure requiring a high degree of technical proficiency. The pilocarpine iontophoresis method is the most widely used and is reliable in all age groups except the newborn.

Examination

Sweat test
❏ Stimulate sweat production over a 5- to 6- minute period.
❏ Rinse the arm with electrolyte-free water and apply preweighed filter paper.
❏ Cover with plastic and seal with plastic tape to avoid evaporation.

Procedure:	Dangers:
check fundi	infection
position back	coning
glove-up	
cleanse skin	
identify L3,4	
local anaesthetic	
use no. 22 gauge needle	
advance at right angle	
to the spine	

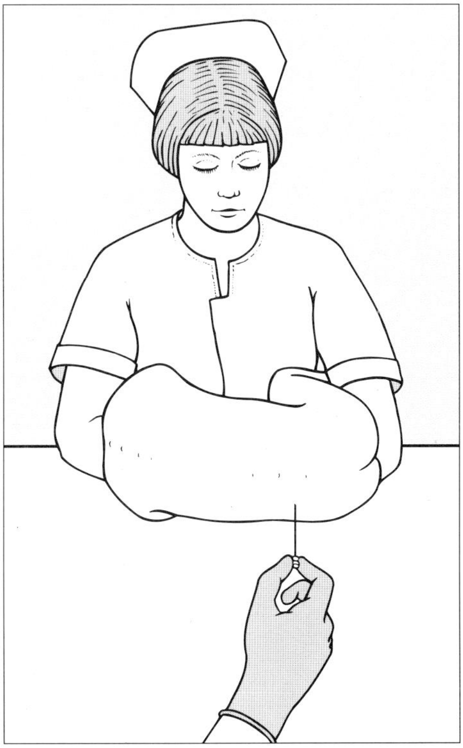

Fig. 10.16 Lumbar puncture.

❑ Remove the filter paper after 30 minutes and determine the amount of sweat collected by reweighing the filter paper. The minimum weight of sweat needed for an accurate test is 100 mg.

The sample is then analysed for sodium and chloride. Normal children under 14 usually have sweat chloride concentrations below 40 mequiv./l. A level over 60 mequiv./l. strongly supports the diagnosis of cystic fibrosis but should be confirmed by repeat testing.

11

Appendix

A SYSTEM OF CASE RECORDING IN HOSPITAL

The emphasis placed on various aspects of the clinical examination varies considerably. The system described here illustrates one sequence of documenting information.

Basic Data

Name: Age: Sex: Status:
Address: Telephone No:
Occupation: Provide that of patient and of partner. In the case of a child give the parents' occupations.
Family doctor:
Date of admission to hospital:
Date of examination:
Source of history (e.g. patient, close relative, etc.).

The history

Present illness

Begin by naming the presenting or principal symptoms and the duration of each. Proceed with a chronological account of the mode of onset and course of the patient's illness up to the day of the examination.

Systemic enquiry. Record the presence or absence of cardinal symptoms (Table 1.1, p. 4). Note any *drugs* taken and any *allergy*.

Previous health

Illnesses, operations, accidents, and their dates. Note any travel abroad, prophylactic medication, vaccination and immunisation. Date and result of any previous medical examination (e.g. for life insurance) or radiological examination. History of birth in the case of infants and children.

Family history

Note age, health or cause of death of parents, siblings, spouse and children (p. 14)

Social and personal history

Record the relevant information about occupation, housing and personal habits including recreation, physical exercise, alcohol and tobacco and, in the case of children, about school and family relationships. In the elderly, describe the level of self-dependence and the available support such as Home Help services.

The physical examination

General assessment

Describe the patient's *demeanour* and *general condition*, i.e. physique, nutrition, state of hydration, posture, gait, personality and mental state. Record height and weight. Note any abnormality not recorded under a systemic heading, for example:

Hands and arms. Information of diagnostic value obtained from inspection of hands and nails. Epitrochlear and axillary lymph nodes.

Head, face and neck. Details of any abnormality such as goitre or enlarged lymph nodes.

Skin. Colour; pallor, cyanosis, pigmentation, jaundice, etc. Specific lesions.

Subcutaneous tissues. Nodules; vascular abnormalities; oedema.

Breasts. Findings on inspection and palpation.

Cardiovascular system

Arterial pulse and pressure. Rate, rhythm, wave form and volume of radial pulse. Blood pressure.

Jugular venous pulse and pressure. Note form of the jugular pulse wave and height of the jugular venous pressure.

Heart

Inspection. Pulsations and deformity of anterior chest wall.

Palpation. Position of apex beat, character of apical impulse and other pulsations; thrills.

Auscultation. First and second heart sounds; added sounds; murmurs.

Peripheral circulation

Arterial. Pulsation of limb arteries; skin temperature and colour; local nutrition; bruits.

Venous. Abnormal vessels; signs of inflammation or occlusion.

Respiratory system

Note cough, character and quantity of sputum, wheeze or other respiratory difficulty.

Upper respiratory tract

Nose; tonsils; pharynx.

Chest

Inspection. Shape and lesions of chest wall; respiration rate and depth; chest expansion; mode of breathing.

Palpation. Range of movement; position of trachea.

Percussion. Anterior, lateral and posterior chest wall; hepatic dullness.

Auscultation. Breath sounds, vocal resonance and added sounds.

Alimentary and genitourinary systems

Mouth.

Lips, tongue, teeth, gums and other mucosae.

Abdomen

Inspection. Scars; veins; hair. Abdominal wall: shape, general and local changes, e.g. hernias and movement of respiratory, peristaltic, vascular or fetal origin.

Palpation. Tenderness; guarding; individual organs and abnormal masses; hernial orifices; inguinal lymph nodes.

Percussion. Fluid, gas and individual organs.

Auscultation. Frequency and character of bowel sounds; vascular bruits.

Genitalia

Inspection.

Palpation. Penis, testes, epididymes and vasa deferentia. Vaginal examination in special circumstances only.

Rectum

Inspection of the anus and examination of rectum.

Nervous system

Speech. Language function, articulation, phonation.

Cranial nerves.

I. Sense of smell.

II. Visual acuity; visual fields; ophthalmoscopic examination.

III, IV and VI. Eyelids, ptosis, palpebral fissures; pupils, size, shape, symmetry and reflexes; eye movements, diplopia and nystagmus.

V. Facial sensation; muscles of mastication, corneal reflex and jaw jerk.

VII. Movements of facial muscles; taste on the anterior two-thirds of the tongue.

VIII. Auriscopic examination; estimation of auditory acuity; tuning fork tests; positional nystagmus.

IX. Sensation of pharynx and of the posterior third of the tongue; palatal and pharyngeal reflexes.

X. Phonation; movements of palate and posterior pharyngeal wall; palatal and pharyngeal reflexes.

XI. Sternomastoid and upper trapezius muscles.

XII. Inspection of tongue and its movements.

Motor system. Inspection of musculature; involuntary movements including fasciculation tone; clonus; power; coordination; fine movements; dyspraxia.

Sensory system. Touch, pain and temperature; position and vibration sense; cortical sensory function, e.g. two point discrimination, stereognosis.

Reflexes. Tendon reflexes; abdominal and plantar responses.

Supplementary tests. Bruits audible in the neck or skull. Meningeal or nerve root irritation.

Locomotor system

Describe any abnormality of gait.

Spine. Shape and movement of neck and trunk.

Joints of limbs. Movements, deformity, swelling, tenderness, temperature.

Muscles. Atrophy, contractures, swelling, tenderness.

Bones. Deformity, tenderness.

The psychiatric examination

The mental state

General appearance and behaviour.

Thought processes. Sample of talk.

Mood.

Delusions.

Hallucinations.

Obsessions.

Evidence of intellectual defect.

    Orientation.

    Memory.

    Attention and concentration.

    General information.

    Intelligence.

Insight and judgement.

Additional information

Personality diagnosis

Urine. Volume, colour, opacity, odour, reaction, specific gravity; microscopy; chemical tests for protein, glucose and other substances as indicated.

Faeces. Inspection. Result of testing for occult blood.
Vomitus. Character and nature.

Clinical diagnosis

Record the differential diagnosis in order of probability.

Further investigations

It is helpful to outline a plan of any further investigations considered necessary at this stage.

Treatment and progress notes

These should be entered from day to day.

Summary

It is advisable to conclude the case recording with a brief summary incorporating the principal symptoms, the main abnormalities on physical examination, the significant findings on further investigation, the final diagnosis or diagnoses, the therapeutic measures employed, the decisions regarding further management and the nature of the explanation given to the patient and the relatives. Alternatively the summary can take the form of a 'problem list' as described below.

PROBLEM-ORIENTATED MEDICAL RECORDS

The traditional method of case recording has been adapted in some centres to incorporate the problem-orientated medical record. The method of collecting the clinical information is the same but its recording is orientated around the patient's problems into four main components, the database, the problem list, the initial plan and the progress notes.

Database

This consists of:

- The principal complaint.
- Relevant social data and the 'profile'; the latter is a description of how the patient spends an average day. Therapeutic goals can be related to this profile.
- The history.
- The physical examination.
- Laboratory and other basic investigations, such as haemoglobin, urea and electrolytes and chest radiography.

Problem list

All the patient's problems, past and present, are named and numbered on a *provisional problem list*. Physical problems may comprise a symptom, such as weight loss, a sign, such as cervical lymphadenopathy, or a pathological condition, such as chronic bronchitis. Other problems may be social, for example cigarette smoking, or psychological, such as a grief reaction. As the clinical situation is clarified, these problems are transposed to a *master problem list*, which is displayed prominently in the front of the case notes. Problems are classified as either active or resolved. The former category includes not only those which have been diagnosed but also any unexplained or ambiguous findings. The master problem is open-ended and is modified as the situation changes. New problems are added as they are recognised. The list serves as a guide to the case notes and provides a summary which helps not only the medical staff but also nurses, physiotherapists, social workers and others to assess the position. An example of a master problem list is given on page 365.

Initial plan

For each active problem an initial plan is organised from three aspects:

- the collection of further data to clarify the situation
- therapy
- education of the patient in active participation in the management of the disease.

Progress notes

The records are kept up to date by entering all additional relevant information, as it is obtained, under the named and numbered title of the problem to which it pertains. The notes are further structured by subheadings:

- subjective data; prominence is given first to the patient's reactions
- objective data
- interpretation; this includes both decisions and impressions
- therapy; this includes education of the patient;
- immediate plans.

These notes can be supplemented by *'flow sheets'* when dealing with fast-moving situations such as diabetic ketoacidosis, shock or acute ventilatory failure. Then the interrelationships of data and therapy are crucial; time, serial measurements, therapy and comment are recorded side by side and repeated as frequently as the situation demands.

Master problem list (1.5.94)
Mrs A.B.C. (date of birth 1.5.38)

Active	*Inactive*
1. Acute abdominal pain	
acute cholecystitis (2.5.94)	
cholecystectomy (10.5.94)	
2. Obesity	
3. Varicose veins	
4. Psoriasis	
5. Left facial pain ? cause	
6. Social deprivation (divorced;	
four children; two rooms)	
	7. Penicillin allergy
	(1982)
	8. Duodenal ulcer
	(1989)
9. Pulmonary embolism (16.5.94)	

Finally a *discharge report* is prepared, summarising each numbered problem on the list; particular attention is paid to any problems which may not have been fully elucidated or which may recur.

Conclusion

Problem-orientated medical records present data in structured ways readily amenable to assessment and audit by others. The methods, however, are initially time-consuming, and this has been a barrier to their widespread acceptance. Many clinicians find the master problem list particularly useful in the follow-up of complicated problems. It provides a flexible, intelligible and up-to-date summary which allows an immediate grasp of the medical and social situation and reduces errors.

KEEPING CASE RECORDS

Any system of case note recording should be designed to give a well-structured and easy-to-follow assessment of a patient's situation, including the working diagnosis and the resulting investigation and treatment plan.

The patient's care may be taken over by other clinicians at any time because of a sudden deterioration in their condition or because of cross-cover arrangements. Accurate, legible and structured case notes containing a record of examination, treatment prescribed, consent to procedures and information given to the patient are the essential prerequisites to effective medical care. Legibility is vital. Although confidential, the patient has access to the case notes, which may be examined by the patient or other medical practitioners, or be exhibited as evidence in a court of law.

Follow-up notes should be entered on a regular basis and should include the performance of investigations and any changes in the patient's management. It is particularly important that concise notes are made as soon as practicable after any emergency treatment such as a cardiac arrest.

Finally, every note entry in the case record should be signed together with the date and time that the record was completed.

DESIRABLE WEIGHTS OF ADULTS

Body mass index (BMI) is derived from the weight in kg divided by the square of the height in metres (kg/m^2) (Fig. 11.1). The 'normal' range is 20–25. Grade I obesity is > 25–30, grade II > 30–40 and grade III > 40.

To use the nomogram, place a ruler or straight edge between the body weight in kg (indoor clothes) and the height in cm (without shoes). The body mass index is read from the middle of the scale.

THE USE OF QUESTIONNAIRES

In a literate society questionnaires constitute an efficient and time-saving method of obtaining information. They can be used in health reviews and as a database in problem-orientated case notes. Questionnaires can also provide detailed information in special situations. They are particularly useful in assessing sexual problems because the questions can be posed without the embarrassment of an interview and the sexual partner can help to answer them.

In sexual problems in the male the questionnaire consists of two parts. In the first the patient provides details about his past and present health, with appropriate reference to:

- conditions such as sexually transmitted disease, mumps and tuberculosis, which may affect the testes

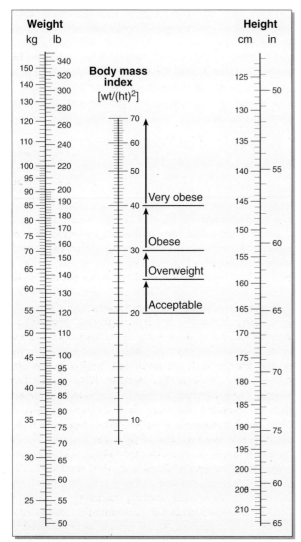

Fig. 11.1 Desirable weights of adults according to body mass index.

Problems with erection

Do you get satisfactory erections of the penis for sexual purposes?

If not please answer the following questions:

1. Which is the situation that most closely resembles your own?
   (i) No erection of any sort at any time.
   (ii) Incomplete erections occasionally but the penis is not firm enough to allow penetration.
   (iii) Firm erections at first allowing penetration but not lasting long enough for completion of sexual intercourse.
   (iv) Firm erections in the morning or during wet dreams but unable to have erections when trying to have intercourse with partner.
   (v) Firm erections but the penis is bent when erect making sexual intercourse impossible.
2. When was the last time you had a normal erection firm enough to allow normal sexual intercourse or masturbation?
3. Do you get morning erections?

Problems with ejaculation

Do you get satisfactory ejaculation of sperm?

If not please answer the following questions:

1. Do you think you ejaculate –
   (i) normally when having sex with your wife/partner,
   (ii) normally when masturbating,
   (iii) sometimes when asleep during dreams?
2. During ejaculation do you feel that –
   (i) the sperm goes the wrong way,
   (ii) ejaculation occurs too quickly,
   (iii) there is no ejaculation?
3. If you ejaculate too quickly, does ejaculation occur –
   (i) before there has been any penetration of the penis,
   (ii) very soon after penetration?
4. If you do not ejaculate at all, do you –
   (i) have no sex because you have no erections,
   (ii) have normal erections but despite much stimulation cannot ejaculate?

• marital status including offspring
• current and previous cigarette and alcohol consumption
• medication and drug abuse
• nature of employment and previous occupations.

The second part of the questionnaire contains explicit questions about sexual activities. A general sexual history is obtained and then more specific information is sought, about such problems as erection or ejaculation. Examples of such questions are given.

In all cases psychological factors are also assessed.

The answers to such a questionnaire usually identify the main problem which the clinician can then clarify at interview.

PROBABILITY THEORY AND BAYESIAN LOGIC

Probability theory

Probability theory indicants are the items of evidence relevant to the probability that a disease is present or not. They include symptoms, signs and laboratory results. A group of indicants is called a *facet*.

Certain indicants are extremely valuable in diagnosis. The term 'pathognomonic' means 'names the pathology'. Unfortunately, few symptoms or clinical signs are pathognomonic, although some narrow the field considerably. The importance of an indicant in the diagnosis of a specific disease (*weight of evidence*) is expressed as *bans*, i.e. the logarithm of the change in the *odds* that the disease is present, given the presence of the indicant. The entire process of diagnosis, from eliciting a set of indicants to decisions on treatment, can be viewed as the selection from a number of facets forming a path down the *diagnostic tree*. The tree begins with a presenting indicant, branches out according to the chosen facets and the outcome of numerous tests and ends with an evaluation of the treatment outcome.

The value attributed by the individual to any state of health has been termed *utility*. Every diagnostic test and form of treatment involves a *cost*, or *negative utility*, in terms both of risk to the patient and of financial outlay. These should be considered when estimating the expected gain in utility. In the ill patient, the clinician's objective is to maximise the increase in utility by avoiding unnecessary risks and by careful choice of treatment. This is known as the *principle of rationality* and can usefully be considered as a measure of the consistency of decision making.

Bayesian logic

The first mathematical approach to probability theory is ascribed to *Bayes*, who derived a formula for combining probabilities. For example, if 50% of patients with appendicitis are female and 50% are age < 20 years then the percentage of female patients aged < 20 is 25%, i.e. 50% × 50%. Similarly, if 75% of patients with diverticulitis are female but only 2% are aged < 20, only 1.5% (75% × 2%) of patients with diverticulitis are females aged < 20. Bayes would conclude that if the patient was a female aged < 20 and the only diagnostic possibilities were either appendicitis or diverticulitis, the probability of having appendicitis would be 95%, i.e. 0.25 + (0.25 × 0.5), and the probability of having diverticulitis would be (0.25 × 0.5) / [0.25 + (0.25 × 0.5)], i.e. 5%. In practice, one would also need to know the prevalence of appendicitis and diverticulitis. If diverticulitis was rare, the patient would be even more likely to have appendicitis. With just three indicants and two diseases, the calculation can be performed on a simple calculator. However, since there are more than 20 common causes of acute abdominal pain and more than 30 symptoms to

analyse, the calculation of the diagnostic probabilities often involves a computer, although the mathematics is the same.

In order to use *Bayes' theorem* and calculate the probability that a patient has a specific disease given a specific indicant, the following data is required:

- the frequency of the symptom in patients with the disease
- the frequency of the disease in the population;
- the frequency of the symptom in other possible diseases
- the frequency of these other diseases in the population.

The frequency of an indicant in a given disease (*likelihood*) is called the *conditional probability* and is obtained by collecting data on a large group of patients with the disease. The frequency of a disease in a population of patients is called the *initial probability*. In a patient with the specific indicant, the *final probability* of having the disease is proportional to the initial probability multiplied by the conditional probability. As more indicants are known, the calculation becomes more precise. In practice, Bayes' theorem has one major drawback. It assumes that indicants are not related to one another. For example, if the patient has a right-sided abdominal pain, the theorem assumes that the patient is no more likely to have right-sided abdominal tenderness than left-sided tenderness. In clinical practice, the sites of pain and tenderness are closely related. In consequence, Bayes' theorem increases the final probabilities, e.g. when the final probability of appendicitis is calculated at 99.9% only 75% of patients may actually have appendicitis.

More advanced probability mathematics (*multivariate analysis*) are necessary to assess the interrelationship between indicants and the usefulness of specific symptoms and signs in helping to discriminate between diagnoses (*discriminant function*).

CONTINUING MEDICAL EDUCATION

The true aim of education should be an understanding of how to learn rather than a knowledge of fact. Once the former has been acquired, it becomes easier to continue to accumulate knowledge which is particularly necessary in a discipline such as medicine in which scientific advances are often rapid.

It follows that all clinicians should continue this process of active medical education throughout their practising years. The ability to keep abreast with developments can be evaluated by self-assessment and medical audit.

Medical audit

There is an increasing awareness of the value of medical audit. This forms one component of resource management and is a method of improving the quality of medical care. It can take many forms. The fundamental requirements are that it involves peer review and that the end result of 'closing the audit loop' should enhance clinical performance.

A simple example of medical audit involves two or more clinical teams. Notes are selected at random from among patients recently discharged from hospital and are then reviewed critically by the other team. Such activity conducted in a friendly atmosphere and in good faith can provide an excellent climate for learning and lead to a general improvement in performance.

Almost any aspect of clinical care can be assessed by audit. Medical audit is not clinical research, but it is a method of evaluating medical care, including the safety and efficiency of treatment regimens and the optimum use of diagnostic and other resources. One method is to compare actual performance with a recommended guideline or protocol devised to standardise care in a common medical condition, such as diabetic keto-acidosis or myocardial infarction. Guidelines for investigation procedures can also be the subject of an audit exercise. For example, it has demonstrated the limited value of routine chest radiographs in patients under 40 years of age without pulmonary symptoms.

Self assessment

This is another aspect of continuing education. It involves making a conscious effort to appraise one's own clinical practice; it should be an integral part of medical care. One simple method involves a written diagnostic analysis of each patient at the time of initial interview, followed by a critical reappraisal once the results of investigations are available. In addition, many self-assessment programmes (SAPs) are now available. These attempt to assess both factual knowledge – a relatively easy task – and judgement. They prove a useful tool for learning and a method of continuing medical education.

INDEX